CW00523783

Tumours
Basic Principles and Cli

Jean, Sally and John

Tumours
Basic Principles and
Clinical Aspects

C. J. Louis
M.B., B.S., Ph.D., M.R.C.Path.,
Senior Lecturer in Pathology (Austin Hospital),
University of Melbourne;
Co-ordinator in Oncology, Austin and Repatriation
Hospitals Clinical School, Melbourne

Foreword by Rupert A. Willis
M.D., D.Sc., F.R.C.P., F.R.C.S., F.R.A.C.P.,
F.R.C.Path.,
Emeritus Professor of Pathology,
University of Leeds;
Consultant Pathologist to the
Imperial Cancer Research Fund, London

CHURCHILL LIVINGSTONE
EDINBURGH LONDON NEW YORK 1978

CHURCHILL LIVINGSTONE
Medical Division of Longman Group Limited

Distributed in the United States of America by
Longman Inc., 19 West 44th Street, New York,
N.Y. 10036 and by associated companies,
branches and representatives throughout the world.

© Longman Group Limited 1978

ISBN 0 443 01703 4

British Library Cataloguing in Publication Data
Louis, C J
  Tumours.
  1. Tumors
  I. Title
  616.9'92   RC254   78–40031

Printed in Singapore by Huntsmen Offset Printing Pte Ltd

Foreword

This book, written particularly for students by an experienced teacher, who is also well-known for his own original work on some aspects of tumour-cell biology, is not just another epitome of the classification, structure and behaviour of tumours; it includes these but much more. It gives an informed outline of the several main hypotheses of the intrinsic nature of neoplastic change, indicating the lines along which current research work is progressing – chemical, radiational, virological and on the complexities of cellular metabolism revealed by modern molecular cytologists. As research increasingly discloses this complexity, with corresponding increase in esoteric chemical, genetic and other terminology, the non-specialist pathologist as well as the student beginner may well feel confused and deterred by the multitude of facts, speculations and names in each of the special lines of research, their seeming lack of relationship to each other, and their inconclusiveness in many respects. Dr. Louis's book, though not pretending to achieve the impossible task of evaluating and integrating the findings and speculations in the several special fields, provides a balanced outline of them, helping the reader to separate established facts from the host of speculations, and indicating points of contact between the several disciplines that might be relevant to the study of the nature of tumours. Two important principles in tumour research are implicit in his discussions, namely (a) that the word 'cancer', or the more general 'tumour', embraces many different diseases, with different extrinsic causes, reflected in differences of age, sex, occupational and racial incidence, and possibly with different fundamental mechanisms of neoplastic change; and (b) that, while there is a broad parallelism between experimental tumours in animals and spontaneous human ones, often shedding light on the extrinsic causes in carcinogenesis, this is not invariably so and may indeed have been misleading in some instances. So, in both the experimental and human fields, each distinct kind of tumour must be investigated as a seperate problem in causation – always with the hope, of course, that light shed on the basic mechanism of carcinogenesis in one kind of tumour may be found to apply to others also.

From his survey of recent laboratory research on the basic problems of neoplasia, Dr. Louis turns to the practical clinical aspects of tumours – their presentation, diagnosis and treatment. These chapters are a discussion of principles only, with, however, some pertinent advice that will remind students and others that accurate and thorough clinical observation plays an indispensable part in human cancer research.

The remaining chapters of the book describe tumours of particular organs and tissues. Though not aiming to be comprehensive or to make every student into an expert histopathologist, these give a well-balanced outline of the structure and behaviour of the main kinds of tumours, stressing the distinctive features and the variants in each regional class. While relatively brief, these chapters provide the average medical student, not aiming to specialize in pathology, as much as he needs to know; indeed their very brevity and succinctness enhance the impact of the essentials that they cover.

Thus, this unusual book, while not neglecting the reader's needs for a factual outline of the structure, functions and clinical aspects of tumours, sets these in the context of current research and speculation. Tumours constitute one of the last of the great classes of diseases of obscure pathogenesis, looming all the larger because of the elucidation of most of the other major classes – parasitic, bacterial, viral, metabolic and genetic. I commend Dr. Louis's book to all students and general pathologists of enquiring minds who reflect on what tumours really *are* and who want to know in what directions we must look for their elucidation.

Heswall, 1978   R.A.W.

List of acknowledgements

First of all, I would like to thank my students who stimulated me to write this book, and Professor E. W. Gault who played a major role in my ability to complete the project.

I am deeply grateful to the following colleagues who have assisted in the preparation of various specialist sections: Dr. J. Stevens (Diagnostic Radiology), Dr. R. A. Smallwood (Colonoscopy), Dr. M. Drake (Cytology), Dr. T. F. Sandeman (Radiotherapy), Dr. S. T. Chou (Tumours of the liver and gall bladder) and Professor H. D. Attwood (Tumours of the female genital tract).

It is a pleasure to acknowledge my indebtedness to many friends and colleagues who have looked over one or more chapters and provided material for the preparation of illustrations: Dr. R. McD. Anderson, Professor H. D. Attwood, Dr. J. M. Blunck, Dr. S. T. Chou, Professor G. S. Christie, Dr. I. D. Gust, Professor E. W. Gault, Dr. H. J. C. Ireton, Mr. R. C. Rivenell, Mr. L. T. Stretton, Dr. F. A. Tosolini, Dr. S. Weiner, Professor R. A. Willis and Dr. J. M. Xipell. In particular, I should like to thank my wife for reading the entire manuscript and proofs. The task of preparing the manuscript at home was made bearable by the support and understanding of my wife and family.

The actual production of this book required much devoted and loyal help. In this regard, I am indebted to past and present members of staff of this department: Gordon Pratt, Helen Makin, Chris Bradley, Robyn Hart, Bryan Lane and Annette Nolan. I am particularly indebted to Miss Edna Bird, whose careful typing and retyping of the manuscript lightened my task. I am also grateful to Dr. S. T. Chou, Mr. Jack Smith and Mr. L. Kont for help with the photographs. Finally, I should like to thank my publishers for their friendly co-operation and for showing every possible consideration and courtesy.

Preface

The changing patterns of disease incidence show that cancer is now responsible for approximately 20 per cent of all deaths and its incidence appears to be increasing. Because of this, the study of cancer is assuming more and more importance in medical education. Whilst a number of books have been written on the pathology of tumours, almost all of these are directed at the specialist; there is no straightforward account suitable for undergraduate students. This book is written in an attempt to fill that gap.

The aim of the book is to give a brief and up to date summary of cancer in terms of morphology, carcinogenesis, classification and clinical correlation. As far as possible, the International System of the Histological Classification of Tumours is used. The material presented has been carefully selected to meet the needs of undergraduate medical students and the size of the book has been restricted so that it can be used as a *vade-mecum* by medical students during their course in histopathology. The information given will also be of value to postgraduate students preparing for higher qualifications and to research students in allied subjects who are now entering the field of cancer research in increasing numbers. A complete set of references is not included and both the macroscopic and microscopic descriptions of tumours are brief, similar to those found in routine biopsy reports. Those who are looking for a more comprehensive bibliography are referred to the sources in the Guide for Additional Reading which is strongly recommended for the interested student.

Melbourne, 1978   C.J.L.

Contents

I

Definition, morphology and classification of tumours

WHAT IS A TUMOUR?

The word *oncology* is derived from two Greek words, *oncos*, meaning a mass or a tumour and *logos*, meaning a dissertation or a special study. Thus oncology is the study of tumours. This definition requires that the word tumour also be defined. Strictly speaking, a tumour is a swelling or a protuberance and in this sense it can be applied equally well to non-neoplastic as to neoplastic nodules. However, in oncology, use of the word tumour is restricted to neoplasms (new growths); here usage rather than logic determines its meaning. In this book, the terms *tumour, neoplasm* and *new growth* will be used synonymously.

There are many definitions of a tumour, but in the absence of precise knowledge of aetiology and pathogenesis none of them is satisfactory. Briefly, a tumour may be defined as *an abnormal mass of tissue or an abnormal cell population with a capacity for progressive growth*. The neoplastic cells are the important component of a tumour. They may be contiguous and localized to a confined space, as in solid tumours, or they may be suspended in a fluid medium as in the leukaemias and ascites tumours. Persistence of growth is the salient feature of tumour cells that distinguishes them from other non-neoplastic cells and, depending on the rate and nature of this growth, tumours may be subdivided into two broad groups – *benign* (simple or innocent) and *malignant*. Malignant tumours composed of epithelial cells are called *carcinomas* and those composed of connective or supportive tissues *sarcomas*. The word *cancer* is a general term which refers to all types of malignant tumours.

The above definition of a tumour is purely descriptive; it excludes any mention of an aetiological agent. Nevertheless, it is a useful definition because it emphasizes the macroscopic, microscopic and behavioural characteristics of tumours.

MACROSCOPIC CHARACTERISTICS OF TUMOURS
(The abnormal mass)

In most cases, the appearance of a mass is the predominant feature that attracts attention and remains prominent in the patient's mind. An accurate diagnosis of this mass is vital because it determines the type of treatment to be given, which in turn influences the clinical course or prognosis of the condition. In making a diagnosis, the macroscopic examination of the mass usually provides valuable information and should be carried out carefully and systematically. The appearance of the cut surface is probably the most important part of the macroscopic examination. It is best assessed on a freshly cut surface and for this purpose the mass is incised in its long diameter. Particular attention is paid to the presence or absence of degeneration, necrosis, haemorrhage, umbilication and ulceration. Evidence of invasion and metastasis should also be noted.

Site
The site where the tumour arises considerably influences the time and type of presentation. Tumours of the skin and of organs such as the breasts and salivary glands that are superficially placed and are readily accessible to examination attract early attention and treatment. Deeply situated tumours, on the other hand, may be overlooked for many years or until their continued growth and development produce symptoms or complications. For example, expanding intracranial tumours may cause local symptoms by irritation and destruction of cerebral tissue or by raised intracranial pressure; a carcinoma of the pylorus may produce symptoms of pyloric obstruction and a carcinoma of the head of the pancreas, by compressing the common bile duct, may present as a case of obstructive jaundice.

Size
Tumours vary considerably in size. The important point to elicit is whether or not there has been a recent increase in the size of the mass otherwise size alone sheds little light on the nature of the growth. Some very large tumours such as those of the ovary are benign, whereas some very malignant tumours are surprisingly small. It is important to realize that, with the present-day emphasis on early diagnosis and treatment, many tumours do not have the opportunity to reach a large size.

Shape

Shapes of tumours also vary considerably depending on whether they grow within the tissue or project outwards from a surface. Tumours growing within tissues may be solid or cystic, or they may show a mixture of solid and cystic areas. A *cyst* is a localized, well circumscribed collection of fluid. Tumours growing outwards, on the other hand, are usually rounded, cauliflower-like growths and are called polyps or papillomas. Those attached to the surface by a stalk or pedicle are described as pedunculated while those that are attached by a broad base as sessile. Pedunculated growths are nearly always benign whereas sessile growths may be benign or malignant.

Colour

Different tissue components give rise to different colours. These are best appreciated on a freshly cut surface:

Colour	Tissue Component
White (glistening strands)	Fibrous tissue
Grey-white	Cellularity (parenchyma)
Blue-grey (gelatinous)	Mucin
Pale yellow-grey	Degeneration/necrosis
Yellow	Lipid
Reddish-purple	Haemorrhage/thrombus
Rust	Iron/old haemorrhage
Black/brown	Carbon/melanin

Because of their cellularity, carcinomas are usually grey-white in colour. Bands of glistening-white fibrous tissue often intersect the tumour parenchyma giving rise to a lobular pattern. Areas of necrosis, haemorrhage, lipid accumulation and mucoid change also produce characteristic colours and when mixtures of these tissue components are present, they impart a variegated colour pattern to the cut surface. Sarcomas, on the other hand, tend to be vascular and are more fleshy in appearance than carcinomas. Their blood vessels are usually thin-walled, friable and easily invaded by the adjacent tumour cells. Thus areas of haemorrhage, necrosis and infarction are common findings in sarcomas.

Other tumours also show characteristic colours. For example, carcinomas of the kidney are yellow because the cells contain large amounts of lipid, choriocarcinoma resembles placental tissue, malignant melanomas that contain melanin are black, carcinoid tumours often turn yellow after fixation in formalin owing to the presence of serotonin and phaeochromocytomas turn brown when the cut surface is exposed to the air.

Capsule

The cut surface should show if the mass is well-circumscribed and if it has a capsule. Encapsulation of a tumour depends on several factors, such as the rate of growth, the ability of the tumour cells to invade and the compressibility of the surrounding tissue. As a general rule, benign tumours grow slowly by expansion and as a result cause pressure atrophy of the surrounding cells. The atrophic cells are gradually replaced by fibrous tissue which eventually condenses and forms a capsule around the mass. Although this capsule is formed largely from fibrous tissue replacement of the peripheral cells, the stroma of the tumour may also contribute to it. Because benign tumours grow by expansion they tend to be sharply demarcated from the surrounding tissue and usually possess a fibrous capsule. Malignant tumours, on the other hand, grow by both expansion and invasion so that their edges are usually poorly defined and a capsule is usually not present. For example, a scirrhous carcinoma of the breast which grows mainly by invasion tends to have scalloped edges from which claw-like fibrous extensions taper out, fixing the mass to adjacent skin and pectoral muscles.

However, not all benign tumours are encapsulated and not all malignant tumours lack a capsule. Leiomyomas of the uterus and the fibroadenomas of the breast, although discretely demarcated, frequently do not possess a capsule whereas encephaloid carcinoma of the breast which grows largely by expansion is usually discrete and may develop a capsule. Thus, while encapsulation is the rule in benign tumours, the presence of a capsule does not necessarily imply that the tumour is benign just as the absence of a capsule does not imply that it is malignant.

Regional lymph glands

Carcinomas frequently metastasize to lymph nodes and the presence of tumour tissue in regional lymph nodes constitutes absolute proof that the lesion is malignant. It is important to realize, however, that lymph nodes commonly respond to diseases by enlargement so that it may be impossible to tell macroscopically whether the enlargement is due to a reactive condition or to a secondary tumour. For this reason, it is essential that all lymph nodes in the catchment area of the tumour site should also be examined microscopically, regardless of whether or not they are enlarged.

Ulcerative lesions

A carcinoma on an epithelial surface may present either as a mass or as an ulcer. Ulceration results from necrosis of the superficial cells which slough off leaving a denuded area or ulcer. Ulcers commonly occur on the skin and in the alimentary canal and many of them are malignant. Although the final decision on whether an ulcer is benign or malignant is made microscopically, the naked-eye appearance of the ulcer frequently reveals characteristics which by experience are known to correspond to certain patterns of behaviour. Thus the site, size and shape of the ulcer should be noted and particular attention should be paid to the edge, base and regional lymph nodes.

Viewed in cross-section, the edge of a malignant ulcer is usually raised or heaped up like an everted lip pouting over the surface of the adjacent normal tissue. Evidence of invasion, when present, is apparent as infiltrating grey-white tissue at the base of the cut surface and the extent of this invasion is an important parameter in the staging of many cancers.

MICROSCOPIC CHARACTERISTICS OF TUMOURS
(The cell population)

Microscopically, tumours are composed of a parenchyma (the cell population) and a stroma. The parenchyma is the neoplastic component which determines (a) the histological characteristics of the tumour, the arrangement of cells and their relation to the surrounding stroma (the cell pattern) and the cytological features of the individual cells (cytoplasmic, nuclear and nucleolar characteristics) and (b) the behavioural properties of the tumour (p. 10). The stroma is a non-neoplastic element derived from the host's connective tissue.

Two major groups of malignant tumours are distinguished according to the two major classes of tissue. Epithelium gives rise to carcinomas, and connective and supportive tissues to sarcomas. Distinction between these two in the adult is relatively easy in most tumours. Usually, epithelium is composed of large, distinct cells with a considerable amount of cytoplasm surrounding a well-defined nucleus. The individual cells are arranged in groups with a very small amount of intercellular cement material. Connective tissues on the other hand are characterized, from the very nature of their function, by a considerable amount of intercellular material.

The individual cells are often small and their outlines may be difficult to recognize, the position of the cell being indicated by the position of the nucleus.

Cell pattern

Great variations are found in the arrangements and appearances of cells of different tumours. In many cases they produce patterns with morphological and functional characteristics which resemble those of the tissue of origin and which make identification of the tumour easy. The histological patterns of benign epithelial tumours are of two principal types:

1. *Papillomas* arise from lining epithelia as finger-like outgrowths from the surface. These outgrowths may be simple or branching and consist of a core of loose fibro-vascular tissue covered by epithelium. Those arising from the skin, mouth, larynx, anus, vagina and cervix uteri are covered by stratified squamous epithelium and are called squamous-cell papillomas, those from the gut are lined by columnar epithelium and those from the urinary tract by transitional epithelium.

2. *Adenomas* occur in solid organs (kidney, thyroid gland and adrenal gland) and are composed of glandular structures such as ducts or acini separated by vascular connective tissue. They usually grow into the tissue and often have a capsule of fibrous tissue. A thyroid adenoma, for example, is composed of closely packed thyroid follicles containing colloid and an adrenal adenoma of cords of cells containing lipid.

Carcinomas are the commonest of all malignant tumours. Some are *differentiated* and their parenchymal cells are frequently arranged into patterns which closely resemble those of the tissue of presumed origin. For example, squamous-cell carcinomas arise from squamous epithelium and are composed of irregular masses of epidermal cells separated by connective tissue. A feature of these cancers is their tendency to reproduce the different layers of normal epidermis so that the central portions of the cellular masses become flattened and undergo keratinization leading to *keratin pearls* (Fig. 11.1a). The adenocarcinomatous pattern shows glandular structures. Here the epithelial cells may form tubules or ducts such as those of the breast and salivary glands, acinar or cyst-like structures such as the follicles in the thyroid gland, or they may consist of cords of cells as in the tumours of the liver and adrenal gland.

Thus the histological patterns of some adenocarcinomas are such that recognition of the tissue from which the cancer has arisen is relatively easy. In other carcinomas, the cells do not form specific patterns but collect into strands, irregular small groups or sheets in which distinguishing characteristics are not present and the site of origin of the tumour is difficult to determine. These are the *undifferentiated carcinomas*.

In connective tissue tumours, the cells tend to lie singly with intercellular material between them which is usually a product of the cells themselves. Fibromas and fibrosarcomas, for example, often show collagen fibres between the tumour cells. Tumours of smooth muscle cells (leiomyomas) are composed of interlacing or whorled bundles of smooth muscle cells without intercellular collagen formation.

In addition to the major tissues, there is a group of tumours which arise from germ cells that are multipotential and can differentiate into a variety of tissues. These are the *teratomas*. A teratoma is a tumour composed of multiple tissues which are uncommon to the part in which the tumour arises. Teratomas may be present at birth or may develop later in life. They must be differentiated from *hamartomas* which are also composed of multiple tissues but these tissues are common to the site where the tumours develop. Hamartomas are not true tumours, they are malformations.

Cell differentiation

In oncology, the term differentiation implies full maturation of morphological and functional characteristics of cells. The degree of differentiation of tumour cells is determined from the most mature and functional representatives such as colloid-containing thyroid follicles, melanin-producing cells and keratin formation. In benign tumours, the cells are usually well differentiated but in malignant tumours cell differentiation tends to vary so that there is usually some deviation from the normal. Generally speaking, the degree of malignancy is inversely related to the degree of differentiation and the terms *well differentiated, poorly differentiated* and *undifferentiated* indicate morphological stages of malignancy. Use of the terms *anaplasia* and *dedifferentiation* is now considered bad practice because they imply a reversal of the physiological processes of maturation. There is no evidence to suggest that differentiated cells can revert to undifferentiated forms. Lack of differentiation is simply an expression of failure of maturation following cell division and it is assessed on morphological grounds, that is, the cell is usually small with a dark staining nucleus and the nuclear/cytoplasmic ratio is increased.

Pleomorphism

This is the morphological variation in the size and shape of cells. Malignant cells often represent a heterogeneous population, they tend to be larger and more irregular in form than the normal parent cells and, because of their high RNA content, their cytoplasm is more basophilic than that of the parent cells. The nuclei may also be large and hyperchromatic because they usually contain excessive amounts of chromatin. The term *aneuploidy* refers to cells with an irregular number of chromosomes and the term *polyploidy* to an excess number of chromosomes.

Mitotic figures

In tumours, rapid growth usually indicates malignancy and attempts have been made to correlate the rate of growth with the number of mitotic figures seen in histological sections. The number of mitotic figures in growing tissues depends on two factors:

1. *The duration of the cell cycle* (p. **00**). In most tumours tested, the regeneration time is slower than in normal comparable cells. This prolongation of the cell cycle is partly responsible for the increased number and abnormal forms of mitotic figures often seen in sections of tumours.

2. *The number of cells undergoing division.* In normal cell division, one daughter cell usually remains as the stem cell and the other differentiates. In tumours, both daughter cells can differentiate and both can remain as stem cells; the latter situation can give rise to a logarithmic type of cell growth. It is generally assumed that the less tendency of cells to differentiate, the worse the prognosis.

Giant cells in tumours

Some malignant tumours are characterized by the presence of giant cells. A giant cell is one that is significantly larger than a normal cell – it may or may not have more than one nucleus. Two types are recognized:

1. *Tumour giant cells* usually contain 2–3 nuclei which vary in size, shape and staining affinities. The nuclei are the result of abnormal mitoses of tumour cells in which there is unequal segregation of chromosomes and failure of cleavage of the cytoplasm. Tumour giant cells are neoplastic cells.

2. *Foreign body or reactive giant cells*, by contrast, are much larger than tumour giant cells. They may contain 100 or more nuclei all of which are regular in form and resemble the nuclei

of the blood monocytes from which the foreign body giant cells are derived. They are not neoplastic cells but constitute a reactive component and when they are present there is usually other evidence of chronic inflammation.

The stroma

Solid epithelial tumours also contain a stroma which provides structural support for the parenchymal cells and carries the nutrient blood vessels. The tumour stroma is composed of fibrous tissue. It represents remnants of normal host connective tissue invaded by the malignant cells as well as newly formed connective tissue which is a result of active proliferation of fibroblasts to keep pace with the growing parenchyma. In developing papillary tumours and intestinal polyps the existing connective tissue support is not adequate and new connective tissue grows outwards with the proliferating epithelium.

The amount of stroma determines the consistency and texture of tumours. Some tumours such as the scirrhous carcinoma of the breast produce large amounts of fibrous connective tissue and collagen and are referred to as *desmoplastic*. They have a firm texture and give a grating sensation when cut. Other cancers are predominantly cellular with very little connective tissue. They give rise to soft masses with a consistency resembling brain tissue or marrow and they are described as *encephaloid or medullary*.

With the exception of the haemangiomas, the blood vessels of tumours are natural concomitants of growth and not a neoplastic component. Newly formed vessels in malignant tumours, especially in sarcomas, are imperfectly developed. They are usually thin-walled and friable consisting of a single layer of endothelium and are easily invaded by tumour cells. These vascular abnormalities explain the general tendency of sarcomas to haemorrhage, degeneration, necrosis and spread via the bloodstream.

Mononuclear cells such as lymphocytes, monocytes and plasma cells are frequently present within the stroma and at the periphery of some tumours. In ulcerating tumours, accumulation of inflammatory cells has been attributed to necrosis of tumour cells, but in other cases, necrosis does not produce an inflammatory reaction. Frequently, no cause can be found to account for the presence of mononuclear cells. Accumulation of lymphocytes near the spreading margin of tumours occurs commonly in some carcinomas of the breast, malignant melanomas of the skin and neuroblastomas. In these cases, accumulation of lymphocytes has been interpreted as evidence of an immune response by the host against the presence of the tumour. In melanoma, there seems to be an inverse relationship between the degree of cellular response and the size and duration of the tumour. In other tumours, such as Hodgkin's disease, the whole stroma of the tumour may be infiltrated with lymphocytes and, in these, the degree of lymphocytic infiltration has shown good correlation with the prognosis of the condition.

BEHAVIOURAL CHARACTERISTICS OF TUMOURS
(Capacity for progressive growth)

The biological behaviour of a cell population determines whether the tumour is benign or malignant. A *benign tumour* is one that grows slowly by expansion, remains well localized and does not recur after surgical removal. In contrast, a *malignant tumour* grows by invasion of adjacent tissues, becomes fixed to surrounding structures, spreads, metastasizes and often recurs locally after removal. Innocence and malignancy are not distinct entities, but represent the two extremes in a broad spectrum of behaviour.

In many tumours, histological differentiation between innocence and malignancy is relatively easy because there is a fairly well established relationship between the behaviour of a tumour and its histological structure. This behaviour can be predicted histologically, even at a very early stage in the development of the tumour. The degree of malignancy can be assessed on the extent of invasion of normal structures that lie in the path of the infiltrating cells and on the degree of differentiation of the tumour cells. Thus a diligent search of the advancing margin of the tumour will often reveal early evidence of invasion. Tumour cells may be seen within capsular or extracapsular vessels, or in lymphatics or perineural spaces. Invasion through the basement membrane of glands and ducts or through the muscularis mucosa of the bowel are also early signs.

However, there is an intermediate group of conditions in which the morphological criteria are confusing. This applies particularly to certain hyperplasias in which some degree of atypical cell growth has occurred. The outstanding examples are hyperplasias of the breast, prostate and thyroid gland. Hyperplasias are localized areas of cell proliferation due to abnormal hormonal activity and differ from carcinoma in that the hyperplastic cells are not permanently changed. They return to their original condition after removal of the stimulus. Though many cases of hyperplasia present no difficulty in diagnosis, some show such extraordinary degrees of proliferation that they present problems in their differentiation from carcinoma. Not only do they show variation in cell size, nuclear form and increase in the layers of cells lining the ducts, but the cellular atypia of the tissue in general makes distinction of such areas from neoplasms difficult. Furthermore, a small focus of malignancy may develop in a relatively large area of hyperplasia and be overlooked.

Histological interpretation is not always the last word in the determination of a malignancy, but it is a most important and valuable means of assessment. Some of the more important histological criteria that are evaluated in determining whether a tumour is benign or malignant are tabulated below. They represent an oversimplification of the biological problem that has to be faced and it should be realized that some tumours do not lend themselves to this approach:

	Benign	Malignant
Parenchyma		
Cell Pattern	Similar to tissue of origin	Variable
Cell Differentiation	Well differentiated	Well, poorly or undifferentiated
Pleomorphism	Absent	Large, pleomorphic, hyperchromatic
Giant Cells	Absent	Often present
Mitotic Figures	Few mitoses	Many mitoses
Invasion and Spread	Absent	Frequent
Stroma		
Connective Tissue	Similar to tissue of origin	May be scanty or excessive
Vessels	Normal	Thin, friable, haemorrhages
Mononuclear Cells	Usually absent	Lymphocytes, monocytes, plasma cells

THE CLASSIFICATION OF TUMOURS

All tumours arise from pre-existing cells. As the tumour grows, the neoplastic cells acquire characteristic morphological features which resemble, to some extent, those of the tissue from which the tumour arises. This resemblance is closer in benign than in malignant tumours. It is on this basis that tumours are classified. As a general rule, the terminology is constructed so as to indicate the histological structure of the tumour, its anatomical site and whether it is benign or malignant. In undifferentiated tumours, normal histological structure may be impossible to determine and such cases are designated *malignant undifferentiated tumours*.

The histological classification of tumours, therefore, depends on the identification of the basic cell type present and on the tissue of origin. The examples listed in Table 1.1 represent only a small cross-section of the tumour spectrum and have been selected to illustrate the principles of terminology. More detailed classifications of tumours of each tissue are presented in the appropriate chapters.

Table 1.1   Classification and nomenclature of some tumours

	Benign Tumour	Malignant Tumour
Epithelium		
Squamous	Papilloma	Squamous-cell carcinoma
Transitional	Papilloma	Transitional-cell carcinoma
Glandular:		
Papillary	Papilloma	Papillary carcinoma
Solid	Adenoma	Adenocarcinoma
Cystic	Cystadenoma	Cystadenocarcinoma
Mixed (cystic and papillary)	Papillary cystadenoma	Papillary cystadenocarcinoma
Connective and Supportive Tissues		
Fibrous tissue	Fibroma	Fibrosarcoma
Cartilage	Chondroma	Chondrosarcoma
Bone	Osteoma	Osteosarcoma
Adipose Tissue	Lipoma	Liposarcoma
Blood Vessels	Haemangioma	Haemangiosarcoma
Muscle		
Smooth muscle	Leiomyoma	Leiomyosarcoma
Striated muscle	Rhabdomyoma	Rhabdomyosarcoma
Nervous Tissue		
Glial Tissue		Glioma
Nerve sheath	Neurilemoma	Neurogenic sarcoma
Meninges	Meningioma	Meningeal sarcoma
Peripheral nerve cells	Ganglioneuroma	Neuroblastoma
Reticuloendothelial Tissue		
Lymphoid tissue		Non-Hodgkin's lymphomas, Hodgkin's lymphomas
Granulocytes		Myeloid leukaemia
Plasma cells		Myeloma
Other Tissues		
Placenta	Hydatidiform mole	Choriocarcinoma
Pigmented cells	Naevus (mole)	Malignant melanoma
Mixed tissues (from germ cells)	Benign teratoma	Malignant teratoma

Benign connective tissue tumours are indicated by adding the suffix -*oma* (i.e. tumour) to the cell-type. For example, *fibroma* is a benign tumour composed of fibroblasts. In malignant connective tissue tumours the suffix -*sarcoma* is added to the cell-type, e.g. *fibrosarcoma*.

Epithelial tumours do not fit the above system of nomenclature as well as connective tissue tumours. Tissues such as gut, respiratory passages, gall bladder and ducts of glands are all lined by a similar type of columnar epithelium which does not permit precise identification of the tissue of origin in tumours of these organs. These tumours, therefore, are classified partly on macroscopic and partly on microscopic features. Again, the suffixes -*oma* and -*carcinoma* indicate benign and malignant tumours respectively. The prefix in epithelial tumours is an adjective which describes the type of epithelium of which the tumour is composed. For example, squamous-cell papilloma and squamous-cell carcinoma describe the benign and malignant tumours that contain squamous epithelium, transitional-cell carcinoma arises in transitional epithelium, adenoma and adenocarcinoma are composed of glandular structures and papillary carcinoma is composed of papillary processes.

FURTHER READING

Adami, J. G. (1909) *Principles of Pathology.* London: Oxford University Press.
Willis, R. A. (1967) *Pathology of Tumours.* London: Butterworth.

The spread of cancer

Malignant cells are characterized primarily by two properties:

1. *Invasiveness*, the ability to infiltrate normal tissues, lymphatics and blood vessels.

2. *Metastasis*, the establishment and growth of secondary tumour nodules at sites remote from the primary growth.

A classical account of the spread of tumours in the human body is given by Rupert Willis (1973). There are five major pathways by which tumour cells may spread.

DIRECT INVASIVE SPREAD

Spread along tissue planes and tissue spaces occurs at the periphery of a growing tumour. The proliferating cells become detached from the main mass and compete for nutriment with adjacent normal cells which are gradually destroyed and replaced by tumour cells.

Detachment of tumour cells from the primary growth is the first step in the spread of cancer. The interrelationship between these cells and the normal cells of the host has been the focus of much research, but it is still the least understood aspect of malignancy. The capacity of malignant cells to invade and destroy normal host tissues has been equated with altered surface properties which render cancer cells less adhesive than normal cells (p. 34). When compared with normal cells, malignant cells growing in tissue culture show increased negative surface charge, increased amoeboid motility, decreased adhesiveness and loss of contact inhibition. Lytic enzymes released by the tumour cells have also been implicated for the destruction of normal tissue.

Direct spread may be an active or a passive process. In histological sections prepared from the periphery of a carcinoma, groups and strands of cancer cells can be seen infiltrating adjacent normal tissues. Although this type of spread tends to occur radially in all directions, cancer cells generally grow more easily in some directions than others. For instance, if the tissue is soft the cells can spread more easily, if there is a layer of fascia, the cells tend to grow along this plane, or if a tumour is in the spinal canal it will grow out more readily through the foramina than through bone. These histological appearances are responsible for the earlier view that growth of malignant cells follows paths of least resistance because they suggest that detached cells are passively propelled along these pathways by tissue movements, gravitational forces and other external pressures such as palpation or injury. Direct spread is also an active process due to the amoeboid movement of cancer cells and to their capacity for progressive multiplication, two properties which confer on these cells considerable survival advantage.

LYMPHATIC SYSTEM

The lymphatic system, a natural drainage mechanism, provides the most common pathway for spread, particularly for carcinoma and malignant melanoma. A prominent feature of spread of carcinomas is their tendency to metastasize to regional lymph nodes and the extent of lymph node involvement is of great prognostic significance following surgical removal of the tumour. Although sarcomas spread less commonly through lymphatics than carcinomas and tend to use the blood route, it is well to remember that both forms of cancer use both routes.

The walls of the lymphatic vessels, normally collapsed and not visible in tissue sections with the light microscope, are attached to adjacent tissue structures by fine fibrous tissue strands. When tissue swelling occurs, whether by oedema fluid or tumour, the strands become taut and act as guy ropes which open up the lymphatic channels and maintain them open against a raised interstitial pressure. Stretching of the walls of the lymphatic vessels creates gaps between the lining endothelial cells and a negative pressure in the lumen. The positive interstitial pressure, the negative intraluminal pressure, the gaps between the endothelial cells and the active amoeboid movement of the tumour cells all contribute to the passage of tumour cells through the walls of the lymphatic vessels and along the lymphatic channels.

Lymph nodes are not effective barriers against the further progress of tumour cells. Tumour cells can consistently be collected from efferent lymphatics following injection of suspensions of tumour cells into the afferent vessel of a lymph node in experiments with animals. Thus, while a lymph node is an effective filter for clumps of tumour cells, it is by no means an impervious barrier to single cells.

The process of tumour spread via lymphatic channels may be orthograde or retrograde. The afferent lymphatics drain into the subcapsular sinuses of lymph nodes where early deposits are seen. Often, in the early stages of spread, histiocytes lining the sinusoids become swollen and may mimic tumour cells in appearance, but such a reactive response can usually be recognized because it is generalized throughout the node and the histiocytes frequently contain phagocytosed material. Malignant cells, on the other hand, usuall· deposit in clumps and are easy to recognize. When the region al nodes are blocked with tumour tissue there is reversal in flow and retrograde spread may occur, involving lymph nodes which do not normally drain the particular area. In carcinoma of the rectum, for example, lymphatic spread is normally upwards to the lymphatics along the superior rectal vessels which drain to the nodes near the bifurcation of the common iliac arteries. When the superior rectal nodes are blocked, downward spread to the nodes along the middle and inferior rectal vessels may occur, involving the external iliac and inguinal nodes. Lymphatic obstruction may also interfere with the normal drainage of interstitial fluid. For example, in carcinoma of the breast, obstruction to lymphatic drainage causes oedema and gives rise to the characteristic *peau d'orange* appearance of the overlying skin.

Careful histological examination of tissues between the primary growth and the regional lymph node containing tumour deposits in a wide variety of tumours may or may not demonstrate tumour cells in the intervening lymphatics. This indicates that spread along lymphatic channels may occur by permeation or it may be embolic in nature.

BLOOD SPREAD

There are three routes by which cancer cells may enter the blood stream:
  1. The lymphatics that communicate with the venous system.
  2. Invasion of the blood vessels.
  3. Intravasation.
Blood spread is the most important pathway of dissemination of cancer cells to distant sites other than lymph nodes.

Invasion of blood vessels
Although tumour cells may enter the blood stream via the thoracic duct, the commonest route is direct invasion of veins. At the edge of a growing tumour there are many capillaries, arteries and veins.

Arteries are rarely penetrated, perhaps because of their thick walls, the arterial pressure and the constant pulsation, but they are not completely immune. For example, the pulmonary artery is frequently involved and, on rare occasions, the wall of a pre-existing aneurysm may become eroded, resulting in a massive and sometimes fatal haemorrhage.

Veins and capillaries, on the other hand, which have thinner walls, are much more vulnerable to invasion by cancer cells than arteries. The factors responsible for venous invasion and the mechanism by which it occurs are vague and uncertain. Obviously, the thickness of the wall of the vein, the low blood pressure and the growth potential of the tumour are important. Unlike the media of arteries, which is a thick, intact, encircling layer, the media of veins is thin with numerous breaks along its length. Tumour cells can infiltrate between these muscle fragments and reach the endothelium. Penetration of the endothelium may cause deposition of platelets which release vasoactive amines and initiate the formation of a thrombus, an ideal growth medium for the tumour cells. If the vein is small, the thrombus may obstruct the lumen and the static column of blood coagulates. Tumour cells may grow and permeate along the lumen of the vein as far as the next tributary where the calibre of the vein becomes larger. At this point, tumour cells may detach from the main column and give rise to emboli. If the vein is large, the thrombus may not obstruct the lumen, but a portion of the thrombus may detach and give rise to emboli, some of which may contain tumour cells.

Certain cancers are noted for their propensity to invade and penetrate veins. Renal carcinoma can sometimes be found growing along the renal vein as a solid column of cells extending up the inferior vena cava and entering the right side of the heart. A carcinoma of the left kidney may invade the spermatic vein and give rise to a varicocele. Carcinomas of the liver also have a similar tendency to invade hepatic and portal veins. Sarcomas have a greater propensity for blood spread than for lymphatic spread whereas malignant melanomas and testicular tumours spread just as frequently by the blood as by the lymphatic route.

Intravasation
Intravasation is the entry of cells into the circulation through defects in the vessel walls. Whether or not cancer cells gain entry by this means remains to be established. Bone marrow, fat, trophoblast and brain have been demonstrated as blood-borne emboli in the pulmonary blood vessels of some accident victims. If normal

cells which do not possess invasive properties can get into blood vessels, it is reasonable to assume that cancer cells also can gain entrance by this means. Should intravasation be a significant mode of entry of tumour cells into the blood stream, one wonders how often clinical palpation and trauma promote blood spread metastases.

Presence of tumour cells in the circulation

In a small number of patients with cancer, it is possible to demonstrate tumour cells in the peripheral blood. If the sample of blood is taken from a vein draining the tumour site, the incidence of finding tumour cells is higher and if it is taken soon after clinical manipulation or a surgical operation, showers and clumps of cells may be found. The presence of cancer cells in the blood of patients appears to have no clinical significance, since no statistical difference can be demonstrated in the survival times between this group and a group of cancer patients with no tumour cells in the blood.

Transport in the circulation

As a general rule, tumour cells in the portal vein go to the liver, whereas those in the systemic circulation, such as the superior or inferior vena cava, find their way into the lungs and, via the pulmonary vein, the cells may be transported to any part of the body. In most cases, the tumour cells are carried in the venous blood, pass through the lungs and are distributed to peripheral organs in the arterial blood. In patients with a patent *foramen ovale*, paradoxical embolism may occur, but this is an uncommon event. In some cases, alternative routes of transport may also occur. For example, in tumours of the prostate, kidney and uterus, tumour cells may be transported through the valveless vertebral system of veins. This occurs when there is obstruction of a vein by a tumour or during periods of increased intrathoracic or intra-abdominal pressure which develops with persistent coughing or straining. In these circumstances, reversal of blood flow occurs in the adjoining paravertebral venous plexus and tumour emboli may be carried to tissues such as the vertebrae, brain and thyroid gland without first passing through the lungs.

TRANSCOELOMIC SPREAD

This route of spread mainly concerns the pleural, pericardial and peritoneal cavities. These cavities are essentially very large tissue spaces which present convenient surfaces along which tumours can grow and spread.

In the gastrointestinal tract, a carcinoma of the stomach arising in the mucosa may invade through the layers of the wall of the stomach to form a subperitoneal deposit. The subsequent growth of this deposit may take one of two courses:

1. It may involve the subperitoneal lymphatics and spread widely through the peritoneal surface giving rise to peritoneal carcinomatosis.

2. It may grow into the peritoneal cavity, in which case groups of cells may detach and escape in the peritoneal fluid.

Gradually, these cells gravitate to the lowest part of the peritoneal sac and may gain a new attachment in a hernial sac, the pouch of Douglas, the broad ligaments, or the ovaries. Occasionally, implantation occurs on the peritoneal coats of the ovaries, giving rise to large bilateral ovarian masses which often show characteristic mucus secreting cells and stromal proliferation and are known as *Krukenberg tumours*. It is not yet established whether Krukenberg tumours arise as a result of implantation, lymphatic or blood spread.

In patients with transcoelomic spread, lymphatic obstruction and vascular invasion often cause inflammation of the serous surfaces resulting in pleurisy, pericarditis or peritonitis, as the case may be. In these patients, the fluid in the serous sac has a high protein content, it is frequently bloodstained and contains tumour cells. The tumour cells can be detected by examining stained smears of a centrifuged deposit of the fluid.

SPREAD VIA NATURAL PASSAGES

Here we are mainly concerned with the respiratory, alimentary and urinary tracts. In a carcinoma of the stomach, additional tumours may occasionally be found in the duodenum and intestines, in a carcinoma of a main bronchus smaller tumours may be found in the more peripheral bronchi and, more commonly, in papillary carcinomas of the pelvis of the kidney, smaller tumours are often found in the ureters and bladder. Such multiple tumours were regarded as implants of cells detached from the primary carcinoma and have contributed to the notion of spread via natural passages.

Three essential prerequisites determine the establishment of tumours following seeding with cancer cells:

1. The detached cells must be viable.

2. The environment into which the cells escape must be conducive to cell survival.

3. There must be a suitable site for the cells to lodge.

Most of our knowledge on the metabolic requirements of

mammalian cells is derived from cells growing in tissue culture. The immediate environment into which the cells lodge is the most important single factor determining growth. Its function is to provide adequate physical conditions of temperature, pH, osmotic pressure and to supply complicated chemical substances such as amino acids, carbohydrates, vitamins and hormones. Maintenance of these factors within very close limits is critical. For example, mammalian cells are rapidly destroyed by temperatures slightly in excess of those at which they operate best (37°C–38.5°C), the osmotic pressure of the medium is critical and the pH has to be maintained close to neutrality, optimum being between pH7.2–pH7.4. Even if the detached tumour cells are viable, it is unlikely that they would withstand either the acidity of gastric juice (pH2) or the high temperatures of ingested food. The presence of bile and enzymes such as proteases and lipases in the intestine would also rapidly digest and destroy any surviving cells.

Assuming that the cells survive the extreme environmental conditions of the respiratory, urinary and alimentary tracts, the chances of lodging at a favourable site are not good. Epithelial surfaces are covered by protective barriers such as cilia, mucin or keratin which separate the tumour cells from the underlying epithelial cells and prevent them from competing for nutrition. If there is an ulcer on the mucosal surface where the cells lodge, the chances of surviving and becoming established would probably be better but still not good.

It is doubtful if implantation metastasis ever occurs, and if it does, it must be an extremely rare phenomenon. The presence of multiple tumours in these areas is now regarded as due to the same carcinogen acting over a large area rather than being due to spread from a primary source. The examples of papillary carcinoma of the renal pelvis that are often associated with multiple similar tumours in the ureter and bladder, and especially when they are bilateral, tend to support the notion of the multifocal origin of these cancers. Cerebral tumours sometimes produce implantation nodules in the walls of the ventricles or meningeal surfaces, but these tumours are a special group. Secondary deposits of these tumours almost never occur outside the C.N.S., even in the most highly malignant glioblastomas.

METASTASES

Sooner or later, tumour cells escape from the main mass of the primary growth. The detached cells may remain in the vicinity of the primary growth or they may gain access to venous and lymphatic channels and then become widely disseminated, lodge in various parts of the body and multiply and grow into new tumours. Such secondary tumour nodules that develop away from the primary growth and have no anatomical continuity with it are called metastases. Cells may escape and start growing at a very early stage in the development of the primary tumour and when such cases are detected, the metastatic tumours may be larger than the primary growth. Indeed, the development of a metastasis is often the first indication of a primary tumour, a finding which has great significance in planning therapy and in the prognosis.

While metastasis is a common complication of cancer, it is a phenomenon which is poorly understood. Studies concerning the tumour cells themselves have provided little information apart from their reduced adhesiveness, low calcium content, high electric surface charge, motility and loss of contact inhibition (p. 34). The role of these factors *in vivo* is of doubtful significance. The type of vessel in which the tumour cells become impacted is probably more important in determining the fate of the cells. If the cells become impacted in a small artery or arteriole with thick walls, they tend to become destroyed. This probably explains the relatively few secondary tumours seen in the spleen. If impaction occurs in a thin walled venule or capillary, the cells are more likely to survive. In these latter cases, most of the tumour cells which lodge in the capillaries and become enmeshed by fine strands of fibrin and platelets die, but a selected few invade through the capillary wall into the perivascular connective tissue, where they undergo mitotic division. Only cells that penetrate the capillary wall appear to have the necessary growth characteristics which enable them to proliferate and give rise to secondary tumours.

Very little is also known about the factors involved in the establishment and growth of metastases. Their distribution can be explained partly on the basis of haemodynamics and volume of blood flow through tissues, and partly on the statistical probability that emboli may lodge at a particular site. But this is not the whole story. For years, pathologists have been puzzled by the fact that metastases are not uniformly spread in the body and that their distribution is not as closely related to blood supply as might be expected. Striated muscles, for example, which constitute a considerable bulk of the body and which receive a large portion of the cardiac output, rarely show secondary tumours. In liver, lungs, lymph nodes, brain and bones, on the other hand, metastases are common and often multiple and large. Certain tumours also show a tissue predilection for the establishment of their metastases; thus bronchogenic carcinoma frequently metastasizes in the adrenal glands and brain and carcinoma of the prostate gland to bone.

In order to explain the inconsistent and unpredictable patterns of metastases and the fact that all circulating cells do not form secondary tumours, attention has been given to the biological properties of the tissues. This is the *fertile soil* hypothesis, first suggested by Paget in 1889 to emphasize that survival and growth of disseminated tumour cells depends to some extent on the site where they lodge. Most of our knowledge on the role of the host in the development of metastases has been obtained from experimental systems by injecting tumour cells into the circulation or peritoneal cavity of animals and studying the factors that influence the development of metastases in specific organs. In the liver, for example, the dose of cancer cells injected, the presence of a thrombus around the cells, trauma at the site of lodgement, the presence of cirrhosis and a high protein and fat diet increased the number and size of metastases. On the other hand, hypophysectomy, adrenalectomy, cortisone administration, heparin and low protein diet resulted in a decrease in the number and size.

It is not possible to provide a plausible explanation for the distribution of metastases in the human body. Large numbers of circulating tumour cells can be seen microscopically in blood vessels but most of these fail to become established as metastatic foci. The *seed and soil* theory suggests that different tumour cells have different metabolic requirements and the availability of these requirements vary from organ to organ, but it seems very likely that other factors such as the immune status of the host (p. 89) are also involved.

FURTHER READING

Abercrombie, M. & Ambrose, E. J. (1962) The surface properties of cancer cells. *Cancer Res.*, **22**, 525.

Easty, G. C. & Easty, D. M. (1963) An organ culture system for the examination of tumour invasion. *Nature*, (Lond.), **199**, 1104.

Fisher, B. & Fisher, R. F. (1967) Metastases of cancer cells. *Methods in Cancer Research*, **1**, 243.

Willis, R. A. (1973) *The Spread of Tumours in the Human Body*, 3rd edn.
    London: Butterworth.
Ziedman, I. (1961) The fate of circulating tumour cells through capillaries.
    Cancer Res., **21**, 38.

3

Biology of the cancer cell

The field of cancer research includes experimentation in all branches of physics, chemistry and biology. The reason for this wide ramification into the basic sciences is that cancer is essentially a disturbance of normal cell growth, and understanding the problems of the origin, nature, development and control of cancer depends on understanding the mechanisms that control normal growth. It is appropriate, therefore, at the outset to mention briefly some of the important characteristics of growth in order to place the biological properties of cancer cells in better perspective.

THE GROWTH OF A TUMOUR

The size of an organ is remarkably constant especially when expressed as a percentage of the total body weight. This stringent control of growth is not a chance phenomenon; it is the result of a delicately balanced replication of cells which is reflected as growth and maintenance of normal organs. The constituent cells multiply in just the right numbers and right relationships to give rise to characteristic structures such as kidney, liver or spleen. Thus normal growth is orderly, controlled and predictable.

The growth of a tumour also results from repeated division of cells, but this type of cell multiplication differs from that of normal cells and precisely how it differs is not known. A clear cut distinction is obviously important if we are to understand the nature of malignancy and to devise methods of treatment that are capable of selecting cancer cells without damaging other body tissues.

A popular theory which is still dogma in some textbooks is that cancer is an autonomous growth and represents a rapid and completely uncontrolled multiplication of cells. This theory, which is supported by the high number of mitotic figures commonly seen in histological sections of tumours, tends to perpetuate the myth of the proliferation of cancer cells outstripping their normal counterparts and reflects a lack of appreciation of the biological behaviour of tumour cell populations.

Laws govern the growth of tumours just as they govern the growth of normal tissues, the essential difference being that in the neoplastic condition there is a disturbance in the homeostatic mechanism which controls the cell mass of a tissue. It is important to emphasize that cancer cells do not have autonomous growth and they do not divide faster than normal cells; if anything, their transit through the mitotic cycle is slower. If the multiplication of cancer cells were autonomous, their potential for growth would be immense. For example, by assuming that a cancer cell replicates once a day and that one gram of tumour tissue contains 10^5 cells, it is relatively easy to show that a single cell in just over three months would give rise to a mass of cells equivalent to the mass of the earth.

Cell kinetic studies have shown that the size of a tumour at any particular instant is the result of a dynamic equilibrium between the rate of cell loss, on the one hand, and the rate of cell replacement on the other. If this equilibrium is reached at an early stage, the tumour will be small, if late, the tumour will be large. The rate of cell replacement depends partly on the proportion of cells that are dividing (the *growth fraction*) and partly on the duration of the *mitotic cycle*. *Cell loss* may result from cell death and from migration of cells outside the original cell population. In other words, three parameters control the overall growth of a tumour at any particular instant, namely, the cell cycle time, the size of the growth fraction and the rate of cell loss (Fig. 3.1).

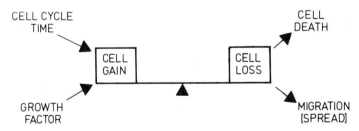

Fig. 3.1 The parameters controlling the growth of a tumour shown in diagrammatic form

THE CELL CYCLE

The cell cycle represents the interval between successive cell divisions and the cell cycle time is the average time that elapses between cell divisions. They are sometimes referred to as the generation cycle and the generation time, respectively. The formulation of the cell cycle concept has been a major breakthrough in studies on the mechanisms of growth control and has had a particular impact on the investigation of cell multiplication and cell differentiation. It has also provided a basis for the rational approach to the treatment of cancer. In conjunction with autoradiography, the cell cycle has played a key role in the development of the science of cell kinetics which is aimed at understanding the dynamic effects that take place in the life history of a cell, that is, its morphology, function, proliferation, differentiation, migration and death.

The mammalian cell cycle consists of four clearly defined periods (Fig. 3.2). Two of these, the period of mitosis (M) and the period of DNA synthesis (S), provide key reference points in the cycle because they can be visualized under the light microscope. The other two periods, in which no specific biochemical event has been demonstrated, represent gaps in our knowledge and are appropriately referred to as G_1 and G_2.

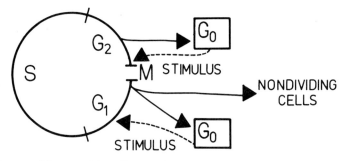

Fig. 3.2 Diagram of the cell cycle of mammalian cells showing the sequence of the phases

Phase G_1

In phase G_1, the cell is basically in a resting state. It synthesizes RNA, protein and probably an initiator protein that activates the enzyme DNA polymerase, which in turn initiates DNA synthesis. The duration of this phase is the most variable and may be prolonged into a resting phase, G_0 (stage of non-proliferation). Events in phase G_1 have a significant bearing on the rate of cell replication and on whether or not the cell will differentiate into a specific phenotype.

S-phase

Once the cell has proceeded into S-phase, it is committed to complete it without a rest period and to progress through to G_2. During this phase, the cell doubles its DNA and histone content to become tetraploid and concomitantly synthesizes RNA, protein and an initiator protein which activates the enzyme *DNA polymerase*. S-phase lasts approximately 6–8 hours in rodents and 10 to 20 hours in man. It is very sensitive to X-rays and cytotoxic drugs.

Phase G₂

Phase G_2 has no specific biochemical function assigned to it, but protein and RNA continue to be synthesized and the microtubules needed for the mitotic spindle are probably polymerized during this phase. Some cells may have a rest period in this phase, especially basal cells of the skin and premalignant cells that have been initiated with carcinogens. It is of interest that immunosuppressants can induce mitosis in G_2-resting cells and that phase G_2 might be an important phase for the action of promotors during carcinogenesis.

M-phase

M-phase represents the morphological process of mitosis and lasts approximately $\frac{1}{2}$ to 2 hours in both man and rodents. Once initiated, mitosis proceeds to completion. In tumours, M-phase varies in duration and abnormal mitoses commonly occur due to unequal segregation of chromatin. If, in addition, there is failure of cleavage of the cytoplasm, tumour giant cells form which are larger than normal cells and usually contain two to five irregular nuclei. Bizarre and grossly abnormal mitoses may result in cell death, an important pathway for cell loss.

TYPES OF CELL POPULATIONS

To place neoplastic proliferation in proper perspective, we should first consider the cycling properties of normal cells. All cells in the body inherit the same genome, because they are derived from the same zygote. Despite their full complement of genetic material, the ability of mammalian cells to proliferate varies from tissue to tissue depending on the cell regenerative capacity of that tissue, so that they move through the cell cycle according to their committed function (Fig. 3.2). Some move continuously around the cycle, others leave the cycle to enter a resting phase (G_0) and others still leave the cycle permanently without ever dividing again. Thus three groups of cells are recognized.

(a) *Continuously dividing (labile) cells* such as the epithelia of the skin, gut and respiratory tract where there is a constant cell turnover.

(b) *Resting (stable) cells*, such as those of the liver, kidney, endocrine and exocrine glands. These cells survive indefinitely but retain their mitotic capacity and only divide to cope with increased functional demands or to replace cell loss.

(c) *Non-dividing (permanent) cells*, in which the growth potential is totally repressed. For example, neurones lose their capacity to divide as they become fully differentiated and highly specialized. These cells respond to excessive demands by hypertrophy, they can synthesize protein and RNA but not DNA, so that their RNA/DNA ratio rises.

Looked at from this aspect, tumours present a mixed cell population which consists of continuously dividing and resting cells. Strictly speaking, only those cell populations capable of cell multiplication should be able to produce tumours. Since nerve cells, for instance, no longer divide in the adult, but do divide in children, neoplasms of nerve cells (neuroblastomas) are found only in young people.

THE GROWTH FRACTION

The cell numbers in any part of the body are kept more or less constant. This *status quo* is achieved by a poorly understood but stringent pattern of events which ensure, in principle, that any cell loss that may have occurred is replaced by new cells.

A good example of a normal tissue that illustrates this maintenance of constant cell numbers is the growing end of a long bone. The ossification plate of a long bone is composed of parallel columns of cells embedded in a stroma of chondromucin. The cells on the epiphysial end of each column are small, dark-staining and contain very little cytoplasm. When these cells divide, one daughter cell remains as the stem-cell. The other daughter cell gradually increases in size, matures, differentiates and then undergoes a degeneration process in which it swells, its chromatin becomes pale and the cell eventually dies, leaving a hole in the diaphysial end of the column into which capillaries grow and enable calcification to occur. The rate at which cells multiply at the epiphysial end of the plate is equal to the rate at which they die at the diaphysial end, so that the cell numbers in the columns and the thickness of the ossification plate remain constant. The thickness of this radiolucent space on X-ray films is an important parameter for the radiologist.

Contact inhibition

If there is an increase in the rate of cell loss, it will result in an increase in the rate of cell production. In the course of healing of a surgical wound of the skin, for example, the first change observed is that the basal layers of cells adjacent to the wound flatten out and start to migrate across the area of defect. As these cells migrate, other cells just behind the advancing cells start dividing and continue to divide until contact is made with adjacent cells from the opposite edge of the wound when cell multiplication ceases. Replacement of destroyed cells by proliferation of reserve cells can only occur in those tissues in which the cells retain the capacity to divide.

Similar changes are observed in cells growing in tissue culture. Normal cells have a great affinity for solid surfaces and readily stick to glass or plastic. As long as there are only a few cells on the glass surface, cell division proceeds regularly once every 24 hours, but once the monolayer has become confluent, cell division and cell motility cease. Certain other alterations also take place, which result in switching off of DNA synthesis, so that further cell division becomes impossible. This inhibition of cell multiplication is known as *contact inhibition*.

This is one way in which tissues may operate in replacing cell loss. Cells appear to have receptors on their surface which register contiguity with adjacent cells and prevent further multiplication. It is likely that the stimulus to cell multiplication is reduction in cell density or cell tension. In contrast, cancer cells in tissue culture do not stop multiplying when a monolayer has formed. Instead, the cells pile up on top of each other forming heaped up masses.

Recent work indicates that this interpretation of contact inhibition could be wrong. One reason why multiplication of tumour cells is not inhibited by contiguity is that they can manage on far less serum and oxygen than normal cells.

Growth inhibiting factors

As a result of such observations, the hypothesis has evolved that cells capable of division would go on dividing except when restrained. If multiplication is inhibited in response to contiguity between cells, something more than mere contact must be involved and the suggestion has been made that inhibition might be brought about by substances such as macromolecules which pass from one cell to another across the areas of contact. In support of this theory, it has been shown that the cells of some tissues are linked by specialized junctions which permit free flow of electrolytes and protein from cell to cell. In cells growing in tissue culture, even cytoplasmic particles have been shown to pass across these intercellular bridges.

Hormone-like substances may be responsible for the phenomenon of contact inhibition. Recently, experimental proof of the existence of an inhibitory substance has been provided by some workers who extracted a factor from epidermis capable of inhibiting cell division in squamous epithelia of a wide variety of animals. They called the substance *chalone*. It is a glycoprotein with a molecular weight of 40 000 and it requires adrenaline as a cofactor in order to exert its effect. Such substances are thought to be elaborated by cells and to inhibit the growth of their own kind.

The theory then is that cells in contact with each other are restrained from multiplying by a constant flow of specific substances through the areas of contact. When tissue architecture is disturbed, the flow is interrupted, the restraint is removed and cell multiplication takes place. When contact is re-established, the flow of these substances is also re-established and multiplication is again inhibited. Cancer cells have fewer contacts than normal cells.

Hormones

The stimulating and inhibiting influence of hormones on cell proliferation has been known for a long time.

1. Eunuchs never develop cancer of the prostate.

2. Growth of carcinoma of the breast and carcinoma of the prostate can be inhibited or enhanced by the administration of heterosexual or homosexual hormones, respectively.

A large proportion of human cancers arise in steroid hormone target organs, namely, the breast, the prostate gland, the testis, the ovary and the uterus. Many tumours of these organs are dependent on hormones for their continued growth; in some cases of carcinoma of the breast, regression of the tumour occurs following bilateral adrenalectomy and oophorectomy which withdraws steroid hormone production, and similarly, carcinoma of the prostate gland regresses following orchidectomy or prolonged administration of oestrogens. However, during the course of further development, these tumours tend to lose their hormone-dependence and start growing again.

The mechanism by which steroid hormones influence cell proliferation has now been worked out in some detail. Steroid hormones are small molecules which interact with specific cytoplasmic receptor proteins, and the complex formed by the hormone and the receptor acts on the genetic material of the cell and controls protein synthesis. Each steroid hormone affects only a few tissues because only the cells of those tissues contain the appropriate receptor proteins. The concentration of receptor proteins in a given tissue controls the cell's response to the hormone, but this concentration is not fixed, it can be influenced by the physiological state of the cell, its age and by the presence or absence of other hormones.

Hormones may also influence cell proliferation via the *cyclic AMP* (*cAMP*)/ *adenyl cyclase* system. Adenyl cyclase is located on the cell membrane and is involved in the formation of cAMP from ATP.

$$ATP \xrightarrow[\text{cyclase}]{\text{adenyl}} cAMP + pyrophosphate$$

This enzyme recognizes specific hormones (adrenalin, glucagon, adrenocorticotrophic hormones and melanocyte stimulating hormone) by their molecular configuration and becomes activated by them. The concentration of cAMP in the cell cytoplasm rises and this in turn stimulates the required response, be it metabolic, contractile or proliferative. In this system, the hormone acts as 'first messenger' by passing on information to the receptor, and cAMP acts somehow by executing the information. The precise mechanism by which these changes are mediated is not clear. An intermediate step involving prostaglandin might also be involved.

These mechanisms of hormonal influence on cell proliferation provide a plausible explanation of how primary and metastatic cancer cells may remain dormant for many years and why spontaneous remissions and regressions of primary tumours occur.

CELL LOSS

Cell loss is an important factor in determining the extent of tumour growth. It is due to random cell death and to migration of cells from the periphery of the tumour via lymphatics and blood to distant parts of the body.

The cause of cell death in cancer is not clearly understood. Nutritional difficulties due to anoxia and poor blood supply in some solid tumours may account for focal areas of coagulative necrosis but they do not explain the more important type of random cell death that commonly occurs, for example, in the leukaemias where no nutritional complications exist. The factors influencing random cell loss are more complex; intrinsic errors in cancer cells are often expressed during mitosis as abnormal and bizarre mitotic figures.

In recent years, isolated necrotic cells have been identified in all tumours, as well as in hormone sensitive tissues undergoing physiological involution, and the mechanism of their removal has been partly elucidated. Initially, the necrotic cell undergoes fragmentation, giving rise to small discrete masses of cytoplasm which may or may not contain fragments of nuclear chromatin. The fragments are phagocytosed by adjacent tumour or histiocytic cells and are digested by lysozomal enzymes. The phagocytosed fragments within cells which can be recognized morphologically have been aptly named *apoptotic bodies* (autophagic vacuoles). Death of cells by apoptosis occurs in both normal and neoplastic tissues and can be augmented by hormones.

Information derived from direct and radiological measurements on the doubling times of over 1 000 tumours in man, and from autoradiographic studies on the duration of the cell cycle, growth fraction and cell loss factor enables certain generalizations to be made.

1. The mean doubling time of human tumours varies widely, but three months is a reasonable working figure.

2. The size of the growth fraction (proportion of proliferating cells) is difficult to assess accurately. It may be as much as 100 per cent in undifferentiated tumours, 35 per cent in squamous-cell carcinoma, 15 per cent in sarcomas and 5 per cent in adeno-carcinoma.

3. Cell loss accounts for approximately 75 per cent of cell production, but also varies from one tumour type to another.

This information has not yet led to any improvements in therapeutic strategy. If the rate of cell loss were made equal to that of cell production, a steady state population would be reached in which no further tumour growth would occur; if cell loss were greater than cell production, it would result in a gradual decrease in population size or tumour regression.

CELL DIFFERENTIATION

Cell differentiation is another important mechanism in the control of cell multiplication. As an embryo develops, its cells differentiate into those characteristic of various tissues such as liver, kidney or brain. It is not known, for example, what dictates that a muscle cell should selectively synthesize contractile protein fibres, a squamous cell, keratin and a melanocyte, melanin. Immediately following cell division the daughter cells are small, undifferentiated and resemble stem cells, but they soon increase in size, their nucleus becomes vesicular, their cytoplasm increases in amount and finally cytoplasmic inclusions and organelles characteristic of the particular tissue become evident. This orderly sequence of changes that takes place in postmitotic cells as they acquire specific morphological and functional characteristics is called *differentiation*. The process of cell differentiation is associated with a decline in proliferative activity and with the elaboration of specific end products.

Mitotic activity is profoundly affected by the functional demands on a particular organ and, as cell output depends on the degree of specialization, it is not surprising that mitotic activity should also depend on the cell's degree of differentiation. It has been suggested that these specialized cell products may operate in a negative feedback circuit to turn off DNA synthesis.

The elaboration of specific end products by differentiated cells is probably a result of selective genetic expression so that the understanding of differentiation is, in a sense, an understanding of how genes function selectively. It is currently thought that differences in protein synthesis arise because only a small fraction of all the genes in a cell is used to make RNA, and because this fraction differs in different kinds of cells. Since all cells in the body are derived from the same zygote, each must contain a complete copy of the genetic information present in the zygote, and the bulk of this information must be constantly suppressed in differentiated cells. Experimental support for this notion came from workers who transplanted an epithelial cell nucleus from the intestine of a tadpole into an enucleated egg. The subsequent development of an adult frog indicated that the differentiated nucleus contained all the necessary information required for the production of an adult frog, even though this information was not being expressed while the nucleus was in the intestinal cell. In other words, the process of differentiation involves selective transcription rather than permanent structural changes in the DNA strand.

THE METABOLISM OF CANCER CELLS

Glycolysis

In his book on the metabolism of tumours, Warburg presented evidence to show that malignant cells consumed less oxygen and produced more lactic acid than normal cells. He attributed this property of malignant cells as an adaptation towards anaerobic respiration. Tumour cells cannot grow without oxygen, but they are able to derive their energy in areas where the partial pressure of oxygen is diminished and, in this way, they have considerable advantage over normal cells. This is in keeping with the finding that many tumour cells have fewer mitochondria and a greater glycolytic activity than normal cells.

The increased anaerobic glycolysis of cancer cells is now well established, but it appears to be no more than a metabolic adaptation of the cells of rapidly growing tumours. In recent studies on the respiratory and glycolytic enzymes of normal and malignant liver cells, the cells of the slow-growing, highly-differentiated *minimum deviation hepatomas* have the same complement of iso-enzymes as normal adult liver, yet the tumours are malignant and kill their hosts.

L-asparaginase

The nonessential amino acid asparagine is readily synthesized by normal cells. Some tumour cells, particularly leukaemias, are unable to synthesize asparagine and die if they cannot acquire it from external sources. The enzyme L-asparaginase cleaves aspara-gine into ammonia and aspartic acid. From the theoretical view-point this property of leukaemic cells has important therapeutic implications. At last we have a metabolic defect in the malignant cell which is not present in the normal cell, and an enzyme which will act specifically against the malignant cell leaving the normal cell unaffected. Although this enzyme is effective in killing some malignant cells in man, resistance to L-asparaginase invariably develops and limits its usefulness.

Other metabolic alterations in tumour cells involve both gains and losses in synthetic activities. Some tumour cells produce hormones (p. 90) others, foetal antigens (α-foetoprotein and carcinoembryonic antigen) which are only present in the foetus (p. 91). The view that malignant cells secrete toxins which are responsible for the *cachexia* (p. 101) seen in patients with advanced cancer has not been substantiated.

THE CELL MEMBRANE

The growth regulation of cancer cells involves a complex and poorly understood chain of events. Extracellular regulators of many types probably interact with the cell membrane and then cytoplasmic mediators appear to transmit signals from the membrane to the nucleus where perhaps they control DNA-binding proteins. The cell membrane, therefore, is being implicated as playing a critical role in cell proliferation. In support of this role, a number of alterations have been demonstrated in the plasma membranes of cancer cells.

1. Increased concanavalin A (Con A) agglutinability.
2. Raised surface electric charge.
3. Decrease in Ca^{2+} concentration.
4. Decreased cell adhesiveness.
5. Increased cell motility.

Much of the work on these properties has been performed on established lines of virus transformed cells so that it has been impossible to unravel which changes are caused by the virus and which have arisen through selection in culture. This is a serious weakness of these studies and one cannot interpret the changes observed in tissue culture as biological properties of cancer cells in the whole animal.

Concanavalin A agglutinability

Con A (lectin), a bivalent agglutinating protein extracted from jack beans, agglutinates tumour cells but not normal cells. If normal cells are pretreated with trypsin, they agglutinate in the presence of Con A just as do transformed cells, suggesting that trypsinization exposes sites on the surface of normal cells which are always exposed in cancer cells. Monovalent Con A, prepared by trypsinization of the bivalent form, also reacts with cancer cells and forms a coat around them, but it does not cause agglutination. The Con A-coated cells behave like normal cells in tissue culture; they continue to divide until a confluent monolayer is formed and then stop dividing. This effect is reversible, because excess of certain substances such as methylglucose compete for Con A.

Alterations in surface electric charge

Normal cells have a negative electric charge on their surface, but tumour cells have a greater negative surface charge than normal cells. Cell electrophoresis shows that tumour cells migrate towards the anode at a faster rate than normal parent cells, a finding in keeping with a higher negative electric charge. Furthermore, there seems to be a relationship between the rate of migration in an electric field and the degree of malignancy, the cells of metastasizing tumours being the most rapidly migrating.

Alterations in Ca^{2+} concentration

According to Coulomb's Law, like charges repel and unlike charges attract each other. Normal cells are ionically bonded together by divalent Ca^{2+} present on their surfaces. Removal of Ca^{2+} with a chelating agent such as EDTA (ethylenediaminetetraacetic acid) results in loss of adhesiveness between adjacent cells and addition of Ca^{2+} restores contiguity. In fact, some embryonic tissues can be broken up and the cells separated by addition of EDTA. The lack of adhesiveness of tumour cells has been linked with a combination of local deficiency of Ca^{2+} and a higher electric surface charge which results in electrostatic repulsion.

Cell adhesiveness

Ca^{2+} bridges are not the only contacts between cells. Normal adult cells secrete substances into the intercellular space which provide the specialized junctions such as desmosomes and intercellular prickles which hold cells together. These adhesions cannot be separated by chelating agents; stronger agents such as trypsin are needed to dissolve them. Normal mammalian cells growing in tissue culture seem to make contact only with their kin, so that in a mixture of liver cells and kidney cells growing together, liver cells will only aggregate with liver cells and kidney with kidney. Tumour cells, on the other hand, cannot recognize each other, intercellular junctions are poorly formed and, in undifferentiated tumours, they may be completely absent.

Cell motility

Interference microscopy and time-lapse photography can be used to study cell motility. Compared with normal cells, tumour cells migrate at a more rapid rate. Continuation of migration and proliferations seems to facilitate infiltration and invasion.

FURTHER READING

Basarga, R. (1971) *The Cell Cycle and Cancer*. New York: Marcel Dekker, Inc.

Boyd, H., Louis, C. J. & Martin, T. J. (1974) Activity and hormone responsiveness of adenyl cyclase during induction of tumours in rat liver with 3′-MeDAB. *Cancer Res.*, **34**, 1720.

Bullough, W. S. (1965) Mitotic and functional homeostasis: A speculative review. *Cancer Res.*, **25**, 1683.

Burger, M. M. (1970) Proteolytic enzymes initiating cell division and escape from contact inhibition of growth. *Nature*, (Lond.), **227**, 170.

Chan, L. & O'Mally, B. W. (1976) Mechanism of action of the sex steroid hormones. *New Eng. J. Med.*, **294**, *1322, 1372, 1430*.

Coman, D. R. [1944] Decreased mutual adhesiveness. A property of cells from squamous cell carcinomas. Cancer Res., **4**, 625.

Furth, J. and Kim, U. (1961) Biological foundation of cancer control by hormones, in *Biological Approaches to Cancer Chemotherapy*, pp. 259–276. Edited by R. J. C. Harris. New York: Academic Press.

Gurdon, J. B. (1962) The developmental capacity of nuclei taken from intestinal epithelium cells of feeding tadpoles. *J. Embryol. exp. Morph.*, **10**, 622.

Iverson, O. H. (1968) Effect of epidermal chalone on human epidermal mitotic activity in vitro. *Nature*, (Lond.), **219**, 75.

Law, L. W. (1969) Studies of the significance of tumour antigens in induction and repression of neoplastic diseases: presidential address. *Cancer Res.*, **29**, 1.

Loewenstein, W. R. (1969) Transfer of information through cell junctions and growth control. *Canadian Cancer Conf.*, **8**, 162.

McNutt, N. S. & Weinstein, R. S. (1969) Carcinoma of the cervix: deficiency of nexus intercellular junctions. *Science*, **165**, 597.

Scott, E. R. & Furcht, L. T. (1976) Membrane pathology of normal and malignant cells – a review. *Human Pathology*, **7**, 519.

Wallach, D. F. H. (1968) Cellular membranes and tumour behaviour: a new hypothesis. *Proc. Natl. Acad. Sci. U.S.A.*, **61**, 868.

Warburg, O. (1930) *The Metabolism of Tumours* (translated by F. Dickens). London.

4

Chemical carcinogenesis

Cancer can be induced in experimental animals and man by many diverse agents. Such agents are known as *carcinogens* and they may be broadly grouped into:

1. Chemical carcinogens
2. Physical carcinogens
3. The oncogenic viruses

In this and the next two chapters, it is proposed to give a brief account of each group of carcinogenic agents and, to round off the subject of carcinogenesis, the possible mechanisms by which neoplastic transformation is achieved will be discussed in Chapter 7. As the chemical carcinogens constitute the major cause of cancer in man, they will be dealt with first, the main purpose being to present instructive examples that may be of relevance to the understanding of the cancer problem.

In addition to the carcinogenic agents are other intrinsic factors such as the genetic constitution of the individual, the hormonal status and the immunological and other defence mechanisms which also confer their own degree of protection or susceptibility. Thus, when a tumour is described as *spontaneous*, it does not imply that the tumour arises without cause, it simply means that the cause or causes are not known.

To prepare the ground for a more detailed discussion of specific chemical carcinogens, a rather brief historical account will be given to illustrate the manner in which present day knowledge of the aetiology of cancer has developed.

HISTORICAL SURVEY

The first clue that cancer might be due to exogenous chemical agents came from Percivall Pott, a Surgeon at St. Bartholomew's Hospital who, in 1775, attributed the high incidence of scrotal cancer in the chimney sweeps of London to prolonged contact with soot and tar. The men who developed cancer of the scrotum had been employed as chimney sweeps since childhood and, as children, they were forced to climb up the chimneys to scrape off the soot from the inside. Pott's observations were not followed up until many years later. In 1895 Ludwig Rhein, a Frankfurt surgeon, was struck by the fact that a number of his patients with cancer of the urinary bladder worked in the German chemical and dye industry. In spite of the limited number of patients that developed cancer, Rhein maintained that prolonged exposure to certain chemicals, mostly aromatic amines and in particular analine, was related to the development of malignancy.

These early clinical observations made by practising doctors set the stage for the epidemiological approach to the study of cancer, an approach which is extensively used today. However, conclusions as to the possible relationship between exposure to chemicals and the subsequent appearance of cancer in man are difficult to prove on the basis of epidemiological evidence alone. Because of this, attempts were made to produce tumours in animals. As a result, the experiments of the two Japanese investigators, Yamagiwa and Ichikawa, reported in Japanese in 1915 and in English in 1918, are one of the classics of cancer research. These workers applied coal tar to the ears of 137 rabbits on alternate days for approximately twelve months and, in this series, they induced seven cases of squamous-cell carcinoma, two of which had lymph node metastases. Thus, a simple experimental model became available for the induction of cancer and for testing carcinogenic substances.

The demonstration that coal tar induced carcinoma of the skin stimulated a search for the nature of the carcinogenic agents in tar. By 1930, Kennaway and Cook had played a major role in the identification of various carcinogenic hydrocarbons and their efforts in isolating pure compounds were comparable to those of the Curies in isolating radium from pitchblende. Cook had two tons of tar fractionally distilled several times at the Municipal Gas Works to obtain 50 mg of a carcinogenic compound which was later shown to be 3,4-benzpyrene. Since then, over 1 000 chemical compounds have been found to have carcinogenic potential and it is likely that many more will be discovered in the next few years.

PARAMETERS OF CARCINOGENIC ACTIVITY

Testing new substances for carcinogenicity

Early experimentalists testing the carcinogenicity of new compounds classified them crudely either as good or bad carcinogens.

A good carcinogen produced many tumours in a short period of time, whereas a poor carcinogen produced one or two small tumours over a long period of time. On this basis, Iball proposed a measure of carcinogenicity which has become known as the *Iball index* (*I*).

$$I = \frac{\text{Tumour Yield}}{\text{Latent Period}} \times 100$$

For many years, the Iball index enabled workers to test and compare the carcinogenicity of many new substances.

A variety of factors are involved in testing new substances for carcinogenicity. Such factors concern the product being tested and the test system, that is, the host and the total environment of the host. It is also important to have adequate controls to completely cover spontaneously occurring tumours. This type of carcinogenicity testing is adequate for powerful carcinogens, but in the case of compounds with borderline carcinogenic activity, the above factors could initially influence the accuracy of the evaluation. For example, the distinction between a compound that is a weak carcinogen and one that is a non-carcinogen can be very difficult indeed. The continuing arguments about the value of the contraceptive pill and the artificial sweetener, *cyclamate*, are two cases in point which illustrate the need for caution before making final decisions.

Dose

The tumour yield or carcinogenicity of a compound depends on the dose. In sensitive strains, large doses produce tumours in nearly 100 per cent of the population. Generally there is an apparent threshold dose below which no tumours develop, but above this level there is a dose/tumour-yield relationship (Fig. 4.1). With repeated subthreshold doses the overall effect is additive, and tumours develop after a long period of time. In other words, there is no threshold dose in the strict sense, the response is related to the total dose. Man is normally exposed only to minute doses of carcinogens, so that tumours take many years to appear.

Latent period

There is always a time-lag between the commencement of carcinogen administration and the appearance of macroscopic tumours. This is the *latent period*. In man, the latent period may vary from seven to 30 years, in rodents it varies from 12 weeks to 12 months. In each case, the latent period represents approximately 10 to 40 per cent of the respective life span. The length

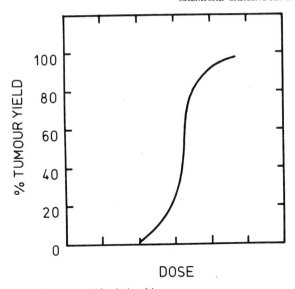

Fig. 4.1 Dose/Tumour yield relationship

of the latent period is dose dependent, the higher the dose the shorter the period. However, there is always a minimum time interval, the *absolute minimum latent period*, that must elapse before a tumour develops. The latent period has both a theoretical and a practical importance. It probably accounts for the rarity of tumours in the foetus and early childhood, and it is of importance in Worker's Compensation litigations in cases where tumours develop 10 to 30 years after the individual has left work.

New developments in screening tests

In modern industrial and agricultural societies, populations are being increasingly exposed to a wide variety of chemicals introduced in response to the pressure for higher living standards. Many of them, such as pesticides, insecticides, fertilizers, petroleum products, plastic precursors, building products and pharmaceutical products are essential components of modern living. Valuable as these substances are, they also carry some risk to health and particularly of carcinogenicity. There is a great need, therefore, for screening tests which can predict quickly and accurately the level of carcinogenic risk that may exist among these thousands of chemicals.

The traditional long-term tests in rodents are still considered to be the penultimate testing system (the ultimate being man himself) but these tests require large numbers of animals, they are time consuming and very costly. New screening tests are now being evaluated which are going to play an important role in identifying potential chemical carcinogens and in the control of environmental pollution. The test depends on the induction of mutations in bacteria such as *E. coli* and *S. typhimurium* by carcinogens which are activated by microsomal preparations incorporated in agar plates. It is extremely sensitive, rapid (results are seen in two days) and relatively inexpensive.

CLASSIFICATION OF CHEMICAL CARCINOGENS

Chemical carcinogens are a diverse group of compounds and can be classified in many ways. They may be sub-divided into those that occur naturally and those that are synthetic or man-made. Also, some chemical carcinogens induce tumours in a wide variety of species and strains of animals, on the other hand others are highly specific and, on this basis, two functional groups are recognized:

1. *Ultimate carcinogens* are compounds that are active as administered and produce tumours at the site of application.

2. *Precarcinogens* are inert compounds as administered. In these cases, the active substance is a metabolite of the original compound given and only the organs which possess the enzyme systems needed to metabolize the original compound to an ultimate carcinogen develop tumours. Precarcinogens, therefore, are remotely acting, they require metabolic activation and they produce tumours in tissues at a distance from the site of application.

Chemical carcinogens may also be classified according to their molecular structure. Whilst such a classification is useful to the organic chemist, it is of little value to the oncologist, because the molecular structure of the compound administered to a test animal is not related to its carcinogenic activity and therefore is of limited usefulness in predicting the carcinogenicity of new compounds. For our purpose, it is more useful and more practical to subdivide chemical carcinogens into those that are synthetic and those that are naturally occurring.

SYNTHETIC CARCINOGENS

The biological alkylating agents

This group comprises a very large number of compounds which are also mutagens. They include the sulphur and nitrogen mustards, epoxides, ethylene imines, certain lactones and many others. All of them are powerful alkylating agents for –OH and –NH$_2$ groups and their carcinogenic activity is thought to be connected with this property. The mustards will be used as key examples of the alkylating agents. Sulphur mustard was used as a war gas in World War I because of its acute cytotoxic effects. It was also found to produce chronic cellular changes similar to those produced by X-rays, hence it was termed a *radiomimetic drug*. Like X-rays, these compounds possess both carcinogenic and tumour inhibiting properties.

Structure
The mustards are organic compounds with a simple chemical structure (Fig. 4.2). Two types are recognized:

(a) *The difunctional* mustards in which both side chains contain reactive halogen atoms. These compounds are used in industry to

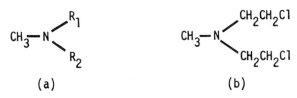

(a)   (b)

Fig. 4.2 The general formula of mustard gases (a) and the structural formula of nitrogen mustard (b)

cross-link wool and cellulose fibres to increase their tensile strength. The difunctional mustards are very cytotoxic, presumably because they cross-link chromosomes prior to mitosis and interfere with the segregation of the chromosomes in metaphase. Because of their cytotoxicity, they are commonly used for the treatment of cancer, for example nitrogen mustard, cyclophosphamide and chlorambucil (Fig. 4.3).

(b) *The monofunctional* mustards represent those compounds in which only one side chain contains a reactive halogen atom while the other is unreactive. These compounds are not as toxic as the difunctional mustards, but they tend to be more efficient carcinogens, possibly because they are good mutagens.

Enzymatic activation
These compounds do not require metabolic activation; they are ultimate carcinogens and act as administered at the site of appli-

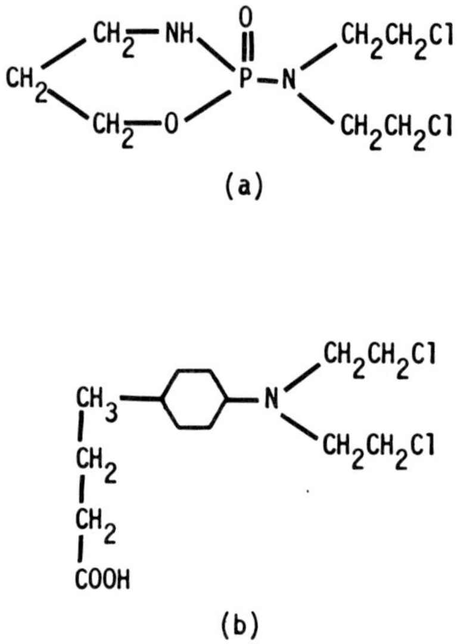

(a)

(b)

Fig. 4.3   The structural formulae of cyclophosphamide (a) and chlorambucil (b) both conforming to the general formula of the difunctional mustard gases

cation. Research with the alkylating agents has proved very successful because of their high reactivity and their capacity to enter into reactions with cellular macromolecules (p. 80).

The polycyclic aromatic hydrocarbons
These were the first compounds shown to possess carcinogenic activity. Common examples of this group are: dibenz(a,h)anthracene; 7,12-dimethylbenz(a)anthracene; benzo(a)pyrene and 20-methylcholanthrene. They were first isolated from coal tar and were tested for carcinogenicity by application to the skin of mice.

Structure
The carcinogenic polycyclic hydrocarbons may be considered to be basically derived from the anthracene nucleus (Fig. 4.4a). Anthracene itself is barely, if at all, carcinogenic. If a benzene ring is added in the *a*-position to form benz(a)anthracene (Fig. 4.4b) it becomes a potential carcinogen. This substitution adds electrons to the *c*-position, raises the electron density of this double bond and renders the compound much more reactive than anthracene. This region of high electron density is the *K-region* (from Krebs = tumour). If another benzene ring is added to block the K-region, carcinogenic activity is lost (Fig. 4.4c). If still another

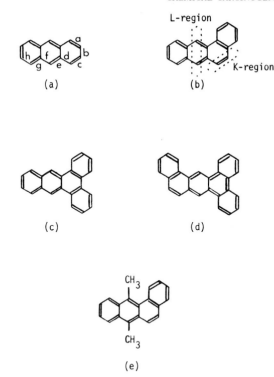

Fig. 4.4 The relationship of the polycyclic aromatic hydrocarbons: anthracene (a), the formation of benz(a)anthracene (b) showing the *K*- and *L*-regions, the inactivation of benz(a)pyrene by adding a benzene ring in the *c*-position (c), reconstitution of a new *K*-region in the *d*-position by adding another benzene ring (d), the structural formula of 7,12-dimethylbenz(a)anthracene (e)

ring is added to the molecule, another K-region is reconstituted and another carcinogenic compound produced (Fig. 4.4d).

If small groups are substituted in the 7,12-position (the *L-region*), the carcinogenicity of the compound is enhanced. CH_3-groups are electron donors and substitution of these groups increases both the electron density in the K-region and the carcinogenicity of the compound. The compound 7,12-dimethylbenz(a)anthracene (DMBA) is one of the most potent polycyclic hydrocarbons known (Fig. 4.4e).

Enzymatic activation

It is now clear that the polycyclic hydrocarbons are precarcinogens and require enzymatic activation. They are metabolized to ultimate carcinogens by the enzyme arylhydrocarbon hydroxylase (AHH) which is an inducible, microsomal, mixed function oxidase present in a variety of tissues. AHH oxidizes polycyclic hydrocarbons to epoxides which appear to be the necessary intermediate reactive forms. The level of activity of this enzyme can be increased by the administration of various drugs, pesticides and by cigarette smoking, as well as by administration of polycyclic hydrocarbons themselves. The induction appears to depend on the formation of new cytochrome P450, which is an essential component of the microsomal enzyme system.

Carcinogenic polycyclic hydrocarbons, particularly benzo(a)-pyrene, are constantly present in man's environment. The major generating sources are heating systems, industrial plants and internal combustion engines, especially aircraft engines, all of which pollute the atmosphere, water, soil and plants. Benzo(a)-pyrene is present in our food at concentrations as high as 25 pg/kg in vegetables, 5 to 20 pg/kg in cooking fats and oils and 5–50 pg/kg on the surface of barbecued meats and smoked foods. Polycyclic hydrocarbons are also released by cooking: fat in the diet heated at temperatures below 270°C is not carcinogenic but if heated above 350°C it is strongly suspect, cholesterol when heated to 430°C may be partially converted to 20-methylcholanthrene. These temperatures may be reached in domestic cooking and at the tips of cigarettes during smoking. Finally, naturally occurring substances such as bile salts and cholesterol might be converted by bacteria in the intestine to carcinogenic polycyclic hydrocarbons (p. 206).

The aromatic amines

Aromatic amines are obtained as by-products in the fractionation of tar. Many of the compounds are widely used as colourings in household products, paper, fabrics and industrial solvents or lubricants. The compounds possessing carcinogenic activity include: analine, auramine, benzidine, magenta, 4-aminobiphenyl, β-naphthylamine, the insecticide 2-acetylaminofluorene and the azo dyes which include *butter yellow*, once used as a food colouring agent.

β-naphthylamine

The compound β-naphthylamine (Fig. 4.5) was formerly used in the dye and rubber industries. It is a potent carcinogen for the urinary tract epithelium of man and dog. The amine itself is not carcinogenic, because it requires to be metabolized to an ultimate carcinogen.

When β-naphthylamine reaches the liver, the aromatic ring is

β-NAPHTHYLAMINE   2-AMINO-1-PHENOL

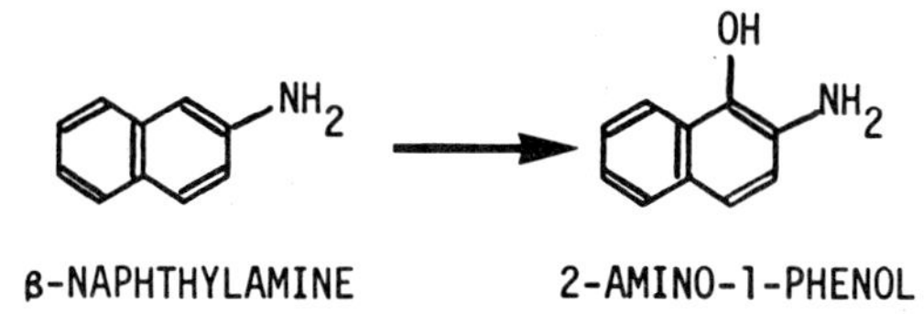

Fig. 4.5 β-naphthylamine and its active form 2-amino-1-phenol by oxidizing the aromatic ring

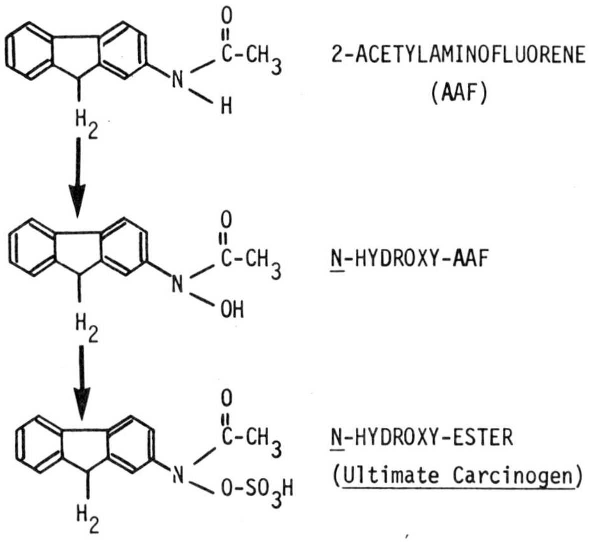

Fig. 4.6 The activation of 2-acetylaminofluorene to an active carcinogen

oxidized and 2-amino-1-phenol (Fig. 4.5) is formed, which is the ultimate carcinogenic metabolite. Normally, the metabolite is inactivated in the liver by conjugation with glucuronic acid and excreted in the urine as an inactive glucuronide, but the urinary epithelium of man and dog secretes the enzyme β-glucuronidase which releases the active metabolite. This metabolite is present in the urine of susceptible species.

2-Acetylaminofluorene (2-AAF)
The carcinogenic activity of 2-AAF (Fig. 4.6) was discovered in 1940 during routine testing before the compound was marketed as an insecticide. It is highly carcinogenic and induces tumours in rats, dogs, cats, rabbits and chickens. When injected, it does not produce tumours locally, but produces tumours in the liver and bladder. The N-hydroxy derivative of 2-AAF is more carcinogenic

than the parent compound and it is carcinogenic for more organs than the parent form. It does appear that the organs which are susceptible to the carcinogenicity of 2-AAF have the ability to N-hydroxylate it. 2-AAF is the first compound in which the oxidative attack on the nitrogen was demonstrated.

Aminoazo dyes

Knowledge of the carcinogenic action of the aminoazo dyes stems from the report by Fisher that injection of scarlet red into the ears of rabbits produced epithelial hyperplasia. These growths regressed when the stimulus was discontinued. Later, Yoshida produced hepatomas and cholangiomas by feeding rats *o*-aminoazobenzene, the active part of scarlet red, and later still it was reported that the isomer 4-dimethyl-aminoazobenzene (4-DAB) was a much more potent carcinogen than *o*-aminoazobenzene. 4-DAB (Fig. 4.7) is commonly called butter yellow because it was used to add colour to butter and margarine.

Like 2-AAF, 4-DAB is inactive as such until oxidized to a carcinogenic metabolite in target tissues. In both cases, the ultimate carcinogens appear to be their N–OH-esters (Fig. 4.7), particularly the sulphuric acid esters. Addition of sulphate to the diet of test animals increases the incidence of liver tumours.

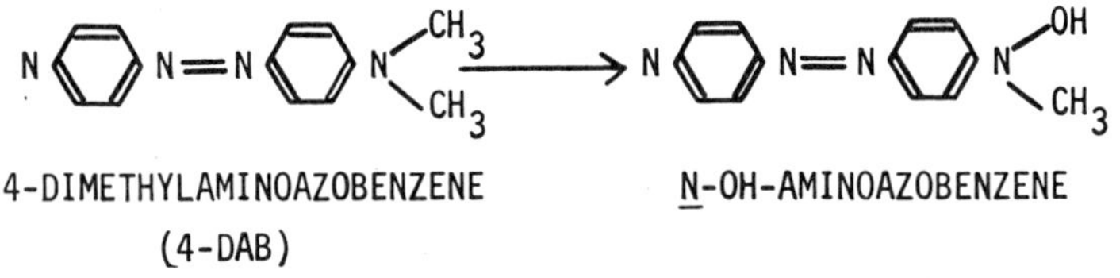

4-DIMETHYLAMINOAZOBENZENE
(4-DAB)

N-OH-AMINOAZOBENZENE

Fig. 4.7 4-DAB (4-dimethylaminoazobenzene) and its N-hydroxy derivative (b)

Very few epidemiological studies in workers exposed to azo dyes have been reported. Except for inconclusive data on certain occupational groups (tailors and hairdressers) bladder cancer rates do not appear to be increased in workers using the azo dyes as opposed to those employed in the manufacture of the dyes.

Film implantation

Subcutaneous implants of impervious plastic and metal films have been shown to be carcinogenic. In general, any solid material having an uninterrupted surface and a dimension greater than 5 mm^2 will cause tumours when implanted in rodents for a long period of time. Since other materials with different chemical structures can also produce tumours at sites of implantation, the term *film carcinogenesis* has been coined. It is assumed that the physical characteristics of the material, and not its specific chemical structure, play the predominant role in tumour induction. Perhaps the presence of a barrier between cells either prevents immunocompetent cells from reaching altered tissue cells or impairs the transmission of signals between cells which maintain contact inhibition. It has also been suggested that these tissues have already been initiated by other carcinogens and that the plastic films are simply acting as promoting agents.

NATURALLY OCCURRING CARCINOGENS

The way in which complex chemical and biological agents in the environment interact to increase or decrease the risk of cancer in man is not known. The food supply represents a major source of exposure of populations to a variety of chemical substances. Food can be contaminated at its source by the use of pesticides or herbicides during cultivation, or intentionally by the addition of chemicals such as antioxidants, preservatives, flavouring and colouring agents for specific purposes during processing. Most of these compounds are man-made and very few of them have been adequately tested for carcinogenicity. In addition, food contamination may be a result of a biological process during storage. Some of these biological contaminants induce liver cancer in mice and other animals when administered under experimentally controlled conditions, but these experiments require large doses, far in excess of those likely to be ingested by man.

The naturally occurring carcinogens are derived from plant and food products and some from mineral products such as shale oil. It is also possible that some carcinogens can be manufactured within the body from harmless precursors, for example, nitrosamines from amines and nitrites in food and 20-methylcholanthrene from the action of bacteria on cholesterol in the gut.

Mycotoxins
Dangers arising from biological contamination of food were first identified in 1961 following the outbreak of Turkey X disease in Britain and the epidemic of liver cancer in rainbow trout in the North-Western lake fisheries of the United States of America. The cause of both epidemics was traced to a groundnut meal contaminated by the common mould *Aspergillus flavus* which produces a

toxin, aflatoxin (Fig. 4.8). This and similar mycotoxins are acutely toxic to animals but, in smaller doses, they are amongst the most potent liver carcinogens known. The fungi are ubiquitous. Serious food contamination can occur, especially in the tropics, thus constituting a potential source of carcinogen for man. Local legislation in most countries prohibits marketing of aflatoxin-contaminated peanut meal.

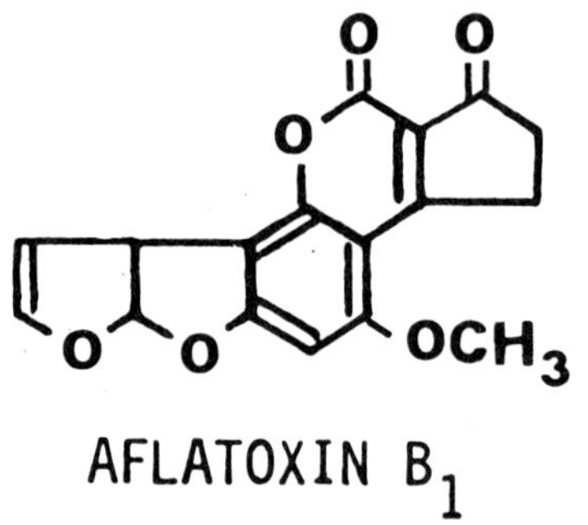

AFLATOXIN B$_1$

Fig. 4.8 The structural formula of aflatoxin B

Enzymatic activation
Recent evidence suggests that aflatoxin is metabolized by microsomal enzymes to form a highly reactive epoxide which is mutagenic to bacteria and carcinogenic to rat skin. The role of other mycotoxins in the induction of cancer in man is currently being investigated in Africa where liver cancer is common and where food crops are stored in conditions which facilitate fungal contamination. Surveys in Swaziland, Uganda, Thailand and Kenya indicate that the risk of hepatocarcinoma in the native populations is increased by exposure to mycotoxins through contaminated food.

N-Nitroso compounds
The nitrosamines comprise a widely acting group of carcinogens which are very potent. Minute quantities of nitrosamine are present in cigarette smoke, alcoholic beverages and certain foods, but their cumulative effect over several years could be an important cause of human cancer. They act optimally via the oral route and have selective carcinogenic action for oesophagus, lung, liver, kidney, bladder and brain.

Structure and synthesis
The nitrosamines have the general formula (Fig. 4.9). In the laboratory they are easily synthesized by mixing a secondary amine with nitrous acid under acidic conditions (Fig. 4.9). Nitrous acid is the acid formed when nitrite salts are dissolved in water. Since acid is an important requirement in the formation of nitrosamines from amine and nitrites the human stomach provides an ideal reaction vessel. Sources of nitrite include crops grown on mineral deficient soil (apparently related to different nitrogen fertilizers) and food cured with nitrite preservatives, and sources of amines include high protein meats and a large number of commonly used drugs such as phenacetin. Tumours have been induced by feeding animals with mixtures of amines and nitrites.

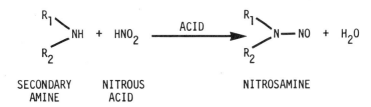

Fig. 4.9 The simple synthesis of nitrosamine by adding a secondary amine and nitrous acid under acidic conditions

The significance of these studies cannot be overrated. The amount of nitrosamine capable of being produced *in vivo* from readily available precursors may be far more significant than the levels of ingestion of preformed nitrosamines. Thus a new carcinogenic hazard is becoming apparent: we not only ingest ready-made carcinogens, but we are probably able to manufacture them in our bodies from harmless precursors.

Enzymatic activation
Dimethylnitrosamine is metabolized by enzymes found predominantly in the liver and in lesser concentrations in the kidney and lung. It is converted to a chemically active product which acts as an alkylating agent.

The compound N-Nitrosomethyl urea, when administered to pregnant rats, produces brain tumours in the offspring. This finding suggests that transplacental carcinogenesis may account for some of the neuroblastomas found in young children. Transplacental carcinogenesis is probably also significant in the development of carcinoma of the vagina in daughters of mothers given diethyl-stilboestrol during pregnancy to prevent abortion.

Pyrrolizidine alkaloids

These are widely distributed in several plant families, especially the *Senecio* (common ragwort) and *Heliotropium* genera. In Australia they are eaten by sheep and cattle and may be responsible for outbreaks of toxaemic jaundice in sheep and for some of the bovine hepatomas. In some parts of the world, such as Africa, the indigenous populations use these plants for food and for the preparation of ritual drinks. Primary carcinoma of the liver is one of the common cancers in these areas.

Cycasin (β-glucoside)

The nuts of the cycad palm which grows in the tropics, are used by many natives as a source of starch. The glycoside is non-toxic but it is hydrolyzed and removed by bacteria in the gut to liberate the carcinogen methylazoxymethanol, a compound whose structure resembles that of dimethylnitrosamine. Methylazoxymethanol is a hepatocarcinogen and, like the other alkaloids and aflatoxin, is responsible for the high incidence of liver cancer in native populations.

Inorganic substances

Many heavy metals can induce cancer. Some of these are radioactive and emit ionizing radiations, others such as chromium, beryllium, silver, copper, lead, nickel and arsenic react with macromolecules to form insoluble phosphates. Metals may, therefore, react with phosphate groups in nucleic acids and thus alter the activity and stability of nucleic acids. Heavy metals also have widespread effects on enzyme systems and may enhance or inhibit the mechanisms controlling cell multiplication.

Asbestos

Of all the varieties of asbestos, chrysotile (blue asbestos) is the most common. Asbestos has become an essential raw material in industry and it is used extensively in electrical insulations, flooring and in the manufacture of brake linings of cars. In man, it is responsible for mesotheliomas (pleural and peritoneal) which are very rare in the absence of asbestos and bronchial carcinoma which, amongst asbestos workers, is several times more common than mesothelioma.

For inhaled particles to penetrate deeply into the lung, they must be of small size (0.5–50 μm). The penetrability of a fibre is related to its diameter and is virtually independent of the length. Those most likely to penetrate to the pleura are thin, short and straight (2 to 5 μm in length and 0.3 to 0.5 μm in thickness). The chemical composition of the fibre seems to be of secondary importance in carcinogenesis. Chrysotile asbestos which produces extremely fine fibres is particularly carcinogenic. Other types of fibre, including fibre glass, produce mesotheliomas when the fibres are as fine as those of asbestos.

Asbestosis has long been known as an occupational disease. Asbestos bodies, which are fibres coated with a yellow-brown substance containing iron and protein, are often found in high concentrations in the lungs of asbestos workers and in the lungs of patients with mesothelioma, and in lesser concentrations in the lungs of city dwellers. The frequent wearing away of brake linings of cars provides a constant supply of asbestos fibres to the atmosphere, and it is difficult to estimate the degree of danger to the general population.

As a race, the Japanese population has a very high incidence of carcinoma of the stomach. A possible explanation for this is that they consume large quantities of raw fish which they coat with a dressing of starch and talc. Talc, a magnesium silicate powder, is frequently contaminated with asbestos fibres which may contribute to the high incidence of carcinoma of the stomach.

FURTHER READING

Ames, B. N. *et al.* (1973) Carcinogens are mutagens: a simple test system combining liver homogenates for activation and bacteria for detection. *Proc. Nat. Acad. Sci. U.S.A.*, **70**, 2281.

Brand, K. G. *et al.* (1967) Carcinogenesis from polymer implants: new aspects from chromosomal and transplantation studies during premalignancy. *J. Natl. Cancer Inst.*, **39**, 663.

Bryan, W. R. & Shimkin, M. B. (1941) Quantitative analysis of dose-response data obtained with carcinogenic hydrocarbons. *J. Natl. Cancer Inst.*, **1**, 807.

Kennaway, E. L. (1955) The identification of a carcinogenic compound in coal-tar. *Brit. Med. J.*, **ii**, 749.

Miller, J. A. (1970) Carcinogenesis by chemicals: an overview – G. H. A. Clowes Memorial Lecture. *Cancer Res.*, **30**, 559.

Ryser, H. J. P. (1971) Chemical carcinogenesis. *New Engl. J. Med.*, **285**, 721.

Wogan, G. N. (1969) Naturally occurring carcinogens in foods. *Progress in Exp. Tumor Res.*, **11**, 134.

Yamagiwa, K. & Ichikawa, K. (1918) Experimental study of the pathogenesis of carcinoma. *J. Cancer Res.*, **3**, 1.

5

Viral carcinogenesis

Until the beginning of this century, viruses were regarded as laboratory curiosities. The discoveries of a filterable agent in some forms of fowl leukaemia by Ellerman and Bang in 1908, and a virus in fowl sarcoma by Peyton Rous in 1911 soon changed this attitude. Subsequently, many other viruses were shown to produce tumours in animals. In 1932, Richard Shope demonstrated that skin papillomas and carcinomas in rabbits were due to a virus; in 1936, Bittner showed that a breast cancer in a strain of mice was transmitted by a virus in the milk and in 1951, Gross discovered the mouse leukaemia virus.

Until this time, all the known viruses were species specific and could be isolated from spontaneously occurring tumours in their natural hosts. The discovery in 1958 that the polyoma virus, which is endemic in mice, was capable of producing tumours in rats, guinea pigs and rabbits illustrated for the first time that viruses are capable of transgressing the species barrier. Further studies showed that other viruses such as simian virus 40 (SV40), endemic in monkeys, and the adenoviruses, pathogenic in man, could produce malignant tumours in rats and mice, but not in their natural hosts.

The experimental approach to the study of the role of viruses in neoplasia led to the development of strains of mice and other animals which showed a high incidence of the disease. These experimental model systems have become an essential component of modern research. Apart from their value as a means of investigating basic problems of neoplasia, it was thought and hoped that they would throw some light on the disease in man.

The role of viruses as causative agents in human cancer has become a controversial and challenging question. The contention that they may cause cancer in man rests mainly on analogy with observations on other species, particularly laboratory animals. There is no good evidence to suggest that human cancer is an infectious disease: for example,

1. Most tumours in man do not occur in clusters characteristic of infectious diseases.

2. Bacteriologists have always adhered to the principle that the cause of any infectious disease is only determined after Koch's postulates have been fulfilled.

3. No virus has definitely been shown to cause cancer in man. Demonstration of viruses in a tumour is insufficient evidence in itself because tumours are a good medium for the growth of passenger viruses. It is understandable, therefore, that there is a general reluctance to accept viruses as aetiological agents in human cancer.

On the other hand, it is difficult to imagine that man is unique among the animals in not having his share of tumour-inducing viruses. If viruses are not implicated in human cancer, then it is also difficult to reconcile the remarkable similarities in the morphological features of some human tumours with those of lower animals which are unequivocally caused by viruses, or the carcinogenic potential of some human adenoviruses in experimental animals. Our failure to prove that viruses cause human cancer is very likely due to our difficulty in finding an adequate experimental system to investigate the viral-human relationship. There has been a recent upsurge in interest in the role of viruses in the induction of various human cancers such as Burkitt's lymphoma, human leukaemia, breast cancer, sarcomas and carcinoma of the cervix.

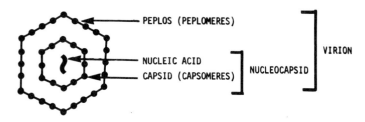

Fig. 5.1   The structure of a virion

THE ONCOGENIC VIRUSES

Viruses consist of a core of nucleid acid surrounded by a symmetrical protein coat (*capsid*) which is composed of identical subunits, the *capsomeres* (Fig. 5.1). The nucleic acid and capsid together form the *nucleocapsid* and this is surrounded by an additional lipid-containing envelope, the *peplos*.

Tumour- inducing viruses can be divided into two major groups with differing physico-chemical and biological properties:

1. The oncogenic DNA-containing viruses.
2. The oncogenic RNA-containing viruses (*oncornaviruses*).

There are no basic differences that distinguish tumour viruses from any other virus. A wide range of DNA and RNA viruses will cause tumours in experimental animals (Table 5.1). Even the vaccinia virus, which is looked upon as a necrotizing virus, has some carcinogenic potential in that administration of vaccinia virus together with a subcarcinogenic dose of a polycyclic hydrocarbon will induce tumours.

Table 5.1 Some oncogenic viruses

Virus	Type	Natural host	Susceptible host	Tumour
Polyoma	DNA	Mouse	Rat, Hamster	Lymphoma, salivary gland tumour
Simian (SV40)	DNA	Monkey	Hamster	Glioma
Epstein-Barr (EB)	DNA	Man	Monkey, Young child	Lymphoma
Rous	RNA	Fowl	Fowl	Fibrosarcoma
Shope	DNA	Rabbit	Rabbit	Skin papilloma
Bittner	RNA	Mouse	Mouse	Breast cancer

THE ONCOGENIC DNA VIRUSES

Typical examples of tumour-inducing DNA viruses are the *polyoma virus* (PV), which occurs naturally in adult mice without apparent ill-effect, the *simian virus 40* (SV40), which occurs naturally in the monkey and the *Shope papilloma virus*, which causes localized tumours of the skin in cottontail rabbits. PV and SV40 contain only a small amount of genetic material, approximately eight genes each, but they possess all the information necessary to replicate and to induce cancer in susceptible hosts.

DNA virus – cell interaction

In susceptible cells, the virus particle becomes adsorbed to the surface, penetrates the cell membrane and sheds its coat. The subsequent fate of the viral DNA depends on whether or not the cell is permissive. *Permissive cells* do not react to the presence of the virus, but allow it to replicate itself freely. The resulting large numbers of virus particles which form eventually destroy the cells and spread to adjacent cells. *Non-permissive cells*, on the other hand, react to the presence of the virus, so that the virus is unable to replicate, but the host cells undergo a process of transformation.

Transformed cells show altered growth properties in that their mode of growth appears to be analogous to the growth of tumour cells. After some time, it is not possible to demonstrate virus particles in transformed cells, but these cells continue to grow as transformed cells and carry some virus-induced antigens. It is assumed that viral nucleic acid (*provirus*) is covalently bound or integrated into the cell chromosomes and replicates synchronously with the cell DNA. The viral genome, therefore, is transferred to daughter cells during mitosis for many generations in this masked form.

If such a virus transformed cell is hybridized with a permissive normal cell by cell fusion, the masked tumour viruses are activated and begin to replicate. It is then possible to observe hybrid cells being filled with virus particles. Therefore, in certain cases, cell hybridization can be used as a means of unmasking dormant tumour viruses in tumour cells suspected to be of viral origin. In the future, this method of study might provide a means of unmasking dormant viruses in human tumour cells.

Transformed cells containing integrated viral DNA carry two important antigens:

1. A *tumour-specific or 'T-antigen'*, which is located in the nucleus and is probably concerned with stimulation of cellular DNA synthesis. It can be identified by immunofluorescence and serves as a marker of viral transformation.

2. A *tumour-specific transplantation antigen* (TSTA), which is localized on the surface of the cell and is probably responsible for the immunological rejection of tumour cells by the host. It is also called a *tumour rejection antigen*.

The immune system in mice does not mature until some days after birth so that, at birth, the body is not able to recognize transformed cells as foreign and the tumour cells are not rejected. This provides a possible explanation why DNA viruses induce tumour in newborn, but not in adult mice. In man, the immune system develops early in uterine life so that the transformed cells at birth would be recognized and rejected.

The polyoma virus
PV occurs naturally in many mouse colonies without producing tumours in these animals. If PV is grown in mouse fibroblast tissue culture, a very high titre of virus preparation is obtained. If this preparation is injected into newborn mice of a colony pre-

viously polyoma-free, typical polyoma tumours in salivary gland, lymphoid tissue, etc. are obtained in 70 to 80 per cent of mice. Occasionally, as many as 10 types of tumours may be found in one mouse, hence the name polyoma (many tumours). If PV is injected into adult mice of the same polyoma-free colony no tumours result, but these adult mice produce antibody to the virus. If the virus preparation is injected into newborn mice of a colony with PV, antibody in the milk protects the newborn mice from developing tumours. So, PV which under strictly artificial experimental conditions is a very potent carcinogenic virus, in nature rarely produces tumours. PV is also carcinogenic for mouse, rat, rabbit and hamster, but not for other species.

Simian virus 40

This virus, called vacuolating virus or SV40 was isolated from *rhesus* and *cynomolgus* monkey kidney cultures in which it grew without causing any cytopathic effect. Although millions of people have been exposed to this virus as a contaminant of polio and adenovirus vaccines, no human disease has been associated with it; yet when SV40 is injected into newborn hamsters, it produces sarcomas.

Shope papilloma virus

Wild cottontail rabbits along the banks of the Mississippi River were seen to have wart-like growths on their skin. In 1933, Richard Shope was able to transmit these tumours to other rabbits by placing a drop of cell-free filtrate on areas of skin after light scarification with sandpaper. In wild rabbits, these tumours grow slowly, they contain free virus and are easily removed without recurring. In domestic rabbits, on the other hand, the tumours grow rapidly, they undergo a malignant change but they do not contain free virus and extracts from these do not give rise to tumours in other rabbits.

The adenoviruses

Adenoviruses are common human viruses which give rise to a wide range of respiratory and alimentary tract infections. They are the first human viruses that have been shown to be carcinogenic in animals. In 1962, adenovirus 12 was found to produce tumours when innoculated into newborn hamsters, and since then, other human adenoviruses and a number of adenoviruses isolated from monkeys have also been shown to give rise to tumours when injected into newborn hamsters.

Herpes viruses

Herpes virus infections are frequent in man causing skin lesions such as herpes simplex, neural lesions such as *herpes zoster* and *varicella* (chickenpox). Both herpes and varicella viruses can remain dormant in the skin or nervous tissue and are subject to reactivation giving rise to cold sores and shingles. These viruses are responsible for a variety of tumours in animals:

1. *Marek's disease virus* causes a lymphoma in chickens.
2. *Lucké virus* causes adenocarcinoma of the kidney in frogs when injected into tadpoles.

THE ONCOGENIC RNA VIRUSES (ONCORNAVIRUSES)

Oncornaviruses are classified into two distinct groups on the basis of the morphology of the virion:

1. *C-type viruses* represent the leukaemia-sarcoma viruses of mammalian, avian and reptilian origin. They have a diameter of approximately 100 nm, a central nucleoid and are identifiable as *C-particles* in electromicrographs.

2. *B-type viruses* represent the mammary tumour viruses of mice and differ from the C-particles in having an eccentric nucleoid and prominent spikes projecting from the viral surface. They are identified as B-particles in electronmicrographs.

In contrast to the DNA tumour viruses, oncornaviruses can multiply in the cells they infect without killing them. The most important biological characteristic of oncornaviruses is that they contain an *RNA-directed DNA polymerase* (reverse transcriptase). This enzyme enables the virus to synthesize DNA which is a copy of the viral RNA. The foreign DNA becomes integrated in the host genome and codes for virus RNA, capsid protein and reverse transcriptase. The newly-formed viral RNA migrates to the cell membrane and, by a process of budding, carries off with it a portion of the transformed cell membrane which becomes the external membrane of the new virus.

Leukaemia viruses

Chronic leukaemia is common in chickens and mice. Chickens suffer from chronic myeloid leukaemia, chronic lymphatic and erythroblastosis, and mice contract predominantly the lymphatic type although the myeloid form does occur. All these forms of the disease can be transmitted by cell-free filtrates.

Sarcoma viruses

In 1910 Peyton Rous, a pathologist at the Rockefeller Institute, was the first to succeed in transmitting a chicken sarcoma with cell-free extracts, thus establishing the viral aetiology of various fowl sarcomas. Some of these tumours contain the virus, others do not. It now appears that two viruses are involved, the Rous sarcoma virus which itself produces tumours but is incapable of replication, and the Rous associated virus which is incapable of producing tumours, but in the presence of which the Rous sarcoma virus can replicate itself. Thus we have three situations:

    1. Rous sarcoma virus that can induce tumours which do not produce virus.

    2. Rous associated virus that does not produce tumours, but merely an infection with no obvious symptoms.

    3. Mixed infection which produces tumours and fresh virus.

Bittner milk factor

Certain strains of mice have a high incidence of breast tumours, other strains less. If a high-incidence mother is crossed with a low-incidence father, offspring with a high incidence of breast cancer are produced. Reciprocal crossing yields offspring with a low incidence. If offspring from a high-incidence strain are foster-fed from birth by a low-incidence strain mother they become low incidence and vice versa. A viral agent is present in the milk of mice of high-incidence strains and suckling from this strain gives a high incidence of breast cancer.

THE ASSOCIATION OF ONCOGENIC VIRUSES WITH CANCER IN MAN

Despite the large number of DNA viruses known to cause cancer in animals, only one group, the herpesviruses, has been consistently associated with human cancer. Of these, the EBV which causes infectious mononucleosis has been implicated as a causal agent in Burkitt's lymphoma and in nasopharyngeal cancer, and the *herpesvirus hominis type 2* (HSV-2) in carcinoma of the cervix.

Burkitt's lymphoma

Burkitt's lymphoma is the best example of a human tumour likely to be due to a virus. It is a malignant lymphoma which occurs in high incidence in malaria endemic regions of East africa and New Gúinea and affects predominantly young children of five to six years of age. These children who have been infected with both malaria and EBV show an augmented antibody production to EBV. The geographic distribution of the disease suggests that an insect vector may be involved and electron microscopy has demonstrated the presence of EBV. The lymphoma cells always carry the antigen and, in tissue culture, they can be induced to produce virus.

Although the evidence supporting a viral aetiology for Burkitt's lymphoma is impressive, it is not conclusive. The disease is not a common sequel of EBV infection, which occurs throughout the world and causes infectious mononucleosis. There is no satisfactory explanation, for example, as to why only 10 per 100 000 children in high endemic areas of Uganda get Burkitt's lymphona, when all the children in that district are infected with EBV and are exposed to malaria. To produce the tumour, a very rare set of circumstances is probably necessary. One could postulate that a mosquito, or some other insect vector carrying the virus, bites a newborn babe and that the baby's mother has no antibodies to the virus in her milk. Under these peculiar circumstances a tumour can result, but most of the population of these areas is either protected by acquired antibodies, or alternatively, contracts the infection later in life and becomes resistant. Burkitt's lymphoma could well be a very rare manifestation of a very common infection. It has been suggested that malaria or some other insult to the reticuloendothelial system, in addition to the virus, is usually necessary to bring about the disease.

Nasopharyngeal carcinoma
This tumour, which is prevalent among Chinese in South Asia, has also been linked with the EBV. It is a squamous-cell carcinoma affecting predominantly males in the 40 to 50 year age group. All cases studied are associated with EBV and their antibody levels against EBV tend to increase as the disease progresses, suggesting that EBV is very likely a passenger virus.

Carcinoma of the cervix
This cancer is rarely found in women who have never had sexual intercourse, but it increases markedly in those women whose active sex lives began before the age of 15, in those with more than five children or in those who have had multiple sex partners. Several studies have shown a serological correlation between HSV-2 and cancer of the cervix. HSV-2 is a venereal infection associated with promiscuity and antibodies to the virus are uniformly high (almost 100 per cent) among patients with carcinoma of the cervix when

compared with control groups (approximately 30 per cent). Results of antibody levels in patients with *carcinoma in-situ* have been equivocal, the most recent being approximately 30 per cent. This finding would tend to exclude HSV-2 as a primary cause of cervical carcinoma, but rather suggests that the virus acts indirectly.

Oncornaviruses

The oncornaviruses have been linked with leukaemia, carcinoma of the breast and various sarcomas, but the evidence incriminating this group as causative agents in human cancer is not as impressive as that incriminating the DNA-containing group.

In man, acute lymphocytic leukaemia of childhood has been most extensively studied from the point of view of attempts to establish a viral aetiology. C-particles have been found in electronmicrographs of leukaemic cells with group specific antibodies for oncornaviruses and, in some leukaemic cells, an enzyme has also been identified which has the characteristics of reverse transcriptase. However, unlike the animal leukaemias, the epidemiological evidence for a viral aetiology for human leukaemia is negative and direct proof that C-particles cause leukaemia is lacking.

Carcinoma of the breast

Human breast cancer is similar to leukaemia in that there is evidence supporting an association between oncornaviruses and the disease. For example, B- and C-particles, similar to those seen in mouse mammary tumours, have been demonstrated in many human breast cancers, similar particles have also been found in the milk from patients with carcinoma of the breast at a much greater frequency than from control patients and the particles from human breast milk possess reverse transcriptase. All this evidence is circumstantial; it provides proof of an association, but not of a causal role. Again, epidemiological evidence provides no support for a viral aetiology of breast cancer in man.

Possible mechanisms of viral carcinogenesis

Until recently there was no basic framework on which to consider how viruses might induce a malignant change. In transformed cells, the viral DNA which is integrated to the cell genome can remain in the cell in a masked form virtually permanently. If the essential lesion that induces the malignant change is due to addition of viral DNA, it might be expressed either as a gain in cellular function or as a loss in cellular function. On this basis, two main hypotheses have been proposed to explain the role of viruses in the aetiology of cancer in man:

The oncogene theory

Huebner and Todaro suggest that all mammalian cells contain an 'oncogene' or 'virogene' integrated into their DNA, presumably derived from some oncogenic RNA virus, which is transmitted vertically during cell division as part of the normal cell genome. Normally this oncogene is suppressed, but it can be switched on by environmental agents such as ionizing radiations, chemical carcinogens or helper viruses secreting a gene product which is responsible for the malignant change. This implies a gain in cell function. Cell-fusion studies (p. 87) have virtually rejected the oncogene hypothesis.

Somatic mutation

If the malignant change is due to a loss in function, then there are at least three types of microscopically visible changes in virus infected cells that could induce it. These changes are:

1. Chromosome breaks are frequently seen in virus infected cells which can induce rearrangements, translocations and deletions.

2. Chromosome pulverization in which portions of chromosomes are severely fragmented.

3. Persistence of the nucleolus during mitosis which holds together the chromatids during anaphase resulting in non-disjunction and producing irregularities in the number of chromosomes – monosomies and trisomies. This variety of mutations in somatic cells could very likely lead to a malignant change.

FURTHER READING

Black, P. H. (1968) The oncogenic DNA viruses: a review of *in vitro* transformation studies. *Annu. Rev. Microbiol.*, **22**, 391.

Burkitt, D. (1958) A sarcoma involving the jaws in African children. *Br. J. Surg.*, **46**, 218.

Goss, L. (1970) *Oncogenic Viruses*. New York: Pergamon Press.

Huebner, R. J. *et al.* (1970) Group-specific antigen expression during embryogenesis of the genome of the C-type RNA tumour virus: implications for autogenesis and oncogenesis. *Proc. Nat. Acad. Sci. U.S.A.*, **67**, 366.

Novinski, R. G. *et al.* (1970) Common properties of the oncogenic RNA viruses (oncarnaviruses). *Virology*, **42**, 1152.

Sabin, A. B. (1968) Viral carcinogenesis: phenomena of special significance in the search for a viral aetiology in human cancer. *Cancer Res.*, **28**, 1849.

Temin, H. M. (1971) The protovirus hypothesis: Speculation on the significance of RNA-directed DNA synthesis for normal development and for carcinogenesis. *J. Natl. Cancer Inst.*, **46(2)**, III–VII.

6

Physical carcinogenesis

The important physical agents associated with cancer are ionizing radiations and actinic or ultraviolet rays. The controversial role of trauma in the development of tumours is also mentioned because it presents an important medicolegal problem of Worker's Compensation litigations.

IONIZING RADIATIONS

The carcinogenic effects of ionizing radiations have been known since the beginning of the century. The first case of X-ray-induced cancer was reported in 1902, only seven years after Roentgen discovered X-rays. Squamous-cell carcinomas developed on the backs of the hands of workers who tested X-ray machines for emission by placing their hands in the radiation field. Even after the carcinogenic potential of X-rays was realized, adequate precautions were still not taken and people continued to receive large doses of radiation in the course of their work or during treatment. Thus, the years that followed showed a significant increase in the incidence of leukaemia and other malignancies in populations exposed to excessive doses of radiation.

PHYSICAL ASPECTS OF RADIATIONS

Isotopes
Atoms are composed of a central nucleus consisting of two types of particles: protons, which are positively charged and neutrons, which are uncharged or neutral. The nucleus is surrounded by a shell of orbiting electrons, each of which carries a unit negative charge. Atoms are identified either by their atomic number which is the number of protons or by their atomic mass which represents the sum of the number of protons and neutrons. Atoms which differ in atomic mass but have the same atomic number are called *isotopes*. As the chemical nature of the atom is determined by the number

of protons in the nucleus, all isotopes of the same element have the same number of protons.

Radioisotopes

Isotopes with nuclei in which the ratio of protons to neutrons approaches unity, are stable. Those with an excess of either protons or neutrons are unstable and tend to decay to a more stable state by the emission of radiations. Atoms may decay by changing a neutron to a proton with the liberation of an electron, or a proton to a neutron with the liberation of a positively charged particle. Such isotopes are radioactive and are called *radioisotopes*. For instance, hydrogen has three isotopes, normal hydrogen and deuterium are stable isotopes, but tritium is a radioisotope which decays to a helium atom by changing a neutron to a proton by the liberation of an electron (Fig. 6.1).

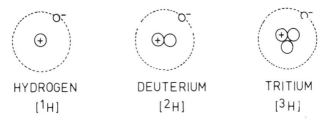

HYDROGEN   DEUTERIUM   TRITIUM
[^{1}H]   [^{2}H]   [^{3}H]

Fig. 6.1   The three isotopes of hydrogen

Individual isotopes are designated by writing the appropriate mass number as a superscript in front of the chemical symbol. For example, naturally occurring iodine is ^{127}I and the commonly used radioisotopes are ^{125}I and ^{131}I.

Some radioactive elements occur naturally. Many more can be produced artificially either by bombarding stable nuclei with atomic particles in a high energy accelerator or by spontaneous fission. They are used extensively in medicine for therapeutic and diagnostic purposes and, therefore, they constitute an important source of radiation exposure.

Rate of decay

The rate of physical disintegration of radioactive isotopes decreases exponentially with time. The time taken to lose half the original radioactivity is known as the half-life. Each isotope has a specific rate of decay (Table 6.1), that of ^{131}I is shown in Fig. 6.2.

Table 6.1   Physical data on some common isotopes

Isotope	Half-life	Energy (keV)
Carbon-14	5.8×10^3y	155
Cobalt-57	270d	270
Iodine-131	8d	250
Iron-59	45d	460
Phosphorus-32	14.5d	1710
Strontium-90	28y	540
Technicium-99	6h	300
Tritium (^{3}H)	12.3y	18.5
Uranium-238	4.5×10^9y	419

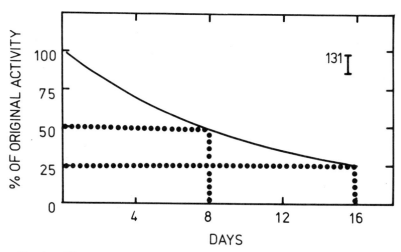

Fig. 6.2   The radioactive decay of ^{131}I

Units of radioactivity

The *Curie (Ci)* is the basic unit of radioactivity. Originally, it was defined as the number of disintegrations emitted per second by one gram of radium (3.7×10^{10}). The current definition of a Curie is the quantity of any radioactive substance which emits 3.7×10^{10} disintegrations per second. A Curie is a very large dose of radioactivity and smaller units such as millicuries and microcuries are commonly used.

$$mCi = 10^{-3} \, Ci$$
$$\mu Ci = 10^{-6} \, Ci$$

Energy and penetrability

The unit of energy commonly used is the *electron volt* (*eV*). It represents the kinetic energy acquired by one unit of electrical charge moving through a potential gradient of one volt. α-particles from a given source have a fairly constant energy, β-particles are emitted at all speeds from near zero to 99 per cent of the speed of light and γ-rays travel at the speed of light.

The relative penetrating power of α, β and γ-rays in tissue depends upon their wavelength and energy, the shorter the wavelength the greater the energy and degree of penetrability. For example, particulate radiations of low energy such as the β-particles from tritium penetrate poorly (2μ) and are absorbed entirely within the cytoplasm of a single cell, whereas by contrast, high energy γ-rays such as those from radium can penetrate the entire length of the human body. The penetration tract of isotopes is measured in water at room temperature and it is the distance a charged particle travels during disintegration. Penetration tracts are specific for each isotope.

The ionizing capacity is also dependent on the energy of the particles. X-rays and γ-rays dissipate their energy over a long distance and are referred to as sparsely ionizing. On the other hand, α- and β-radiations, because of their shorter tracts, produce higher ionization densities.

Radiation doses

The exposure dose of X-rays or γ-rays is measured in roentgens. The amount of radiation delivered is not the same as the amount that is absorbed by the tissue. Though dose is important, the effect depends more on the amount of radiation absorbed, so that in radiotherapy, the major objective is to measure the amount and distribution of absorbed energy within the absorbing mass of tissue. Three units are used in practice:

1. A *roentgen* (*r*) is the quantity of X- or γ-radiation required to ionize 1 cm^3 of dry air at standard temperature and pressure. Dose rates are delivered in roentgens or milliroentgens per hour (mrh^{-1}).

2. The *rad* is the unit of absorbed dose and represents the deposition of 100 ergs per gram of tissue. In general, exposure of tissue to 1 r of X- or γ-rays delivers an absorbed dose of slightly less than one rad.

3. The *rem* (roentgen equivalent man), a new unit, is now used in radiation protection. It is the product of the absorbed dose in rads and the quality factor of the radiation. The quality factor indicates the damaging capacity of the particular radiation.

SOURCES OF EXPOSURE

Man is exposed to ionizing radiations from many sources. Some of these are occupational hazards, others are the result of atomic explosions, but the most significant source of radiation exposure is related to medical practice. Cosmic rays constitute another source of exposure, but these are screened out mostly by the atmosphere.

Occupational radioactivity

Some radioactive elements such as uranium and thorium compounds in rocks and soil occur naturally and constitute an important industrial hazard. There are many examples of radiation-induced tumours which illustrate a close relationship between exposure to naturally occurring radiation and the development of malignancy. A classical correlation was demonstrated in the uranium miners in Czechoslovakia and in the cobalt mines in Saxony. Both groups were exposed to radioactive dust and developed a high incidence of lung cancer after a latent period of approximately 16 years. Another example is the high incidence of osteosarcoma that was reported in New Jersey among a group of young girls employed painting watch dials with luminous paint. These girls tipped the points of their brushes with their tongues and lips and, as a result, swallowed significant amounts of radioactive material which was selectively retained in bone.

Diagnostic and therapeutic radiation

The cancer risk from diagnostic and therapeutic radiation has also been apparent for many years. The high rate of skin cancer and leukaemia among former radiologists, radiotherapists and patients with ankylosing spondylitis treated with X-rays is well recognized. Local irradiation of the thyroid area for therapeutic purposes has also been implicated in a subsequent increase of tumours of the thyroid gland. In particular, children treated with X-ray in infancy for thymic enlargement showed a high incidence of carcinoma of the thyroid gland, osteosarcoma and salivary gland tumours. Irradiation during pregnancy, even with very small doses, raises the incidence of leukaemia in children by a statistically significant amount. In early pregnancy, the foetus is believed to be particularly susceptible to irradiation and necessary diagnostic radiological procedures are kept to a minimum at that time.

In diagnostic radiological examinations, the background level of radioactivity is greatly increased but, provided normal precautions are taken and normal exposures used, the risk of malignancy is not increased. It is important, however, to realize that the benefits derived from these investigations far outweigh any theoretical risk of increased cancer incidence.

Radioactive fallout

There has been much concern over the possible carcinogenic and other effects on man of radioactive fallout from nuclear weapon testing. The concern has become so intense and so world-wide that the United Nations has established a special Committee, the United Nations Scientific Committee on the Effects of Atomic Radiation (UNSCEAR), which meets twice a year and produces general reports which provide the main source of information on the effects of radiation on man and the environment.

Following nuclear explosions, many hundreds of radioactive substances are released in the atmosphere. The large particles fall out close to the site of the explosion, but small particles remain airborne in clouds, they are carried over the earth's surface and are deposited mainly by rainfall.

1. *Iodine-131* (^{131}I) is the predominant isotope in the early fallout and it is taken up selectively by the thyroid gland.

2. *Strontium-90* (^{90}Sr) is one of the fission products of uranium and has a half-life of 28 years. It is deposited chiefly by rain, ingested by grazing cattle and, being similar to calcium, it appears in high concentration in cows' milk and in the milk of lactating mothers. In this regard, infants whose staple diet is cows' milk are particularly at risk. Strontium-90 accumulates in growing bones and delivers a relatively high radiation dose to adjacent tissues.

3. *Caesium-130* (^{130}Cs), also a fission product of ^{235}U, has a half-life of 30 years and is a β- and γ-emitter. It is found chiefly in soft tissues, particularly muscle.

4. *Carbon-14* (^{14}C) is another isotope which may be naturally occurring or produced in atomic explosions. It is important because it has a very long half-life (5 800 years) and makes up approxi-

mately 37 per cent of DNA. It is, therefore, well placed to produce gene mutations.

The increased incidence of leukaemia, carcinoma of the thyroid gland, carcinoma of the lung, carcinoma of the breast and osteosarcoma among the atomic bomb survivors both in Hiroshima and Nagasaki during the past 30 years is related to radioactive fallout. The increase in the incidence of leukaemia showed the best correlation with the dose of radiation received as estimated by the subject's distance from the hypocentre (Table 6.2). The induction period (latent period) was also shorter in the more heavily irradiated subjects.

Table 6.2   Incidence of myeloid leukaemia among survivors of the atomic bomb in Japan

Distance from hypocentre (in metres)	Incidence of leukaemia (per 100 000)
0– 999	146.0
1 000–1 499	38.0
1 500–1 999	5.7
2 000–9 999	2.9
10 000 +	1.3

BIOLOGICAL AND CARCINOGENIC EFFECTS

The ionizing radiations to which man is exposed are:

1. Electrically charged α- and β-particles.
2. Electromagnetic radiations (X-rays and γ-rays).

Radioactive emissions are called ionizing radiations because they are able to cause the formation of ions in tissues by removing electrons from atoms or molecules in their path. Ionization may be the result of direct collisions of charged particles with molecules, or it may be indirect, in which case radicles are first produced in intracellular water and these in turn ionize important macromolecules. Highly reactive radicles are formed instantaneously, initiate complex interactions within cells and result in biochemical disturbances which lead to morphological and functional lesions. The chief role of radioactivity in carcinogenesis is traceable to these ionizing effects.

Knowledge of the biological effects and means of measuring ionizing radiation enables us to evaluate the radiation hazard for human populations. The marrow is particularly sensitive and leukaemia is the chief neoplastic disease induced by ionizing radiations. By assuming that the dose/response ratio to radiation is linear, a whole body exposure dose of one rad per year would result in four cases of leukaemia per 100 000 population per year.

Effect on cell survival

Any cell can be killed or sterilized by irradiation if exposed to a large enough dose, but with smaller doses, there are variations in the susceptibilities of different cells. Cells may be classified broadly into three groups according to their sensitivity:

1. *Labile cells* may be injured or killed by doses less than 2 500 r.
2. *Stable cells* are killed by 2 500 to 5 000 r.
3. *Permanent cells* require doses greater than 5 000 r.

Knowledge of the radiosensitivity of neoplastic cells is of great importance in planning treatment of malignant tumours by ionizing radiations.

Effect on the cell cycle

The position of a cell in the cell cycle at the time of exposure considerably influences its response to irradiation. Certain phases of the cell cycle are more sensitive than others and, more importantly, cells not in the cycle, such as resting cells and permanent cells, are more resistant than cycling cells.

Irradiation of cells synchronized at various phases of the cell cycle results in different degrees of susceptibility. The general pattern seems to be an increase in sensitivity as cells progress from phase G_1 through phases S and G_2. Phase G_1 is a period of relatively low sensitivity, S is twice as sensitive as G_1, and G_2 twice as sensitive as S. This implies that ionizing radiations act by affecting specific intracellular targets and the relatively high sensitivity of cells after chromosomal duplication (late S and G_2) might be attributed to the increase in the number of sites at risk.

Chromosomal aberrations

There is a wealth of evidence linking radiation exposure in man, animals and bacteria with the appearance of mutations. Mutations may be either genetic, at the molecular level of the DNA (point mutations) and not visible microscopically, or chromosomal, in which case the structural alterations in the chromosomes can be demonstrated in photomicrographs. The distinction between the two types of mutation is not always easy in practice.

The nature of the initial lesion is not understood, but the damage may lead to breaks in chromosomes involving one or both strands. Normally, the broken ends unite with restoration of normal structure and function; however, with repeated or continuous irradiation the broken ends may unite with other fragments causing exchange aberrations and inversions. Furthermore, the fragments may remain unjoined, in which case the fragment without a centromere becomes lost at anaphase, giving rise to deletions. The number of radiation-induced chromosomal aberrations is dose-dependent and may lead to death of cells, loss of their reproductive capacity or to genetic mutations. Large doses may lead to giant cell formation, a change that is common in human tissues following therapeutic radiation. It is likely that giant cells and cells with visible chromosomal aberrations may represent sterile cells in which the genetic apparatus has been permanently and irreversibly damaged. Such cells may not be able to complete the process of mitosis and consequently would be incapable of contributing further to the growth of the tumour. Smaller doses which produce fewer breaks and fewer aberrations are more efficient mutagens and better carcinogens, possibly because more altered cells survive. The findings of some workers that high doses of radiation produced more chromosome aberrations in liver cells, but fewer hepatomas than low dose irradiation, are in keeping with this view.

It is generally assumed that the carcinogenic effect of ionizing radiations is bound up primarily with their ability to induce mutations (heritable changes) in the genetic material of the cell and secondarily with their ability to cause cell death and to suppress the immune system. The mutations produced appear to play an important role in the initiation of the carcinogenic process (p. 89), whereas cell death and immunosuppression are considered as promoting factors. Radiations are also thought, especially with the leukaemias, to activate latent viruses.

It was near the turn of the century when both the somatic mutations theory of carcinogenesis and the viral theory of carcinogenesis were elaborated. For many years, and to some extent still today, these two theories were considered to be opposing, but with the realization that both agents produce a variety of mutational changes, the common ground between the two hypotheses is apparent.

SOLAR RADIATION

Fair-skinned people are much more susceptible to carcinoma of the skin than dark-skinned, and coloured people are virtually immune to the disease. The condition is particularly prevalent in outdoor workers in countries like Australia where the sun beats down for long periods of time. This relationship between skin cancer and sunlight has been confirmed experimentally and the causative agent has been narrowed down to the ultraviolet component.

Sunlight consists of rays with a broad range of wavelength. Rays of the visible spectrum with wavelengths from 390 nm to 780 nm have few physiological and pathological actions on human tissues. Infrared rays (780 nm to 50 000 nm) give out heat and when absorbed by the skin, they may cause oedema, blistering or even necrosis (burns). Ultraviolet (UV) rays, on the other hand, have short wavelengths (290 nm to 330 nm) and are responsible for a variety of skin reactions. They have a low penetrating power and a low energy output and are not capable of causing ionization but they can shift electrons from an inner to an outer shell of an atom. Certain macromolecules such as DNA can utilize this energy and give rise to specific photochemical reactions. Photosynthesis in green plants, vitamin D formation in the skin, skin pigmentation and various other photosensitivity reactions are examples of ultraviolet light-induced chemical reactions.

The carcinogenic properties of ultraviolet light are not in dispute but the mechanism by which they induce malignant transformation is not understood. A connection between UV-induced DNA damage and cancer development has been demonstrated in patients with xeroderma pigmentosum. This condition is an autosomal recessively transmitted disease in which the skin in these patients shows a hypersensitivity to sunlight. Exposed areas of skin first become inflamed, then warts form in the inflamed areas and finally skin cancers develop, namely, squamous-cell carcinomas, basal-cell carcinomas, melanomas, fibrosarcomas and angiosarcomas. Cells from xeroderma pigmentosum patients show no obvious chromosomal abnormalities but they are deficient in an enzyme of the DNA repair system and are unable to repair damage in DNA induced by UV light. The abnormal cell lines probably represent one step in the process of cancer development, and one may well ask whether malignant transformation results from the primary photochemical lesion or from an error in the repair of this lesion.

Prolonged exposure to sunlight over many years is responsible for degenerative changes in the skin. These changes are seen in fair-skinned elderly people as multiple lesions on exposed areas of skin particularly the face, backs of hands and the mucocutaneous junction of the lower lip. They consist of wrinkling, excessive pigmentation and scaly thickening of the skin and are responsible for the familiar weather-beaten complexion or *solar keratosis*. Often the lesions become hyperkeratotic and may develop into

cutaneous horns. Malignant transformation of areas of solar keratosis into squamous-cell carcinoma or basal-cell carcinoma can
occur and the incidence of this event has been estimated at
approximately 20 per cent.

TRAUMA

It is neither possible to prove nor to disprove that trauma causes
cancer. The claim that a single incident of trauma can cause cancer,
particularly in bone, breasts and testes, although important in
Workers' Compensation litigations, may be dismissed as un-
founded. In such cases, trauma merely draws attention to a pre-
existing tumour.

In view of the thousands of serious war injuries and innumerable
bruises, lacerations and fractures occurring in civil life and the
rarity of cancer following such injuries, it is illogical to assume
that a single injury plays any significant role in the causation of
the disease. Before accepting a single injury as an immediate cause
of cancer certain postulates should be fulfilled, namely, a definite
evidence of injury, identical sites of injury and tumour development, a logical time interval between the date of injury and the
appearance of the tumour, the absence of pre-existing tumours at
the same site and the histological type of tumour should be consistent with the site of origin.

On the other hand, repeated trauma in the form of chronic
irritation for many years would cause an increase in cell loss by
cell death and also decrease the life span of the cells. Such a
situation would also result in increased cell regeneration, which
may act as a promotor to tumour development. The irritation of
the tongue or cheek from ill-fitting dentures, the pressure of pipe
stem on the lower lip and the daily irritation of the oesophagus
by swallowing wines, spirits and hot food are common examples of
promoting agents of cancer. All these sites, however, have been
initiated or transformed by chemical carcinogens such as polycyclic
hydrocarbons present in food and tobacco.

FURTHER READING

Bacq, Z. M. & Alexander, P. (1961) *Fundamentals of Radiobiology*. London:
Pergamon Press.
Behrens, C. F. & King, E. R. (1964) *Atomic Medicine*. Baltimore: Williams
and Wilkins.

Cleaver, J. E. (1969) Xeroderma pigmentosum: a human disease in which an initial stage of DNA is defective. *Proc. Nat. Acad. Sci. U.S.A.*, **63**, 248.

Upton, A. C. (1968) Radiation carcinogenesis. In *Methods in Cancer Res.* Ed. by Bush, H. Vol. 4, pp. 53–82. New York: Academic Press.

Wallace, B. & Dobzhansky, Y. (1963) *Radiation Genes and Man*. New York: Holt, Rinehart and Winston, Inc.

7

The pathogenesis of cancer

Regardless of whether tumours are induced by chemical agents, viruses or radiations, they all have one feature in common – a capacity for progressive growth. Because of this uniformity in their behaviour, it is felt that there might also be some uniformity in the mechanism of their induction through a final common pathway. Thus, even if the initial actions of carcinogens are dissimilar the subsequent changes leading tö the development of cancer might be the same.

GENERAL FEATURES OF THE NEOPLASTIC PROCESS

Many authors have suggested that carcinogenesis is a multistep process. Berenblum and Shubik, in their experiments demonstrating the co-carcinogenic action of croton oil in mice, suggested that at least two steps may be distinguished, namely initiating and promoting actions. Such a view was subsequently supported by the statistical studies of Armitage and Doll who, from a mathematical relationship of cancer distribution and age, suggested that from five to seven different mutations occur in the same cell or its progeny before malignant transformation becomes evident. Later, Armitage and Doll reviewed their results and considered that only a two-step process may be involved.

Berenblum then showed that a single application of a sub-carcinogenic dose of a polycyclic aromatic hydrocarbon to the skin of a mouse (*initiation*) followed by repeated applications of croton oil (*promotion*) resulted in the development of tumours (Fig. 7.1). The tumour yield was not decreased when the same promotion procedure was carried out months later, after initiation. He also showed that reversal of the initiation and promotion procedures did not yield tumours, indicating that the combined effect of carcinogen and oil is not additive.

Much subsequent work has been carried out on this subject and

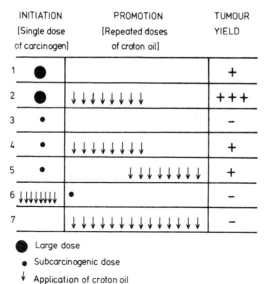

INITIATION [Single dose of carcinogen]	PROMOTION [Repeated doses of croton oil]	TUMOUR YIELD
1 ●		+
2 ●	↓↓↓↓↓↓↓	+++
3 •		−
4 •	↓↓↓↓↓↓↓	+
5 •	↓↓↓↓↓↓↓	+
6 ↓↓↓↓↓↓ •		−
7	↓↓↓↓↓↓↓↓↓↓↓↓	−

● Large dose
• Subcarcinogenic dose
↓ Application of croton oil

Fig. 7.1 Initiation and promotion in mouse skin: a single large dose produces tumours (1) and repeated applications of croton oil give a larger yield of tumours (2). A single subcarcinogenic dose does not produce tumours (3), but promotion with croton oil results in tumour formation (4). Tumour yield is not decreased if promotion is carried out months after initiation (5). Both reversal of the procedures of inititiation and promotion (6) and promotion in the absence of initiation (7) do not give rise to tumours (from Ryser, H. (1971) *New Eng. J. Med.*, **285**, 72)

the active principles in croton oil have been isolated and identified as phorbol esters. When these extracts are used alone in very high concentrations, they may produce a low tumour yield, but when used in association with carcinogenic initiators, they produce more tumours in a shorter time. Phorbol esters also lower the threshold of action of initiators and enable the detection of new carcinogens. Being lipophilic/lipophobic agents, they probably interfere with cell-to-cell contacts releasing cells from contact inhibition; so that their most likely action in carcinogenesis is to stimulate cell proliferation.

The two-stage theory of carcinogenesis has provided an impetus to cancer research. It has demonstrated that the initiation process is rapid and irreversible whereas promotion is nonspecific, prolonged and reversible. The number of initiated cells is very small and it is not possible to identify them histologically. Pathologists find this notion difficult to accept because application of a carcinogen to a tissue often produces obvious changes in many cells, but this difficulty merely represents one facet of the problem because carcinogens exert both toxic and neoplastic effects.

THE INITIATION STAGE OF CARCINOGENESIS

The nature of the changes occurring in cells during the trans-formation stage and concomitant with the development of malig-nancy are not fully understood but they appear to be irreversible and heritable. Therefore, they must involve the genetic material of the cell.

The study of the chemical carcinogens has contributed more to our understanding of the initiation process of carcinogenesis than any other experimental approach. Most carcinogens that have been adequately investigated are converted, either by spontaneous breakdown in the body or by enzymatic reaction, to ultimate carcinogens. The molecule of the ultimate carcinogen contains a positively charged reactive centre, that is, it has an electron-deficient atom (*electrophilic*) which binds covalently to relatively negative groups (*nucleophilic*) such as amino acids in proteins and bases in nucleic acids. The reaction is shown in schematic form (Fig. 7.2) where A is the precarcinogen, A^+ the ultimate carcinogen of A, B^- is the relatively negative group in macromolecules and A–B the covalently-bound complex. Most experimental work on carcinogen binding measures covalent binding but, it is also possible that other less stable interactions might be just as important.

If, for example, a tritium-labelled carcinogen is injected into an animal, the cells of the target organ fractionated and the com-ponents examined for radioactivity, it is found that (Fig. 7.3):

1. A high level of radioactivity is bound to protein.
2. Less radioactivity is bound to RNA.
3. Trace amounts of radioactivity are bound to DNA.

At present we do not know which, if any, of these complexes is essential in the neoplastic process but, whichever it is, it would have to alter the expression of information that controls normal growth. Thus, identification of the critical target attacked by carcinogens would mean better understanding of neoplastic trans-formation.

Protein binding

Protein binding might be important in carcinogenesis. In favour of this concept we have, in at least some instances, a highly specific protein involved. For example, the carcinogenic azo dyes are preferentially bound to a special electrophoretic class of basic

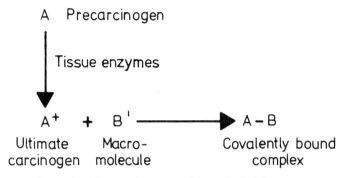

Fig. 7.2 Conversion of precarcinogens to ultimate (active) forms

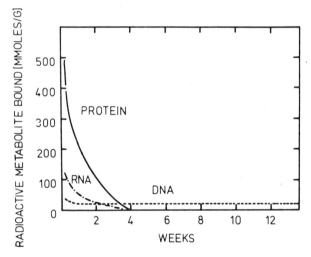

Fig. 7.3 Binding of radioactive metabolites from tritiated 4-DAB to liver DNA and RNA and cytoplasmic protein (from Warwick, G. P. and Roberts, J. J., *Nature*, **213**, 1206, (1967)

protein (h_2-protein) in rat liver, which is the target organ. There is a clear correlation between the extent of binding and the carcinogenicity of the compound and, more importantly, both h_2-protein and bound carcinogen are greatly diminished or absent from the tumours that subsequently develop. These findings led to the development of the *protein deletion hypothesis* of carcinogenesis in which it was suggested that loss of certain proteins with growth-regulating properties was followed by the development of malignant tumours.

A major defect in the protein deletion hypothesis was that it did not provide an explanation for the heritable nature of neoplastic transformation. Protein not being self replicating, would not be expected to store the altered information during the long latent periods, so that any effect protein binding could have would be transient. Studies on genetic regulation in bacteria have provided a theoretical basis for a possible mechanism by which the interaction of a carcinogen with a soluble protein fraction could produce heritable changes in somatic cells by inactivating repressor proteins and impairing gene transcription.

Protein deletion appeared to be a critical step in the carcinogenic process and the theory initially received widespread support. It was considered that if h_2-proteins were growth regulators, then administration of these substances should inhibit the growth of certain cells. In fact, concentrated extracts of h_2-proteins did inhibit the growth of tumour cells in tissue culture and, moreover, when the h_2-proteins were removed from the culture medium the tumour cells started growing again. Recent work suggests that the inhibitory effect of h_2-proteins may be due to arginase which breaks down arginine, an amino acid essential for cell growth. Addition of arginine to the tissue culture medium compensated for the inhibitory effect of the h_2-proteins. However, chicken liver extract which does not contain arginine is also able to inhibit cell growth. It is therefore likely that there are several growth controlling factors with similar electrophoretic properties. Some of these proteins may be enzymes that activate carcinogens and their absence in tumours would explain the resistance of tumour cells to the toxic effects of the carcinogen.

The problem then, is whether these alterations in soluble cytoplasmic proteins play a causative role in the carcinogenic process or whether they are secondary phenomena. If deletion of h_2-proteins is essential in carcinogenesis, one would expect to find demonstrable changes in the soluble proteins of human tumours. Some recent data from various types of lung cancer are of interest. In contrast with experimental tumours in rat liver and mouse skin, there is no decrease in basic proteins in bronchogenic carcinoma in man, relative to normal bronchial mucosa; in fact, there is an increase. Furthermore, the more undifferentiated oat-cell tumours show a greater increase in the proportion of basic protein than the squamous-cell and bronchiolar carcinomas. These findings in human tumours imply that loss of basic protein is not a general phenomenon of carcinogenesis.

RNA binding

Changes in RNA are also capable of altering cell behaviour. RNA provides important links in the process of regulating transcription and translation and alteration in its structure may produce temporary functional changes in the cell. For example, RNA may code for new proteins which in turn may induce new functional changes, it may interfere or compete with other RNAs of cell or viral origin, or it may repress or depress cellular DNA.

The demonstration that reverse transcriptase in RNA tumour viruses can synthesize new DNA in infected cells emphasizes the potential of RNA as a source of new genetic information.

DNA binding

Binding of chemical carcinogens to DNA was not demonstrated in many early reports. This is because very few molecules of carcinogen bind to DNA and their detection requires isotopic labelling techniques and very extensive purification procedures. Despite the low levels of bound carcinogen, DNA binding seems to fit in well with the somatic mutation theory of carcinogenesis (p. 83) because DNA is the genetic material of the cell and any structural damage to it would necessarily be transmitted to the daughter cells unless it was repaired by DNA repair enzymes.

Unlike protein and RNA-bound carcinogen, DNA-bound carcinogen persists for a long time because DNA turnover is slow. If DNA binding is important in carcinogenesis, it would be consistent with the cumulative effect of carcinogens and the long latent periods required for the development of tumours. Thus, more and more attention is being focused on DNA because it is believed that DNA damage interferes with the expression of information and might be a key lesion in the conversion of a normal cell to a tumour cell.

Sites of DNA binding

Since it is believed that all carcinogens may act *via* a common pathway, attempts have been made to determine the sites in DNA proteins at which they bind. Most carcinogens so far investigated become covalently bound to bases in DNA of target cells. The positions in which substitution occurs *in vivo* are N–3, N–7, O–6 and C–8 of guanine; N–1, N–3 and N–7 of adenine and N–1 of cytosine. In fact, there are very few positions not attacked by chemical carcinogens. The N–7 position of guanine appears to be the most reactive atom and alkylation in this position increases the ionization of N–1 in guanine and results in mispairing of guanine with thymine instead of cytosine in the Watson–Crick model of DNA replication. This type of mispairing results in the production of a nonsense type RNA and eventually in depurination of DNA. Alkylation in the O–6 position correlates best with carcinogenesis. In proteins, methionine is selectively attached by azo dyes and 2-AAF.

These findings have now become more meaningful with the recognition that most carcinogens require metabolic activation to interact with DNA and suggest that genetic alterations in somatic cells are fundamental to the initiation process. Alterations in informational content of chromosomes involves alterations in DNA structure which can be brought about by either:

1. Damage of existing DNA by chemical carcinogens or radiation.

2. Addition of new information by RNA viruses.

Somatic mutations probably represent alteration in base sequences of the DNA molecule. Since, as mentioned above, reactions between DNA and chemical carcinogens occur *in vivo* through alkylation, it is assumed that somatic mutation must be a causal factor in some, if not all, carcinogenic reactions.

DNA repair

Carcinogens may also interfere with DNA repair mechanisms. Normally, if segments of altered DNA occur, the cell is apparently able to excise the altered portion of the DNA strand and repair the defect. Thus, a single application of a carcinogen does not cause a permanent alteration in DNA. If the carcinogen inhibits the repair mechanism, continued administration of carcinogen maintains the altered base. Acridines inhibit the repair mechanism of certain bacteria and administration of a single subcarcinogenic dose of a carcinogen followed by repeated administration of acridine will produce tumours. DNA repair is also inhibited by exposure to UV-irradiation, ionizing radiations and to co-carcinogens such as croton oil. Croton oil may not only inhibit DNA repair but, by stimulating cell proliferation, may decrease the time available for repair.

NATURE OF HERITABLE CHANGE

Regardless of whether or not carcinogen binding is important in carcinogenesis it is clearly evident that initiation alters the information content of some cells and renders them insensitive to growth control. The nature of the alteration is not understood but it is permanent and heritable. In principle, there are three lesions that may induce a heritable change in cells:

1. It might be a mutational change involving alterations in the structure of DNA. These mutations are not in the sex or germ cell line but in the somatic line of cells in the body, hence the term *somatic mutation*.

2. The lesion might be a stable *epigenetic change*, rather than genetic, which might induce a change in the cell analogous to differentiation. This type of change would then become heritable in the same way as differentiation becomes heritable, but it would not involve any changes in the mutation rate.

3. There could be a specific causative agent such as a virus which parasitizes the cell and induces a particular type of multiplication, and it would be the persistence of this virus in all the cells of the tumour that would be responsible for the continued growth of the tumour.

Somatic mutation

A somatic mutation may be dominant or recessive. If it is a dominant mutation, one that is expressed as a normal dominant mutation, there would be certain difficulties in accommodating what is already known about the natural history of cancer. A dominant mutation would mean that every time a specific mutation occurs it would give rise to a tumour, and implies that cancer occurs at a mutational frequency and is independent of age. This implication is not in keeping with the statistical incidence of cancer distribution. There are some Mendelian dominant conditions in man that are sometimes associated with cancer, such as retino-blastoma, but these conditions are extremely rare.

On the other hand, if the lesion is recessive, it would not be expressed. For every chromosome there is a homologous chromosome carrying the dominant trait which prevents expression of a recessive mutation. In order to have expression of this recessive gene the mutation must be either homozygous with two recessives at the same locus, or the cell would have to be hemizygous (mono-somal) for that lesion by having lost either a relative part or all of the homologous chromosome by deletion. In other words, in order for a recessive mutation to be expressed, something must have happened to the homologous gene on the other chromosome set.

This means that the initiation of malignancy requires at least two independent lesions, one to generate the necessary mutation and one to generate hemizygosity at the locus. This process must occur very infrequently in somatic cells; however, the fact that many tumours are of clonal origin (arise from single cells) fits in with the theory. Examination of chromosomes of developing tumours shows that this is precisely what happens. First, there is a stage in which there are a lot of chromosomal abnormalities – irregularities in number, translocations, breaks, inversions, deletions – a whole battery of abnormalities. This situation may persist for a long time, but, when eventually the tumour forms, the chromosomes of the tumour show a very strict range of changes, presumably corresponding to those changes from which the tumour arose. Thus there is an initial run of genetic instability and somewhere within this unstable population there are a few cells with the prerequisite genetic changes which give rise to the tumour.

Cell fusion studies
The nature of heritable change is being investigated at the cellular level by fusing tumour cells with normal cells by adding inactivated Sendai virus to a mixed cell suspension. In this process, hybrid cells form which contain the chromosomes of both parent cells (Fig. 7.4). The malignant potential of these hybrid cells is tested by inoculating the cells into newborn irradiated mice or into thymus-deficient (*nude*) mice. Malignant hybrids show progressive growth and give rise to tumours which kill the animals. Non-

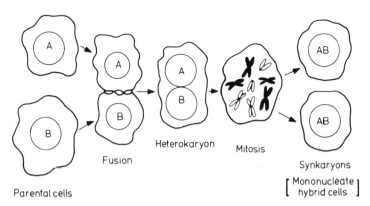

Fig. 7.4 Formation of binucleate heterokaryon by fusion of cells A + B using Sendai virus. After mitosis the heterokaryon gives rise to two mononucleate hybrid cells (synkaryons). Each of these cells contains one set of A-chromosomes and one set of B-chromosomes (tetraploid)

malignant hybrids fail to grow. These studies showed that:

1. Fusion of malignant with non-malignant cells gives rise to hybrid cells which are non-malignant.

2. Occasionally, tumours do arise from these hybrids, but such tumours have reduced chromosome complements – there is particularly a reduction in the number of chromosomes from the non-malignant parent cell.

3. Fusion of two malignant parent cells always gives rise to hybrids which are as malignant as the parent cells.

Initially, these observations suggest that malignant cells have lost something which can be replaced by the genetic complement from a non-malignant cell and that the same genetic locus is probably affected in different tumours, thus supporting the view that non-tumorigenecity is dominant to tumorigenecity.

The role of viruses

A recessive lesion implies loss of function. If the malignant change is a result of loss of function then what is the role of the tumour viruses? Assuming that the virus particle causes cancer in the simplest way, that is, the virus enters the cell and makes a gene product which, in turn, gives rise to a tumour, one would expect the lesion to be dominant, because such a change would be a gain in function. Cell fusion studies clearly show that this is not how viruses act. If a virus-induced tumour cell which carries the virus and which expresses all the antigens of the markers characteristic of the particular virus is fused with a normal non-malignant diploid cell, it is found that the hybrid still carries the virus and still expresses all the antigens, but it is not malignant. The cell fusion experiments indicate that the virus does not act *trans* (directly) by making some gene product, it acts *cis* (indirectly) by producing a cellular loss of function which can be made good by fusing the malignant cell with a normal cell.

Other gene models support this notion. It is possible the virus integrates at a site in the DNA strand and stops transmission of the adjacent genes with which it has integrated. The Rous phage, for example, can integrate at any site of the bacterial chromosome and, at each site, it produces a loss of function at the site in which it integrates by stopping transcription at that locus.

Therefore, regardless of whatever else viruses do when they infect cells, it seems very likely that their key role in malignancy is to integrate at a particular site of the chromosome and stop those genes from transmitting.

Epigenetic change
Instead of malignancy being the result of somatic mutation, it has been suggested that it could be an epigenetic change similar to the phenomenon of differentiation. In other words, the malignant change might be likened to the changes involved in determining the formation of an organ like the liver, that is, a change produced without any mutational change in the strict sense. The difficulty in this theory lies in our lack of understanding of the changes involved in differentiation; it is not a clearcut phenomenon – a whole series of changes are induced under certain conditions before differentiation occurs.

The model proposed (p. 82) of carcinogens binding to repressor proteins was suggested as a possible example of a stable epigenetic change. The theory is that carcinogens create new environmental conditions that impose changes in expression but not in the structure of genes. Such a comparison between carcinogens and differentiation has many pitfalls. For example, in cancer many diverse agents produce the same end result whereas differentiation is induced by specific stimuli.

It is also clear from cell fusion experiments that the expression or non-expression of the malignant phenotype is chromosomally determined. Furthermore, in assessing the role of epigenetic factors and loss of differentiation in the initiation of malignancy, one should keep in mind the frequent observations that the cells of many cancers preserve many features of their parent cells in the organ of origin. This applies both to morphological and functional features. Should loss of differentiation be of causal significance in carcinogenesis it might be expected that total loss of morphological and functional peculiarities of the tissue of origin would also be a feature of most cancers.

THE PROMOTION STAGE OF CARCINOGENESIS

Little is known about the sequence of events occurring during the promotion stage of carcinogenesis. In contrast to the initiation process which is rapid in onset, irreversible and requires a relatively small amount of carcinogen, the promotion process is reversible and requires repeated application of promoting agent for a considerable period of time. In addition, the proliferative capacity of the tissue and host factors such as diet, hormones and immunological status are important, but the way in which they exert their effect is not understood.

Cell proliferation

Obviously the tumour cells must arise from dormant initiated cells which, somehow, have escaped rejection by the usual host elimination mechanisms. In the first place, the genetically altered cell must enter mitosis. In some organs such as the epidermis, the epithelium of the gut and bone marrow, where mitotic activity is normally great, this would occur as a natural event. In other organs such as the liver, breast, prostrate and endocrine glands in which mitoses are sparse, most cells remain dormant (G_0-phase). In the latter group, a variety of agents may play an important role in stimulating initiated cells into mitotic activity. Substances that enhance cell proliferation and have been demonstrated to act as co-carcinogens include phorbol esters, phenols, hormones, viruses, stimuli to regeneration and wound healing, and repeated application of carcinogens. Thus, Virchow's irritation theory that regenerating processes and increased cell division play an important role in carcinogenesis, is now placed in better perspective.

Once the initiated cell enters mitosis, the tumour may be regarded as having commenced its progression, hence the definition 'a population of cells capable of progressive growth'. In this regard, the duration of the latent period raises interesting speculations. Since the latent period is considerably shortened by promoting agents, it is possible the *absolute minimum latent period* represents the minimum time required for a critical number of cells to form before the tumour becomes apparent macroscopically. Viewed in this light, it appears that the essential role of promotors is to induce cell proliferation and conversely, any stimulus that leads to cell proliferation should enhance the carcinogenic process.

Initiated cells are not the only targets of promoting agents, normal cells also are affected. The difference in response between normal and initiated cells becomes apparent when the stimulus is removed, normal cells cease to proliferate and the resultant hyperplasia regresses whereas initiated cells continue to multiply and may invade the adjacent tissue. These changes are commonly seen in the breast, prostate, bronchus, cervix and skin.

Host immune mechanisms

The theory of *immunological surveillance* in neoplasia is based on two concepts:

1. That tumour cells are antigenically different from normal cells and, in the host, they behave as foreign and transplanted cells.

2. That the host mounts an immune reaction against these cells.

Tumour specific transplantation antigens (TSTAs) are found on the surface of most tumours. All tumours that are virus-induced carry common antigens (p. 58) which are coded by nucleic acid derived from the particular oncogenic virus. Chemically-induced tumours, on the other hand, have different antigens that do not cross-react. Each of these chemically-induced tumours carries its own TSTAs, even though several tumours are produced by the same chemical compound in one animal. This difference between viral-induced and chemically-induced tumours might be explained on the basis of multifocal binding of chemical carcinogens to DNA, giving rise to random mutations which in turn produce different kinds of protein molecules. As it is unlikely that each cell will be hit in exactly the same locus by a carcinogen, one would not expect tumours arising from different cells to carry the same TSTAs.

The immunological surveillance concept implies that, throughout life, mutant somatic cells with malignant potential are constantly emerging, but they are recognized by the TSTAs and eliminated by the immune mechanisms.

1. The T-cell mediated immune response is the most effective cytotoxic mechanism. T-cells may also release a factor which stimulates macrophages to participate in the recognition and destruction of tumour cells.

2. B-cells may co-operate with T-cells by producing humoral antibodies and fixing complement. In some cases, however, this antibody may block the T-cell mechanism and thus enhance the growth of the tumour.

3. K-cells, a recently described group of lymphocytes, may bind to antibody-coated tumour cells and produce a cytotoxic effect.

Obviously, the host response is not sufficiently strong to inhibit cell proliferation or reject incipient tumours, as evidenced by the large number of tumours that develop. This inefficiency in the immune response might be a result of many factors: immunodeficiency, immunosuppression or blocking factors. More importantly, most carcinogens, whether chemicals, viruses or radiations are immunosuppressive.

In addition to TSTAs, cancer cells also exhibit certain *oncofoetal* antigens which are re-expressed embryonic proteins. They are expressed on the cell surface, but they are readily liberated into the circulation. These antigens are present in the normal foetus and usually absent in the adult; they are not antigenic, but they are so common that they are proving useful as diagnostic aids in human cancer. Two important examples detected in the serum of patients are:

1. The *carcinoembryonic antigen* (*CEA*), produced by tumours of the gastrointestinal tract.

2. *Alpha-foeto protein* (*a*-FP), which is a foetal ablumin produced by hepatomas.

Selection

Of the vast numbers of cells exposed to carcinogenic agents, only a rare selection give rise to tumours. Since cancer can arise from a single cell, proliferation must play a role in selecting cells as well as hastening neoplastic expression. If the stimulus causing cell proliferation is withdrawn, carcinogenesis may be interrupted or prevented, on the other hand, if the cells continue to divide the growth advantage of the initiated cells becomes expressed.

Chemical carcinogens also have the capacity to select initiated or dormant cells because these cells are resistant to the toxic effects of the compounds. The toxic side effects of the carcinogens suppress the activity of the immune system and the proliferations of normal cells, creating an environment which increases the chances of survival of tumour cells. For example, benzo(a)pyrene is toxic to normal fibroblasts in tissue culture, but not to benzo(a)-pyrene-induced fibrosarcoma cells. Many other examples could be cited.

In experimental animals given repeated applications of carcinogen, selective resistance to the carcinogen is the obvious explanation for the outgrowth of cancer cells. In tumours induced with a single dose of carcinogen, the situation is more complex; in these cases, there is a very long latent period, so that tumours arise when the animal is in an advanced age. With advanced age there is an associated weakening of the host's immunological surveillance which might allow initiated cells to escape the immune defence mechanisms.

Tumour progression

So far we have been dealing with changes which might be involved in the generation of a heritable line of cells which have the capacity for progressive growth and continue to multiply. Once this situation is reached, these cells can accumulate secondary mutations which may confer an even stronger advantage for growth. During the growth of the tumour, therefore, there is a constant selection for the cells that would do best in a particular situation.

The subsequent progression of the tumour appears to depend

on a process of repeated selection of mutants. There is morphological and chromosomal evidence within developing tumours of sub-populations of cells growing outwards from the main mass. These cells, already insensitive to the growth control factors, give rise to new populations of cells with additional secondary mutations, some of which confer a further survival advantage. Along with this, there is loss of certain differentiating markers which also confer advantage for growth. For example, the tumour starts off having certain gross characteristics of the tissue of origin, such as tumours of endocrine glands secreting hormones, but as time goes on sub-populations arise which have lost this specificity.

We are not dealing here with dedifferentiation in the sense that the cells which are already specialized revert to embryonic cells, what is happening, is the population which is generating more cells varies and cells with no specialized function (undifferentiated) progressively increase in number because of survival advantage. Thus once the tumour cell population gets going, it will continue to produce all sorts of changes and one of the most important changes that occurs is metastasis. It is possible that specific mutations may determine the population of cells which attack blood vessels and metastasize.

Conclusion
Fig. 7.5 attempts to summarize these concepts on the pathogenesis of cancer in schematic form. Somatic mutation may be considered the *final common pathway* by which chemical carcino-

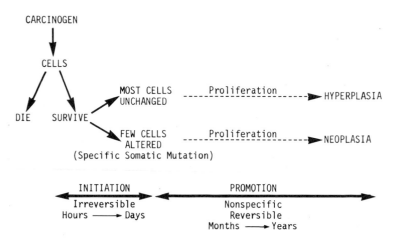

Fig. 7.5 Proposed sequence of events and related factors in carcinogenesis

gens, viruses and ionizing radiations initiate the malignant change. When applied to tissues, these carcinogens cause death of many cells. However, some cells survive and of these, some remain unaltered, whereas others are changed in such a way that, at some time later, they escape whatever it is that controls normal growth and give rise to tumours.

The nature of these changes that occur in the cells and concomitant with the development of malignancy are not precisely defined, but they are heritable and have all the characteristics of a recessive somatic mutation.

It is equally important to emphasize that these carcinogens can influence the development of overt malignancy and its subsequent progression at several stages. Like promoting agents, they can act as nonspecific stimuli to cell proliferation, they can induce secondary mutations and they can suppress both the immune system of the host and the growth of normal cells by their toxic effects.

FURTHER READING

Berenblum, I. (1941) The carcinogenic action of croton resin. *Cancer Res.*, **1**, 44.

Burnet, F. M. (1970) The concept of immunological surveillance. *Proc. Exp. Tumor Res.*, **13**, 1.

Editorial (1973) Environmental nitrosamines. *Lancet*, **2**, 1243.

Grover, P. L. & Sima, P. (1970) Interactions of the K-region epoxides of phenanthrene and dibenz(a,h)anthracene with nucleic acids and histone. *Biochem. Pharmacol.*, **19**, 2251.

Harris, H. (1974) *Nucleus and Cytoplasm*, 3rd edn. Oxford: Clarendon Press.

Heidelberger, C. (1973) Current trends in chemical carcinogenesis. *Fed. Proc.*, **32**, 2154.

Kellerman, G. *et al.* (1974) Aryl hydrocarbon hydroxylase inducibility and bronchogenic carcinoma. *New Eng. J. Med.*, **289**, 934.

Louis, C. J. & Blunck, J. M. (1971) Alteration in the distribution of basic soluble rat liver proteins during azo dye carcinogenesis. *Cancer Res.*, **31**, 2110.

Louis, C. J. *et al.* (1973) Agarose gel electrophoresis of soluble proteins from bronchial mucosa and bronchogenic carcinoma. *Oncology*, **27**, 324.

Louis, C. J. & Kushinsky, R. (1977) The effect of cigarette smoke on aryl hydrocarbon hydroxylase and cytochrome P450 content in rat liver and lung microsomes. *Oncology*, in press.

Loveless, A. (1969) Possible relevance of O–6 alkylation of deoxyguanosine to the mutagenicity and carcinogenicity of nitrosamines and nitrosamides. *Nature*, (Lond.), **223**, 206.

Pitot, H. C. & Heidelberger, C. (1963) Metabolic regulatory circuits and carcinogenesis. *Cancer Res.*, **23**, 1694.

Sorof, S. (1969) Carcinogen-protein conjugates in liver carcinogenesis. In *The Jerusalem Symposium on Quantum Chemistry and Biochemistry*. Ed. by Bergman, E. D. and Pullman, B. Vol. 1, *Physicochemical Mechanisms of Carcinogenesis*, pp. 208–217. Jerusalem: The Israel Academy of Sciences and Humanities.

Van Duuren, B. L. (1969) Tumor-promoting agents in two-stage carcinogenesis. *Progress in Exp. Tumor Res.*, **11**, 31.

8

Complications and clinical implications of tumours

Tumours, even the very malignant varieties, do not necessarily produce symptoms themselves. Symptoms are due to complications, such as pressure and obstruction on essential organs to such a degree that they fail to function. Benign tumours produce serious effects only when they occur at an important site or when they secrete hormones. Malignant tumours also produce local effects because of their size and location, but, as they differ from benign tumours in their more rapid growth, in their ability to spread and to form metastases and in their capacity to invade and destroy normal tissues, they may have additional risks of haemorrhage, ulceration and secondary infection. In many instances, death from cancer is related to one or more of these complications. Thus a patient with cancer may be examined and found apparently well and expected to live for several years, but because of some unexpected complication, his condition may rapidly deteriorate. The importance of a particular tumour, therefore, lies in its ultimate effect on the patient.

LOCAL EFFECTS OF TUMOURS

The mere presence of a growing tumour, irrespective of whether it is solid, cystic, benign or malignant can give rise to a variety of mechanical effects. These effects are determined primarily by the size and location of the tumour.

Anatomical disfigurement
Tumours of superficial tissues such as skin, thyroid gland, breasts and bones may cause conspicuous swellings and create important cosmetic problems. If ulceration also occurs, secondary infection and persistent discharge add to the disfigurement.

Obstruction
Tumours are a common cause of obstruction in tubular organs.

The obstructing lesion may be located within the lumen, within the wall or outside the wall of the tube. The consequences of obstruction in various parts of the body and their accentuation by superimposed infection are well recognized.

1. Oesophageal obstruction gives rise to dysphagia, initially to solids, but later to liquids also, and interferes with nutrition.

2. Pyloric obstruction is characterized by projectile vomiting immediately after eating, dehydration and electrolyte imbalance, dilatation of the stomach and reflux oesophagitis.

3. A polyp in the small intestine may form the apex of an intussusception, which results in acute intestinal obstruction.

4. Bronchial obstruction is followed initially by absorption collapse of the lobe distal to the obstruction, followed by infection and possibly abscess formation. Bronchiectasis is also a common sequel.

5. In urethral obstruction there is hypertrophy, trabecular and diverticular formation in the wall of the urinary bladder, infection and urinary calculus formation.

6. Ureteric obstruction results in hydroureter, hydronephrosis, superimposed infection and renal calculus.

7. A small tumour, even less than 1 cm in diameter, in the region of the ampulla of Vater may cause complete biliary obstruction, preventing bile entering the duodenum. This causes obstructive jaundice with clay-coloured bulky stools which contain excessive amounts of fat, dark urine due to excess urobilinogen, pruritus due to increased amounts of circulating bile salts, a bleeding tendency due to failure of absorption of the fat-soluble vitamin K and various degrees of liver damage. In the absence of other disease, the gall bladder may become distended and, if there is a superimposed infection, ascending cholangitis might result. Obstruction to the common bile duct produces similar changes.

Pressure

A tumour is a space-occupying lesion. Concomitant with its growth, there is a corresponding increase in pressure within that space. The effects produced by the compression are again determined by the size and location of the tumour and the diversity of these effects is illustrated in the spinal cord and skull.

In the spinal cord, compression usually develops gradually and the most frequent presenting symptoms are sensory, particularly pain, which may be localized over the spine or it may be of root distribution. Motor symptoms usually appear later than sensory and may vary in degree from a mild muscular weakness to a com-

plete paralysis. Posterior root pressure results first in hyperaes-
thesiae and later sensory loss over the appropriate dermatome,
whereas anterior root pressure produces a lower motor neurone
lesion at the corresponding level. Interruption of ascending fibres
cause sensory loss below the level of the lesion and interruption
of descending tracts give rise to upper motor neurone signs below
the level of the lesion.

In the case of intracranial tumours, because we are dealing with
an expanding space occupying lesion within a rigid box, the clinical
features are determined by the level of intracranial pressure and
by the degree of compression and displacement of brain tissue.
Sometimes, changes within the tumour such as haemorrhage or cyst
formation may produce a rapid increase in volume of the intracranial mass with an acute onset of symptoms. In general, three
major groups of symptoms occur:

1. *Cerebral oedema*, which is the result of a chain of circulatory
disturbances, namely, venous stasis, arteriolar congestion and
increased capillary permeability caused by the increase in the
volume of the mass.

2. *Hydrocephalus and dilatation of the ventricles*, which are the
sequelae to the obstruction of the flow of C.S.F. through the
foramen of Monro and the aqueduct of Sylvius.

3. *Herniation of brain tissue and splaying of sutures.* In children,
increase in the volume of intra cranial contents leads to splaying of
the cranial sutures and to a consequent increase in the size of the
skull. In adults, the expanding mass may cause (a) herniation of
the uncinate process beneath the free edge of the falx, (b) herniation
of the hippocampal gyrus in the tentorial notch between the brain
stem and the free edge of the tentorium cerebelli and may be associated with pressure disturbances of the III and IV cranial nerves,
(c) herniation of the cerebellar tonsils in the foramen magnum
causing compression of the medulla with respiratory and cardiac
arrest and death, (d) compression of the regional arteries and veins
causing infarction in the territory of the posterior cerebral artery,
or brain stem haemorrhages, and (e) herniation of the inferior
surface of the frontal lobe under the lesser wing of the sphenoid.

HORMONAL EFFECTS

The hormonal effects of tumours of endocrine glands on the host
are of particular interest (Chapter 18). In general, benign tumours
are more likely to be functional than malignant tumours. Benign
tumours, even when small, may produce excessive amounts of

hormone; the size of the tumour is not necessarily related to the degree of functional activity. Occasionally, malignant tumours of non-endocrine origin, especially lung cancer, may produce a variety of hormones, but the mechanism of production is not understood; perhaps it may be a re-expression of suppressed genes. Tumours may arise from any one of the endocrine glands and the diversity of their effects on the host are shown in Table 8.1 and, in order to give a concise and comprehensive picture of the hormone secreting tumours, both benign and malignant tumours are included in the table.

GENERAL EFFECTS OF MALIGNANT TUMOURS

Anaemia

Anaemia is a frequent accompaniment in patients with certain forms of cancer. Its development is the result of three major groups of causes:

1. Blood loss
2. Impaired erythropoiesis
3. Haemolysis

Blood loss

Haemorrhage is probably the most important cause of anaemia in malignancy, especially in cancer of the gastro-intestinal tract. The source of bleeding is commonly an ulcerating or fungating lesion. In most cases, the bleeding is mild and the anaemia is not evident in the early stages, but it gradually progresses in severity during the course of this disease. The persistent bleeding depletes the body of its iron stores and results both in hypochromic microcytic anaemia and in a mild elevation of the reticulocyte count.

The exact source and amount of bleeding is difficult to estimate. In carcinoma of the stomach, the blood is usually mixed with gastric contents which alter the colour of the blood and, when vomited, the vomitus has a *coffee grounds* appearance. In the intestine, blood presents in two forms, depending on the level of the bleeding source: (a) in lesions located in the distal parts of the large bowel, sigmoid and rectum the blood is usually bright red, (b) in more proximal lesions, such as those originating in the stomach, small intestine or proximal part of the large intestine, the blood is partly digested along its passage through the rest of the bowel and altered to give a dark tarry appearance (*melaena*). Small amounts of bleeding are common in malignancy and may not be macroscopic-

Table 8.1 Some hormone-secreting tumours and the syndromes they produce

Tumour	Hormone	Syndrome
Pituitary		
Acidophil adenoma	Growth hormone	Gigantism – (children)
		Acromegally – (adults)
Basophil adenoma	ACTH, TSH, FSH, LH	Cushing's syndrome
Thyroid		
Adenoma	(Usually non-functional) Thyroxine	Thyrotoxicosis
Medullary carcinoma	Calcitonin	Nil
Parathyroid		
Adenoma	Parathormone	Osteitis fibrosa (von Recklinghausen's disease)
Adrenal		
Phaeochromocytoma	Noradrenaline, adrenaline	Paroxysmal hypertension
Cortical adenoma	Steroid hormones	Cushing's syndrome
	Aldosterone	Conn's syndrome
Ovary		
Granulosa-cell tumour	Oestrogens	Endometrial hyperplasia and bleeding
	Androgens	Virilization
Placenta		
Hydatidiform mole	Gonadotrophic hormone	Nil
Choriocarcinoma	Gonadotrophic hormone	Nil
Testis		
Interstitial-cell adenoma	Androgens or oestrogens	Feminization
Intestine		
Carcinoid	5-HT	Carcinoid syndrome
Kidney		
Carcinoma	Erythropoietin	Polycythaemia
Lung		
'Oat-cell' carcinoma	Parathormone, ACTH, ADH	Hypercalcaemia, Cushing's syndrome, Diabetes insipidus
Carcinoid	5-HT	Carcinoid syndrome
Mesothelioma	Insulin	Hypoglycaemia
Pancreas (islets)		
α-cell adenoma	Glucagon	Diabetes mellitus
β-cell adenoma	Insulin	Hypoglycaemia
δ-cell adenoma	Gastrin	Zollinger–Ellison syndrome (peptic ulceration)

ally visible in the faeces, but it can be shown to be present by tests for occult blood. The possibility of a malignancy of the gastro-intestinal tract should always be considered in a patient over 40 years of age with an iron deficiency anaemia without obvious cause.

Bleeding occurs in other tumours in the body such as tumours of the uterus, skin, lung and urinary tract. Here also, small amounts of unaltered blood may not be evident with the naked eye, but can be detected by microscopic examination.

Impaired erythropoiesis

Lack of nutritional factors is usually the result of anorexia, dysphagia and vomiting, which impair intake, and diarrhoea, which interferes with absorption of factors essential for erythropoiesis. In carcinoma of the stomach, lack of intrinsic factor may lead to a macrocytic anaemia and lack of hydrochloric acid to impairment of iron absorption. Decreased erythropoiesis may also be secondary to toxins resulting from infection and renal insufficiency. Chemo-therapy and radiotherapy usually produce a transient depression of marrow activity, but large doses of radiotherapy may cause a permanent marrow aplasia.

Haemolysis

Acute and chronic haemolytic anaemias are occasionally seen in malignancies of the lymphoreticular system. In a series of cases of chronic lymphatic leukaemia studied by the author, approxi-mately six per cent of the patients suffered from auto-immune haemolytic anaemia, in which the red cells showed a positive response to the Coombs' test. Splenomegally is invariably present in these patients. Hodgkin's disease also augments haemolysis. Occasionally, auto-immune haemolytic anaemia is seen in carci-nomas of the stomach, prostate and in metastatic bone disease.

Tumour metastases frequently occur in bone, especially in sites occupied by red marrow. Infiltration at these sites either by tumour or other abnormal tissue may cause an anaemia with the appearance of primitive red and white cells in the peripheral blood —*leuco-erythroblastic anaemia.*

Infection

Secondary infection is a common complication in certain malignant tumours. It is particularly common in bronchogenic carcinoma with bronchial obstruction and in carcinomas of the bladder and uterus which cause urinary obstruction.

Patients with malignancies of the lympho-reticular system are more particularly prone to infections with pathogenic organisms than the general population. Moreover, when such infections develop, they take on a rapid and often fatal course. For example, tuberculosis is more frequent in patients with Hodgkin's disease and the development of pulmonary, meningeal and miliary forms of this disease may determine the cause of death. These patients have also an increased liability to certain fungal infections, such as cryptococcosis (torulosis), candidiasis, aspergillosis and histoplasmosis that are normally non-pathogenic or very weakly pathogenic to the general population. The increased proneness of patients with lymphomas and leukaemias to these so-called *opportunistic infections*, as well as to infections with pathogenic organisms, is attributed to two major groups of predisposing factors:

1. *Disturbances in Leukocytes.* The ganulocytes may be increased or decreased in number. In granulocytopoenia, which may be due either to the disease process itself or secondary to therapy, there is an insufficient number of granulocytes in the peripheral blood to help combat the infection. On the other hand, granulocytes in acute and chronic myeloid leukaemia, despite their increased numbers, are generally incapable of responding to infection.

2. *Disturbances in Immunoglobulins.* Immunoglobulin levels in the serum also may be decreased by either the disease process or by immunosuppressive therapy. Alternatively, high levels of abnormal globulins in patients with multiple myeloma are ineffective against infection.

Fever

Infection is the commonest cause of fever in patients with cancer. Apart from infection, fever is an infrequent accompaniment. The fever in Hodgkin's disease is usually of a low-grade irregular type, but, in some cases, there are remittent bouts of pyrexia of 38° to 39°C for several days, alternating with afebrile periods (*Pel-Ebstein fever*). This type of fever is associated with cases in which the spleen and retroperitoneal lymph glands are affected and, when present, the fever can be a particularly distressing symptom. Often it is the persistence of a low-grade fever that prompts the patient to seek medical attention.

Cachexia

The term cachexia refers to a state of anaemia, debility and emaciation commonly seen in patients with advanced cancer but it is not specific to malignancy. The progressive wasting that leads to a state of cachexia is so characteristic that any unexplained substantial loss of weight should always raise the suspicion of cancer. The cause of this wasting is not clear, but it can be attributed to secondary factors such as loss of appetite, vomiting, malabsorption, anaemia and infection. The likelihood that cancerous tissues liberate toxic factors has not been substantiated.

Carcinomatous neuropathy

A number of neurological and muscular disorders are now recognized to be associated with the presence of a primary tumour elsewhere in the body. Almost all types of cancer have been implicated, but the most common are those of the lung and ovary. Degenerative changes may occur in the central nervous system with progressive demyelination of various tracts and, sometimes, with myopathies such as severe muscle weakness and dermatomyositis. In some cases, the neurological symptoms appear as early as one to two years before the tumour becomes clinically evident, but more often they appear after the primary has been detected. The pathogenesis of these complications is not clear but the course tends to be progressive. It is not due to direct invasion of the nervous system by metastatic deposits, but there is some evidence that abnormal immune mechanisms may be involved. Occasionally, the symptoms disappear when the primary is removed.

Pulmonary osteodystrophy

This is characterized by clubbing of the fingers and toes and it is accompanied by cyanosis, curving of the nails and pain and swelling of the wrists and ankles. Histologically, there is subperiosteal bone formation and synovitis. The underlying cause of these changes is not understood. The condition is associated particularly with carcinoma of the lung, bronchiectasis, lung abscess and congenital heart disease with cyanosis.

In cases of operable lung cancer, removal of the tumour results in a rapid amelioration of the condition.

Thrombotic complications

Occasionally advanced cancers, particularly of the stomach, pancreas and lung are complicated by thrombophlebitis migrans of superficial or deep veins. The cause of this is not known, but cases have been reported where removal of the tumour leads to improvement of the phlebitis.

FURTHER READING

The bibliography for Chapters 8 and 9 is incorporated in that of Chapter 10.

9

Principles of diagnosis

The present survival rates of patients with cancer do not engender complacency, in fact, the outlook for many patients is grave. The problem then, is how to improve this situation? Since the survival rates of patients with cancer is directly related to the stage of the disease at which treatment is instituted, one method of reducing the cancer death rate is to treat the disease as early as possible. Nowadays, therefore, emphasis is placed on the early diagnosis of cancer. This objective is usually achieved by a collation of data derived from the history of the patient, a complete physical examination and from various specialized methods of investigation that are available, particularly radiology, endoscopy and cytology.

There are few symptoms that cannot be directly or indirectly caused by some form of neoplasia. These are too numerous to be mentioned individually, but the American Cancer Society has for many years emphasized seven danger signals of which the public should be aware. These are:

1. A change in a wart or mole.
2. A lump in the breast.
3. A sore in the skin, mouth or elsewhere which does not heal.
4. Unusual bleeding or discharge from any source.
5. A persistent cough.
6. Indigestion or difficulty in swallowing.
7. Changes in bowel or urinary habits.

Knowledge of these points often brings the patient to the doctor at a much earlier stage than if he were unaware of their possible significance. Once the patient presents, there are many points to be elicited in the history and physical examination. The history is probably the most important part of the examination and should be taken methodically, bearing in mind the known causes of cancer and the symptoms produced by the different types of the disease. A complete physical examination is also essential and special attention must be given to the detection of the early phase of the disease which, in many patients, is asymptomatic and will not be discovered unless special techniques are employed.

DIAGNOSTIC RADIOLOGY

Radiology is probably the most important early investigation in the diagnosis of neoplasia. Radiation images form because X-rays are absorbed to different degrees by different substances whose absorptive capacity is related to the following major factors:

1. *Atomic number*. Barium and iodine have a higher absorption co-efficient than calcium in bone, and bone higher than other organic tissues.

2. *Density concentration* (the number of atoms per unit volume). Soft tissues are more absorbent than gases.

3. *Thickness irradiated*.

4. *Wavelength of the radiation* (a function of the kilovoltage applied across the X-ray tube). In many circumstances, the composition of tumour tissue, or the changes produced in adjacent normal tissues, provide a sufficient contrast in density for accurate identification of a tumour to be achieved on the plain radiograph. In other instances, where there is insufficient contrast between normal and neoplastic tissue, additional techniques can be employed to enhance the contrast and increase the radiologists' ability to make a diagnosis. However, it is well to remember that, although X-ray images are very useful, they do have severe limitations and important features such as size, shape and internal structure are frequently in doubt. Notwithstanding these limitations, it is still often possible to distinguish between neoplastic and non-neoplastic lesions, between benign and malignant and between primary and secondary tumours.

PLAIN RADIOGRAPHY

No radiological investigations of a patient suspected of suffering from neoplasia is more important than a plain film. Tissues such as blood, bile, muscle, fibrous tissue, parenchyma of solid organs and tumours all have similar densities and effective atomic number, and their opacities are indistinguishable on the plain radiograph. They are *opacities of water density*. Adipose tissue, on the other hand, has a lower density and casts a shadow which is somewhat less dense than a water dense shadow and which, under favourable conditions, can be distinguished. Thus on the plain film one can expect to distinguish between air, fat, bone (including other calcified tissues), and a range of tissues classified as water dense.

Air contrast

Neoplasms of the lung are often seen as clearly marginated shadows against a background of aerated pulmonary parenchyma. Less frequently, abdominal tumours may become definable against gas contained in stomach or colon, or the mass may displace loops of gas filled intestine which enfold it and give some indication of the size and shape of the tumour.

Bone contrast

Tumours involving bone frequently cause demineralization of bone tissue which is easy to see. This may take the form of a discrete or irregular destructive lesion or a well marginated pressure erosion.

Fat contrast

Neoplasms of the breast can frequently be discerned in the surrounding fibro-fatty stroma, and mammography is a very useful aid in diagnosis and management of breast lumps. On rare occasions, a retroperitoneal mass such as carcinoma of the kidney can be seen because of its vague encapsulation of extraperitoneal fat. Infiltrating tumours of the posterior abdominal wall may efface normal fat shadows such as perinephric fat which defines the lateral margin of psoas major muscle and the renal outlines; however, tumours are an uncommon cause of such effacement in practice.

THE INTERNAL STRUCTURE OF TUMOURS IN PLAIN FILMS

Fat

Adipose tissue is often recognizable in plain films of tumour masses. Lipomata can frequently be diagnosed in favourable sites, such as renal hamartomas and teratomas of the ovary.

Calcification

Dystrophic calcification is common in some tumours, especially in chondromas and chondrosarcomas, and shows up as fine punctate deposits of amorphous calcification in a homogeneous background of water dense opacity. A particularly coarse form of calcification is occasionally seen in the cartilage of pulmonary hamartomas, often described as *pop-corn* calcification. Numerous other neoplastic tissues may show variable patterns of dystrophic calcification and even ossification, but only a small part of the tumour mass is usually involved. Those that commonly calcify include meningioma, neuroblastoma, carcinoma of the breast, synovioma and several others. In addition to calcification, the rare osteogenic tumours often produce recognizable osseous tissue which clearly indicates the origin of the tumour. Some teratomas also produce a characteristic radiological appearance because of their cartilage, osseous and dental tissue content. However, it should be emphasized that the type of dystrophic calcification seen in most tumours is non-specific and too variable in appearance to be of much help in diagnosis.

Air

Air may occasionally enter the necrotic core of a bronchogenic carcinoma which has produced a bronchial sinus. Secondary neoplasms of the lung such as metastatic squamous-cell carcinoma may also cavitate, but this feature is more common in primary lung tumours. Neoplastic cavities in the lung tend to have thick, irregular walls which helps to distinguish them from lung abscesses and cavitating granulomas. However, the latter still can cause confusion, but in the older age group, neoplasia is far more common than these lesions.

PATTERNS PRODUCED BY THE BEHAVIOUR OF TUMOURS

Obstruction

Bronchostenosis is frequently caused by bronchial carcinoma or adenoma. Retained secretions distal to the obstruction tend to become infected and air in the related alveoli becomes replaced by fluid and pus (*consolidation*); resorption of air in the remaining aerated alveoli results in *partial atelectasis* of the involved region of the lung. Segmental consolidation with variable atelectasis is an important radiological sign of carcinoma of the lung. Less commonly, a bronchostenotic lesion may result in *air-trapping* rather than atelectasis, for the obstruction in these cases is presumably complete only during expiration. The involved area of lung, therefore, becomes hyperinflated and is seen as increased lucency, especially if the film is exposed in full expiration.

Large bowel obstruction is frequently caused by an annular carcinoma of the descending or sigmoid colon. The radiological pattern shows:

1. Multiple gas-distended loops of small and large bowel.
2. Conspicuous caecal distention.
3. Multiple fluid levels in erect and lateral decubitus films.

Pyloric stenosis is usually caused by peptic ulceration, but occasionally it is the result of antral carcinoma. In these cases, the pattern is of a large distended stomach with gastric residue and air together with a relatively gasless abdomen.

Invasion and perforation

Infiltrating neoplasms such as carcinoma and malignant lymphoma may thicken the walls of hollow organs and make then rigid. Rapid invasion, as seen occasionally in squamous-cell carcinoma of the oesophagus, may be followed by necrosis and perforation. In such a case, air may be seen in the mediastinum as lucent streaks around the heart and great vessels, often extending into the neck, and hydrothoraces are usually present. Perforation of a colonic neo-plasm usually results either in a localized abscess in the peritoneum, which may be recognized as an extra-lumenal pocket of air, or in an internal fistula.

METASTASES

Blood spread

Blood-borne metastases to lung and bone are readily detected radiologically, especially if they exceed 1 cm in diameter. In the lung, a variety of patterns may be seen: (a) Most commonly, there are multiple rounded opacities exceeding 1 cm in diameter but rarely cavitating; (b) less commonly, there may be a diffuse infil-trate of *miliary nodules*, 2–3 mm in diameter, and (c) rarely, the metastases may take the form of a diffuse linear infiltrate with thickened septal lines known as *lymphangitis carcinomatosa*. In bone, the lesions are usually osteolytic, but occasionally they may be osteoblastic and produce areas of increased bone density. Osteo-blastic metastases are characteristic of carcinoma of the prostate, but, occasionally, they may also be produced by Hodgkin's disease, carcinoma of the breast, carcinoma of the bladder and malignant carcinoid.

Lymphatic spread

Lymphatic spread results in enlargement of draining lymph nodes. This is often well seen in the bronchopulmonary nodes in cases of carcinoma of the lung, where enlarged lymph nodes may be more conspicuous than the primary tumour. Indeed, *oat-cell* carcinoma of the lung most commonly presents radiologically as a mediastinal mass, effacing the profile of the hilar vessels, aortic arch and heart shadow. Enlargement of abdominal lymph nodes is not recognized unless it is gross. Similarly, secondary deposits in the liver, which

are a common pathological finding, are seldom recognized radiologically; their presence may be suspected only if liver enlargement
is marked and if the metastases are subphrenic in location. In such
cases, the right cupola of the diaphragm may be elevated and its
outline, nodular.

DISPLACEMENT OF NORMAL STRUCTURE

In the skull, raised intracranial pressure may be produced by
tumours which obstruct the normal flow of C.S.F. Distortion of
the aqueduct of Sylvius, tentorial and tonsillar herniations are the
usual precipitating mechanisms.

1. *In adults*, the signs of raised intracranial pressure that may be
recognized in plain films are: (a) increased convolutional markings,
(b) demineralization of the *dorsum sellae* and erosion of the
posterior clinoid processes, and (c) enlargement of the emissary
foramina.

2. *In children*, sutural diastasis and excessive digitations of the
sutures are the conspicuous features.

3. *The pineal gland* and related structures commonly calcify after
the age of 20 years and displacement of the centre of this structure
in excess of 3 mm from the midline in all frontal projections of
the skull is an important sign of intracerebral space-occupying
lesions, be it blood clot or neoplasm.

Many other organs, such as the trachea, kidney, stomach, duodenum and subcutaneous fat are characteristically displaced by
tumours. These displacements, particularly of the trachea, may
be detected on plain films of high kilovoltage exposures of the
chest. Such films may also display certain mediastinal lines defined
by pleural reflection plains lying tangential to the incident X-ray
beam, of which the easiest to see are the right and left paraspinal
lines. Posterior mediastinal tumours, such as neurofibromas and
lymphomas, displace these lines laterally away from the vertebral
column.

REACTIVE CHANGES

Invasion of a serous surface by tumour cells frequently produces
a serosanguinous exudate containing proteinaceous fluid, tumour
cells and blood cells.

1. *Pleural effusions* formed in this way typically produce water
dense opacities at the lung bases in the erect position. The
opacity has a hazy upper margin and a meniscus at the costal and

mediastinal margins. Smaller effusions can only be detected in erect films by obliteration of the posterior and lateral costophrenic recesses.

2. *Peritoneal effusions* (*ascites*) are usually recognized only when large and, in such cases, the plain film tends to show a uniform grey appearance of poor contrast with wide separation of loops of gas filled bowel. The loops tend to lie centrally in the abdominal cavity leaving broad zones of water density in each flank and tending to give a lateral convexity to the extraperitoneal fat lines visible above each iliac crest.

3. *Osseous tissue* may show reactive sclerosis at the margin of a destructive neoplastic lesion. This reaction usually takes the form of thickening of pre-existing trabeculae and commonly indicates a benign or slowly progressive process; it is not seen in malignant neoplasms of bone. Osteoid osteoma and benign osteoblastoma are good examples of this reactive process. Meningioma often produces dense thickening of the inner table of the calvarium beneath its site of attachment to the dura mater.

4. *Malignant neoplasms involving bone*, especially the rare primary bone tumours, frequently cause a reactive change called a *periosteal reaction*. Malignant cells eroding through the cortical lamellae multiply beneath the periosteum and elevate it several millimetres from the cortex. The periosteal osteoblasts proliferate and form new bone which appears in the space between the periosteum and the cortex and which can easily be recognized on radiographs. The pattern of new bone formation is variable: (a) it may be linear or lamellar, and sometimes resemble *onion peel*, or (b) it may show *sunray spiculation* with streaks of calcification radiating out from the cortex. Such periosteal reactions are however nonspecific, and are more frequently seen in inflammatory lesions of bone.

5. *Desmoplasia*, the fibrous tissue response to a neoplasm, is also occasionally visible radiologically. This is best seen in mammograms of scirrhous carcinoma of the breasts and gives the tumour its characteristic *crab-like* appearance.

6. *Vascular hyperaemia* that is often associated with neoplasms can occasionally be suspected on plain radiographs. For example: (a) the vascular grooves of the middle meningeal artery on the calvarium may enlarge and show abnormal tortuosity, and (b) the foramen spinosum may be expanded and seen in the basal view of the skull. These are important radiological signs of intracranial meningiomas.

CONTRAST STUDIES

The elements iodine and barium have atomic numbers of 53 and 56 respectively. At the wavelengths of X-rays used in diagnostic radiology these elements show unusually good absorption with a minimum of radiation scatter and, therefore, they are ideal substances for use as *positive contrast media*. Nowadays, they are the sole elements used for this purpose. In some situations, gases are used as *negative contrast agents*; these include atmospheric air, carbon dioxide and oxygen. A full account of the techniques and range of patterns seen in the various contrast studies is far beyond the scope of this chapter. Only a few salient points on each will be mentioned.

Barium meals and enemas
Neoplasms of the stomach and colon produce filling defects, stenoses and ulcers, all of which can often be clearly defined in the barium. Moreover, infiltrating tumours produce rigid aperistaltic segments, efface mucosal folds or, occasionally, accentuate them. These changes can also be detected in small bowel.

Intravenous pyelography
This examination defines renal outlines and pelvi-calyceal shapes, both of which may show characteristic deformities by renal neoplasms. Displacement of kidney or ureter by extra urinary tumours and obstruction of the ureter by neoplasms of the bladder or cervix may also be seen.

ANGIOGRAPHY

Preshaped, flexible catheters are inserted percutaneously and placed in almost any selected artery or vein under image intensifier control. Contrast material can be injected to define the vascular pattern and blood samples removed for analysis.

In selective arteriography, many tumours may be defined by the abnormal vascular patterns they produce. For example: (a) displacement of vessels in the form of circular stretching around the margin of a tumour, (b) reactive dilatation and decreased circulation time, (c) diffuse tumour staining (tumour blush), (d) contrast pooling in portions of the tumour mass, (e) early venous filling due to aterio-venous fistulae, and (f) new vessel formation. Neovascularization consists of poorly formed vessels lacking organized walls. In certain benign tumours, the new vessels may resemble normal vessels, although frequently forming fistulae, but, in malignant tumours, they are irregular in calibre and bizarre in their branching pattern. New vessels in malignant tumours usually do not respond to adrenergic stimulation and their appearance may be enhanced by selective cortical injection of adrenalin, which constricts the surrounding normal vessels and makes them relatively less conspicuous.

PERCUTANEOUS TRANSHEPATIC CHOLANGIOGRAPHY

The treatment of patients with jaundice depends on whether the jaundice is obstructive or hepatocellular. Generally, the history and physical examination can distinguish between the two types of jaundice, but occasionally, the clinical picture is confusing and in these cases a liver biopsy or percutaneous transhepatic cholangeogram are needed to make a distinction. Cholecystographic preparations are ineffective in the presence of jaundice with serum bilirubin levels exceeding 85 μmol/l.

A fine needle is passed through the liver and a dilated intrahepatic bile duct is injected with contrast medium under fluoroscopic control. In favourable circumstances, excellent visualization of the biliary tree can be obtained, and the common bile duct defined. In the absence of obstruction contrast material flows through to the duodenum whereas in the presence of obstruction, the passage of contrast material is arrested at a point which is easy to see in the presence of proximal dilatation of the duct system which is invariably present. The technique is of particular value in management of carcinoma of the head of the pancreas, ampulla and carcinoma of the bile ducts.

ENDOSCOPIC RETROGRADE CHOLEDOCHO-PANCREATOGRAPHY (ERCP)

ERCP is occasionally attempted in some centres in the diagnosis of space occupying lesions of the pancreas. The pancreatic duct is directly cannulated and injected with contrast via a flexible duodenoscope. However, the technique requires the services of an experienced gastroscopist, and its role in management of pancreatic lesions is still being evaluated.

LYMPHANGIOGRAPHY

This investigation involves the intralymphatic injection of contrast material. A dye such as methylene blue is injected into the web spaces of the toes and within 30 minutes the lymph channels can be seen through the skin. A lymphatic can then be dissected free and cannulated and an oily contrast medium slowly injected into the vessel over a period of approximately one hour. Early films taken at the end of injection show lymphatic vessels, and those taken 24 hours later show the actual lymph nodes themselves. Lymphatic involvement by neoplasia may be seen as filling defects in the normal granular pattern of the node, as uniform or irregular enlargement of nodes or as non-filling of nodal groups. Lymphangiography is used most frequently nowadays in the staging of lymphomas preparatory to treatment.

OTHER METHODS OF MEDICAL IMAGING

Although traditional radiology still occupies a prominent position in the diagnosis of tumours, there have been several recent developments which have changed the emphasis of radiological investigation.

Computerized axial tomography

This is perhaps the most exciting new development in medical imaging in recent years. Using specific orientations of a single X-ray beam in multiple positions over a period of approximately 10 to 20 minutes, absorption co-efficients of small cubes of tissue in a given anatomical plane within a patient can be directly computed. This produces a composite image of a body section of surprising contrast and clarity, but with limited resolution. The equipment is so sensitive that it can distinguish, for example, quite clearly between brain tissue and cerebrospinal fluid. The technique has enormous potential for studying difficult tumours, such as carcinoma of the pancreas. Currently, the technique is used in the diagnosis of cerebral lesions, and it has already revolutionized the diagnostic approach in this field. However, the equipment is elaborate and expensive, factors which limit the extent of its application.

Radioisotope scanning

Radioisotope scanning is now firmly established as a valuable aid to the diagnosis and management of tumours. In some areas it has distinct advantages over conventional X-ray techniques. The method involves the administration of radioisotope (*radionucleide*) in a suitable inert preparation (*radiopharmaceutical*) which will be selectively accumulated by the organ of interest. The radionucleide most commonly used is metastable *technicium-99* (^{99}Tc) because it has a high enough energy to make counting or screening possible, yet a short enough half-life (6 hrs) to reduce any radiation damage to an absolute minimum. Other radionucleides are used in some circumstances.

Detecting devices are of two main types:

1. *Rectilinear scanner*. This is a moving scanning head which systematically scans an area and maps out an emission pattern, which is recorded on X-ray film. Areas of increased emission show as dark spots, squares or lines.

2. *Gamma-Camera*. Here the recording head is stationary and a large detecting crystal is used. The instrument is a far more sophisticated piece of equipment and images the scintillation pattern of the entire area simultaneously. The result is recorded on polaroid film as a negative, where areas of increased emission show as light patches.

Tumours show up either as areas of reduced emission or areas of increased emission. This depends upon the nature of the radiopharmaceutical used and its binding in the organ under examination; it also depends to some extent on the type of tumour. For example:

1. *Brain Tumours*: ^{99}Tc invariably shows up as areas of increased emission, but this depends upon their vascularity and the integrity of the blood-brain barrier. Less vascular tumours are not detected.

2. *Liver Tumours*: ^{99}Tc-sulphur colloid show up as areas of reduced emission because the radiopharmaceutical is taken up by the reticuloendothelial cells. It is in metastatic carcinoma of the liver that this technique has its most useful applications and far surpasses conventional radiography.

3. *Kidney Tumours*: ^{99}Tc-chelate is taken up by the cells of the renal tubules. Well differentiated renal cell carcinomas, therefore, show up as areas of increased emission.

4. *Thyroid Tumours*: ^{131}I is taken up by active thyroid tissue. Follicular adenomas concentrate the nucleide and show up as an area of increased emission (*hot nodule*). Secretion of thyroxine by the adenoma results in suppression of the rest of the gland which is then unable to concentrate iodine to a detectable degree. The remainder of the gland therefore shows reduced emission. Some

adenomas and most carcinomas have no affinity for ^{131}I (*cold nodules*) at all and appear as zones of reduced emission in an otherwise normal thyroid emission pattern.

5. *Bone Tumours*: ^{99}Tc-labelled phosphorous compounds are *bone-seeking* and accumulate in areas of bone where there is greatest cellular and metabolic activity. Bone tumours, therefore, show up as areas of increased emission and this increased activity is seen in both osteolytic and osteoblastic bone tumours and appears long before any changes are detectable by conventional X-ray techniques. Bone scanning is a preferable technique to radiological skeletal surveys when the extent of metastatic bone carcinoma needs to be assessed.

Ultrasound

Ultrasound probing or *echography* is done by an electronic instrument which detects and records echoes of sound reflected at the interfaces of tissues of different densities.

Ultrasound waves are used because they are more penetrating than audible sound waves. The B-ultrasonogram produces a longitudinal or transverse section of the part examined and records the result on polaroid film. Cystic structures have no boundaries and are devoid of internal echoes whereas solid structures show internal echoes at high gain and can thus be distinguished Cystic lesions are more likely to be benign or non-neoplastic than solid ones and valuable information about a mass can, therefore, be obtained.

Xeroradiography

This technique employs conventional radiography for the production of the radiation image, but instead of radiographic film, a semiconducting plate such as *selenium* is used. The conducting properties of the charged plate are altered to a variable degree by different intensities of X-rays, and if this plate is dusted with fine charged particles after exposure, an image can be produced. The method provides good contrast and good detail and has provided a major advance in soft tissue radiography. Its principle application is in mammography, where the added advantage of increased film latitude and reduced radiation are further commendations.

ENDOSCOPY

In recent years, technical advances in the field of endoscopy have revolutionized the investigation of the gastrointestinal system. With the present flexible fibreoptic instruments, it is possible to view the whole of the oesophagus, stomach, duodenum, colon and terminal ileum and, with help from the radiologist, the pancreatic duct and biliary tract can be cannulated and visualized. The only area of the gastrointestinal tract which cannot be completely examined is the small bowel. Not only can the gastrointestinal tract be viewed directly, but a biopsy or cytological specimen can be obtained from any suspicious area and greatly increase the accuracy with which the diagnosis of cancer can be established or, more importantly, ruled out.

Fibreoptic endoscopy is a valuable adjunct to radiology in diagnosing tumours of the gastrointestinal tract. Where radiology raises a suspicion of a neoplasm, endoscopy can usually confirm or refute that suspicion. On the other hand, where radiology shows no lesion, despite a strong clinical suspicion, then diagnostic evaluation must be regarded as incomplete until endoscopy has been performed.

Endoscopy of the upper gastrointestinal tract

The indications for upper gastrointestinal endoscopy are the clinical signs or symptoms which would prompt a radiological examination. These include dysphagia (for solids in the first instance), epigastric pain, anorexia, nausea and vomiting, weight loss, haematemesis or melaena, iron deficiency anaemia and a palpable epigastric mass. A barium meal examination is customarily performed first, since it is a simpler procedure and may serve to direct the endoscopist to a particular area of the stomach or oesophagus.

The examination is performed on a fasting patient who is sedated, but able to co-operate. Discomfort to the patient is minimal and he generally dozes quietly throughout the investigation. One of a variety of instruments may be used, but the most commonly used is the forward viewing *panendoscope* which allows a complete examination of the oesophagus, stomach and duodenum to be made in 10 to 20 minutes. In most cases, a complete panendoscopy is performed, since it is not uncommon to find more than one lesion.

Carcinoma of the oesophagus

This is usually seen as a constricting lesion which narrows the lumen of the oesophagus and often prevents the endoscope from passing beyond the tumour. Differentiation from a benign oesophageal stricture may be difficult and biopsy may only show inflammatory tissue even though a carcinoma is present. In such a case, brushing the lesion to obtain cells for cytological examination will greatly improve diagnostic accuracy.

Carcinoma of the stomach
Endoscopically, carcinoma of the stomach may present as a polypoid or irregular mass, an ulcer, or as an infiltrating lesion. A localized mass presents no diagnostic difficulty, but benign and malignant ulcers can look the same. A malignant ulcer is suggested by a nodular base, irregular margins and thickening or heaping up of the surrounding mucosa. It is important that all ulcers in the stomach are biopsied from several sites and that brush cytology is taken. An infiltrating carcinoma is the most easily missed, endoscopically, because it masquerades as thickened folds without obvious mucosal abnormality. An infiltrating lesion should always be suspected if the stomach wall seems inflexible, not easily distended and if peristalsis through the area is abnormal.

Other tumours of the stomach and duodenum
1. *Leiomyoma or a leiomyosarcoma* presents a characteristic submucosal, smooth, rounded tumour which bulges into the stomach lumen and which is often surmounted by a small ulcer. Biopsy does not help because the tumour is always covered by normal mucosa.

2. *A fibroma or lipoma* may have appearances similar to those of leiomyomas. It is usually not possible to tell whether the lesion is benign or malignant until the surgical specimen is examined.

3. *Lymphoma of the stomach* has no characteristic endoscopic appearance; the diagnosis is usually not made until the stomach has been removed surgically.

4. *Carcinoma of the ampulla of Vater* is readily seen by the duodenoscope and carcinoma of the head of the pancreas is suggested by an irregular fixed medial wall of the second part of the duodenum.

Colonoscopy
With the present instruments, it is now possible to view the whole colon and terminal ileum. The colon needs to be carefully prepared so that no faecal material is present in the lumen. Colonoscopy is a more prolonged and technically a more difficult procedure than upper gastrointestinal endoscopy, so that it is not generally available and its place as a diagnostic tool is not yet clearly established.

Sigmoidoscopy and barium enema are still the two most important examinations in the diagnosis of carcinoma of the large bowel.

Colonoscopy may contribute to the diagnosis in the following situations: (a) when there is a strong clinical suspicion of a lesion but sigmoidoscopy and barium enema are negative, and (b) when the barium enema shows a suspicious but ill-defined lesion. It is also possible to take a biopsy from the lesion. The colonoscope will occasionally identify a small tumour that has been missed radiologically and, undoubtedly, it increases the evidence with hich a tumour can be ruled out.

CYTOLOGY

Diagnostic or clinical cytology is concerned with the study of individual cells for evidence of a variety of disease processes with particular emphasis on the diagnosis of malignancy. Such a diagnosis is based on the recognition of cells which display certain structural abnormalities that indicate that they have come from a malignant neoplasm. These abnormalities are referred to as the cytological criteria of malignancy. These are:

1. Variations in the chromatin pattern of the nucleus.
2. Irregularities of the nuclear membrane.
3. Enlargement of the nucleus relative to the total cell size, i.e. an increased nuclear/cytoplasmic ratio.

By the use of these criteria it is possible, in most cases, to establish a diagnosis of malignancy and in some cases to indicate the type of carcinoma from which the malignant cells are derived. This may be of considerable importance in localizing the area for further investigation, particularly in a patient in whom the carcinoma is small and not clinically apparent. To determine the type of carcinoma, or its differentiation, the cytoplasm of the malignant cell is examined for evidence of specialized activity. For example: (a) keratinization of the cytoplasm indicates a squamous-cell carcinoma, (b) secretory vacuoles suggest an adenocarcinoma, (c) bile, a hepatoma and (d) melanin pigment, a melanoma. Finally, in the case of cervical cytology at least, if a carcinoma is detected, it may be possible to predict whether or not the lesion is invasive.

In addition to detecting established cancer in asymptomatic patients, cytological examination may reveal lesions that are generally regarded as being *precancerous*. This feature of cytology is the basis of cytological screening programmes aimed at controlling certain forms of cancer. The possibility that some cancers may be controllable is based on the belief that they develop slowly, in stages, and cytological techniques may be used to recognize these stages and to enable appropriate treatment to be instituted. In order to conduct an effective cytological screening programme for a particular type of cancer, certain conditions must be satisfied:

1. It must be possible to define a *high risk* group at which to aim the screening programme.

2. The area under consideration must be accessible to cytological examination.

3. There must be facilities for follow-up procedures so that the presence of a carcinoma or precancerous lesions, detected cytologically, can be histologically confirmed and treated.

Diagnostic cytology is now accepted as a sensitive and extremely accurate technique for the investigation of patients in whom malignancy is suspected on clinical grounds. Although virtually any system of the body is amenable to cytological examination, the method is most useful in the investigation of the female genital tract, respiratory system, oesophagus and stomach, lower urinary tract and the serous cavities of the body. In addition, the fairly recent development of fine-needle aspiration cytology provides a valuable method of non-surgical examination of a variety of body tissues, notably prostate gland, breast, lymph nodes and subcutaneous masses.

The female genital tract

A variety of specimens may be examined, but the most valuable is a direct scrape of the cervix, particularly of the endo-ectocervical junction and adjacent tissues. This may be supplemented by material from the posterior vaginal fornix, from the endocervical canal and, in special circumstances, by washings of the uterine cavity. The presence of cervical cancer can be detected with a high degree of accuracy and it is usually possible to predict whether the carcinoma is still limited to the surface epithelium (*in situ* or pre-invasive carcinoma) or whether it has invaded the underlying tissues. Cells shed from the carcinoma of the endometrium or of the ovary may also be detected in the cervical smear although the technique is much less sensitive for these areas. It is also possible to assess the patient's hormonal status and, in cases where there is evidence of inflammation, to detect a variety of micro-organisms, especially *trichomas vaginalis* and *monilia albicans* (candida).

The respiratory system

The specimens usually submitted for examination are sputum and bronchial washings, the former being preferable. At least three specimens of sputum should be examined before a negative report is issued and it is essential that the material is sputum coughed up from the bronchial tree, not saliva. Various inhalational techniques are available if a patient has difficulty in producing sputum, or a physiotherapist may be of assistance. Provided adequate numbers of good quality specimens are examined, it should be possible to make a diagnosis of primary bronchogenic carcinoma, if present, in approximately 70 per cent of cases. Metastatic carcinoma of the lung is less suitable for cytological diagnosis.

In addition to detecting the presence of a bronchogenic carcinoma, the type of carcinoma present is usually apparent. Thus, squamous-cell carcinoma, adenocarcinoma and undifferentiated carcinoma (both small cell and large cell) each have their characteristic cytological appearances. Cytological typing of bronchogenic carcinoma may be of considerable practical importance since, with the increasing use of cytotoxic drugs for inoperable cancers, the regime of therapy may be determined by the type of carcinoma present.

Oesophagus and stomach

With the recent improvements in endoscopic instruments, it has been possible to wash or brush gastric lesions under direct vision. The specimen thus obtained is then examined cytologically for tumour cells. Whilst these methods have considerable advantages, they should be regarded as complementary to the technique of blind lavage, since the latter technique may result in the detection of unsuspected cancer or confirm the diagnosis of cancer where the lesion is inaccessible to other diagnostic methods. Both oesophagus and stomach may be washed vigorously with a physiological solution, such as saline or Ringer's solution, with or without mucolytic agents. The washings are then retrieved and centrifuged, and the centrifuged deposit is examined for malignant cells. Carcinoma of the stomach is particularly amenable to detection in this way.

Lower urinary tract

Cytological examination of a freshly voided specimen of urine is a sensitive and accurate method for the diagnosis of carcinoma of the renal pelvis, ureter and urinary bladder. However, problems of interpretation may arise in the presence of a urinary tract infection or renal calculi. The fragments of tissue dislodged by instrumentation, such as ureteric catheterization, may also be misleading, hence it is important that information regarding such procedures be made available to the cytopathologist. A cytological problem peculiar to this area is the evaluation of material shed from a very well differentiated papillary transitional cell carcinoma or a papilloma of the bladder. In these cases, the nuclei lack criteria of malignancy, but the lesion may be suspected if epithelial cells with tapering cytoplasmic processes or tails are seen. Occasionally, a renal parenchymal carcinoma may be diagnosed by cytological examination of the urine. However, this type of carcinoma does not invade the pelvi-calyceal system of the kidney until a relatively late stage and the carcinoma cells, if present in the urine, are usually very degenerate and hence difficult to identify.

Serous cavities
The cytological evaluation of pleural and peritoneal effusions is difficult and very prone to diagnostic error. The main reason for this is the reactive changes manifested by mesothelial cells in a variety of non-neoplastic conditions. These may be seen particularly in the pleura overlying an area of infarcted lung or in both pleural and peritoneal surfaces in association with inflammatory conditions. The occurrence of *false positive* diagnoses of malignancy can be minimized if the cytopathologist bases his diagnosis on tissue fragments only and assesses single cells, no matter how abnormal, with extreme caution. It is important that the clinician recognizes the difficulties in the cytology of serous effusions and is prepared to discard the cytological diagnosis if it is not in accord with other clinical laboratory data.

FURTHER READING
The bibliography for Chapters 8 and 9 is incorporated in that of Chapter 10.

10

Principles of treatment

In accord with the general scope of this book, this chapter is not intended to serve as an exhaustive review of cancer therapy. Rather, it is intended to serve as a guide to the principles of treatment based on a knowledge of the biological behaviour of cancer cells and on sound pathological and clinical observation.

The treatment of any disease depends essentially on the methods available and on the goal to be achieved. The methods available include surgery, radiotherapy, chemotherapy, hormone therapy and possibly immunotherapy. Each of these may be used singly or in combination yet, at the present time, there is no completely satisfactory method of treating cancer. Surgery is effective in the treatment of many primary tumours and is still the treatment of choice when the disease is localized, but it is ineffective against disseminated cancer. Radiotherapy can accomplish the same effect in certain radiosensitive tumours and chemotherapy is mainly indicated in the management of widespread malignancies yet both forms of treatment are carcinogenic and toxic to tissues and can cause serious side-effects. Immunotherapy has yet to be shown to be effective in the treatment of cancer. The aim of the treatment varies with each tumour. Ideally, the doctor aims for a cure. If this is not possible, he attempts to procure some regression of the tumour with the object of returning the patient to useful active life, but if the tumour is disseminated and not responsive to treatment, palliative therapy is necessary.

Planning of treatment

As a preliminary to any form of treatment, the following information should be obtained:

1. The histological characteristics of the tumour, as this alone may determine the choice of treatment.
2. The site and extent of the disease process.
3. The general state of health of the patient.

This information is assessed by a team consisting at least, of a pathologist, a surgeon, a radiotherapist and a physician to choose and plan the treatment. The information also provides a baseline for assessing the patient's response to the treatment.

Staging of the tumour

There are basically two stages to malignant disease irrespective of the primary site of the tumour. The disease is *early* if the tumour is localized and potentially curable by local surgery, or *advanced* if it is disseminated and local surgery alone cannot improve the prognosis. An accurate assessment of the extent to which the tumour has advanced is of primary importance in its treatment.

The International Union against Cancer (UICC) has proposed the *TNM* system of notation for staging malignancy, which can be adapted to fit almost any tumour and which is now generally accepted throughout the world. The basis of this system is straightforward: the letters T, N, M, stand for *tumour, lymph nodes* and *metastases*, respectively, and the numerals attached to these letters indicate the extent of spread. This information is obtained from physical, radiological and endoscopic examination and, in deeply situated tumours, from surgical exploration. Applied to the breast:

T1 – Small tumour (less than 2 cm in diameter)
T2 – Large tumour (greater than 2 cm in diameter)
T3 – Fixation to muscles or greater than 5 cm in diameter.
T4 – Fixation to chest wall.
N0 – Axillary nodes not palpable (when accessible).
N1 – Axillary nodes palpable but mobile.
N2 – Axillary nodes palpable and fixed.
N3 – Supraclavicular nodes involved.
M0 – No metastases.
M1 – Metastases have occurred.

In other words, the TNM system provides a form of shorthand notation to describe the important features of the tumour. For example, a carcinoma of the breast designated *T3 N2 M0* indicates that the tumour is more than 5 cm in diameter, it is adherent to the pectoral muscles, the axillary nodes are palpable and fixed but there is no clinical evidence of metastases. The purpose of this system is to categorize all tumours when first seen and to systematically add subsequent information as it becomes available.

The histological type of tumour

The manner in which a specimen is obtained for cytological or histological examination is important:

1. *Needle aspiration* is possible in tumours close to the surface. A needle attached to a syringe is inserted into the mass, the cells and tissue fluid are aspirated and smears are immediately prepared on glass slides.

2. *Needle biopsy* provides a small core of tissue, approximately 2 mm in diameter and 1 cm long, which can be used to prepare paraffin sections.

3. *Wedge biopsy* of the tumour edge provides a larger sample than a needle biopsy which can be used for both frozen and paraffin sections. This is an *incisional biopsy* used when the tumour is too large to remove completely prior to establishing a diagnosis.

4. *Excision biopsy* involves removal of the whole tumour together with a margin of normal tissue. The whole specimen should be sent to the laboratory.

5. *Lymph node biopsy* (p. 172).

Needle aspiration and needle biopsy are simple to perform and there is little danger of haemorrhage. The main disadvantages are poor sampling of the lesion and the risk of spilling tumour cells along the needle tract. In both cases, a positive diagnosis is acceptable, but a negative diagnosis is not and merely implies that the sample is inadequate. A wedge biopsy provides a more representative sample adequate for both paraffin and frozen sections. A frozen section can be prepared quickly and, in many cases, the histological detail is adequate for diagnosis.

SURGICAL TREATMENT

There is rarely a problem with the aim of surgery in the treatment of primary tumours. Its purpose is to remove the tumour with adequate precautions to prevent spread of the disease at the time of operation. Surgery does not attempt to alter the course of the disease process, it simply cuts it out, and the extent of the excision is determined by the histological type and clinical stage of the tumour.

Despite adequate technical precautions during surgical operations, tumour cells somehow manage to escape and can often be demonstrated in the circulation. The presence of tumour cells in the circulation is not of itself important, what is important is the host-tumour relationship. The risk of developing metastases appears to be dependent partly on the degree of differentiation of the tumour cells and partly on the efficiency of the host's defence mechanism. Factors such as stress, adrenocortical depletion, injury to tissues, lipaemia, heparinaemia etc. (p. 22) can modify the host's receptivity and may enable migrating cells to become established. Correction of these factors should be an essential component of the preoperative treatment.

Local resection

The rapid diagnosis of tumours provided by the frozen section technique is extremely valuable in informing the surgeon whether the lesion found at operation is benign or malignant. If the tumour is benign, local excision is adequate, if it is malignant, local excision might still be possible but the line of excision might have to be extended.

The best and perhaps the only opportunity of eradicating a malignant lesion is at the first operation, when the limits of the growth can usually be recognized. At a second operation, the edge of the tumour might be obscured by inflammation and fibrosis. Where possible, therefore, it is preferable to excise the tumour immediately following the biopsy. When the diagnosis is in doubt and the results of the operation likely to be mutilating, it is advisable to temporarily close the wound and postpone the operation until good quality paraffin sections are available when the pathologist can decide whether the tumour is benign or malignant.

In certain superficial lesions such as a malignant melanoma, an *excisional biopsy* is done which serves both as a diagnostic and therapeutic measure. For this to be successful, the lesion should be excised with a wide margin of normal tissue, the wider the margin of tissue between the line of excision and the edge of the tumour the more likely the removal to be complete. The whole surgical specimen is sent to the laboratory and the subsequent biopsy report should clearly indicate the type of tumour and whether or not the line of excision has cleared the lesion both peripherally and on its deep aspects.

Radical resection

The notion that carcinomas spread by permeation through lymphatic channels has led to complicated radical resections with *en bloc* excision of the lymphatics in the hope that surgery might offer improved prognosis in established neoplastic disease. Such resections encompass the lesion, the lymph nodes and the intermediate tissues containing the lymphatics which are in continuity with the primary tumour. Based on this principle, a number of standard operations have been designed. For example:

1. *Myer-Halsted's operation* for breast cancer involves removal of the breast, the pectoral muscles and the axillary lymph nodes.

2. *Wertheim's operation* for cancer of the *cervix uteri* involves removal of the uterus, tubes, ovaries, upper third of the vagina, broad ligaments, parametrium and the external, internal and common iliac and obturator lymph nodes.

3. *Miles' operation* for carcinoma of the rectum involves removal of the rectum and mesorectum together with the lymph nodes as far as the origin of the inferior mesenteric artery.

Management of regional lymph nodes

There is some doubt concerning the treatment of regional lymph nodes either by surgery or radiotherapy. The problem arises because of evidence suggesting that there may be an immunological reaction against the tumour occurring principally in these nodes and this could, theoretically, be of value to the patient. This alleged defensive role of lymph nodes in man has evolved from results obtained by inference from artificial experimental models.

There is no good evidence that surgical removal or irradiation of the regional lymph nodes has any aggravating influence in man; in fact, in certain well-defined situations the opposite is true. For example, with testicular seminomas, if the treatment is resection of the primary tumour only, approximately 40 per cent of the patients would be alive five years after surgery but, if the drainage lymph nodes are also irradiated, the five year survival rate is increased to 95 per cent. However, there is still a controversy concerning the role of lymph nodes in carcinoma of the breast and in malignant melanoma; more information is needed in these cases before any hard and fast rule can be made.

The decision on whether or not to remove regional lymph nodes depends on:

1. *Tumour size*: Tumours greater than 2 cm in diameter carry a higher risk of lymph node spread than small tumours.

2. *Anatomical site of the tumour*: Tumours of the tongue and floor of the mouth carry a 50 per cent risk of lymphatic involvement, whereas the risk for tumours of the lip is less than 10 per cent.

Adjuvants to surgery

Whilst surgery is the most effective form of treatment for malignancy, there appears to be a need for adjuvant chemotherapy or radiotherapy, even for patients with localized disease in whom the primary tumour has been removed. This is an area of tremendous importance because it is now widely accepted that the outcome for early cancer is predetermined by the extent of subclinical distant metastases at the time of presentation.

Unfortunately, the current modes of adjuvant therapy tend to suppress non-specific and specific immunological responses of the host against the tumour. Therefore, efforts have been made to devise treatment regimes that will produce maximal toxicity in tumour cells and a minimal immunosuppressive effect. Results achieved so far in clinical trials using long-term chemotherapy, support the concept that intermittent chemotherapy is preferable to continuous chemotherapy. This preference is based on a better balance between the desired tumour inhibitory effect and the undesirable immunosuppression.

RADIOTHERAPY

Radiotherapy may be defined as the therapeutic use of ionizing radiations. Radiations most commonly used clinically are:

1. *Electromagnetic emissions* (X-rays or γ-rays) generated by X-ray machines or artificial radionucleides.

2. *Charged particles* (π-mesons, electrons, protons and β-particles) derived from naturally occurring radioactive elements such as radium, radon or uranium, or from artificially activated isotopes such as cobalt, caesium, gold, phosphorus and iodine).

3. *Uncharged particles* (neutrons) derived from the interaction of deutrons (^2H) accelerated in a cyclotron with either a berrylium or a tritium target.

Radiations interact with cells causing ionization and production of highly reactive radicles which, in turn, affect essential macromolecules. The effects on cells include suppression of mitosis, giant-cell formation, prolongation of interphase, induction of mutations and chromosomal aberrations (p. 72).

As water is the major constituent of the cell, hydrogen and peroxide are the predominant radicles formed. Their formation is dependent on the supply of free oxygen and, for this reason, the degree of oxygenation of the tissue governs the extent of radiation injury. The biological effects of proton irradiation are less dependent on the presence of oxygen than are X-rays or γ-rays. Maximum ionization occurs just as the radiation is brought to rest at the end of its tract (Fig. 10.1).

Sources of radiation

A tumour may be irradiated either from external or internal sources, the choice of which is determined by a number of factors: availability, the site of the lesion to be irradiated and the need to protect normal tissues.

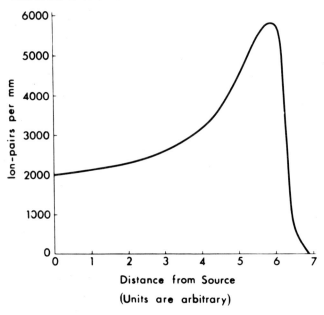

Fig. 10.1   The Bragg peak showing that ionization occurs predominantly just before a charged particle is brought to rest in tissue

External irradiation

A beam of radiation from a suitable generator of X-rays or from a large amount of radioactive material such as cobalt-60 is projected through the patient so as to encompass the tumour and its extensions.

1. *Low energy X-rays* up to 120 000 volts (120 KeV) confine their effects to the skin with little penetration into the deeper layers.

2. With *orthovoltage X-ray machines* (200 to 400 KeV) penetration is much greater, but the ionization is still mainly on the surface and gives rise to skin reactions. The penetrating rays are absorbed by the calcium in bone. While the effects on bone are increased, the organs behind bone are shielded.

3. *Megavoltage machines* generate X-rays with energies greater than 1×10^6 volts (1 MeV). This beam does not cause scatter easily because the secondary electrons that are produced are carried in a forward direction. With megavoltage treatment, there is less absorption in skin and bone and so large doses can be given to deep-seated tumours with less damage to skin and bone. Linear accelerators which work at energies of 4 to 6 MeV, or higher, are now used in some large centres.

4. *Cobalt-60 emission.* A simpler method of obtaining mega-voltage radiation is to utilize the emissions of radioactive cobalt, but this has certain disadvantages. Beam definition is poorer because the source of the radiation is of finite size compared with the point source of an accelerator. The beam energy is also fixed and treatment times must be continually adjusted to allow for the decay in the intensity of the source.

5. Radioactive sources may be brought into close contact with tumours by applying them in the form of *moulds* (usually 5 mm away from the tumour) to accessible surfaces such as the skin, mouth or sinuses.

Internal irradiation

Radioactive elements such as radium, cobalt, caesium, iridium, gold or tantalum, enclosed in protective housings, can be inserted into accessible tumours or into the cervical canal and uterine cavity in the form of needles, wires, tubes or seeds. This form of therapy can be used to boost the local dosage above the maximum permissible dose that can be delivered by an external beam because of the proximity of sensitive structures such as rectum or bladder. The inserts are removed after an interval of three to seven days.

Unsealed radioactive isotopes may be injected into the lymphatics or body cavities such as the pleura or bladder. This is an uncommon method of treatment because the isotopes tend to concentrate unevenly and give rise to *hot* and *cold* spots. Systemic absorption by mouth or intravenous injection is commonly used with isotopes that are preferentially taken up by one type of cell. For example, ^{131}I is taken up by the thyroid gland and used in the treatment of certain types of thyroid cancer and ^{32}P is taken up by the marrow and used in the treatment of leukaemia.

Therapeutic aspects

Radiotherapy, except when used in the form of systemic radio-isotopes, is local in its therapeutic effects. Its primary aim is to destroy sensitive malignant cells and its primary place is in inoperable tumours and in patients who are unsuitable for operation.

As a general principle, the sensitivity of a tissue to radiation goes hand in hand with the rate of cell turnover in that tissue. Sensitivity is also inversely related to the degree of cell differentiation. Thus, rapidly growing poorly differentiated tumours are generally more radiosensitive than slowly growing well differentiated tumours. However, rapidity of growth and lack of differentiation reflect the capacity of the tumour to metastasize so that the most radiosensitive tumours are also those least likely to remain in the field of tolerable field sizes.

Radiation doses are measured in rads (p. 69) and the doses required to destroy tumour cells are usually slightly less than those required to destroy normal cells. The ratio of these two doses is called the *therapeutic ratio*; it is a measure of the degree of radiosensitivity of a tissue and provides the basis for clinical radiotherapy. The therapeutic ratio can be controlled to some extent by increasing the oxygen tension (*hyperbaric oxygen*) and the temperature, and also by the concomitant administration of anti-tumour drugs. In this way, radiation damage can be manipulated so that it is maximal in tumour cells and minimal in normal cells.

In this connection, the effect of radiation in depressing local and general tissue immunities must be borne in mind. On the positive side, some tumours are rendered more susceptible to the host immunological defence system by reducing the bulk of the tumour and hence its ability to soak up antibodies. This leaves more anti-bodies to deal with smaller volumes of neoplastic cells in micro-metastases. On the negative side, high local doses of irradiation may leave the area more susceptible to invasion by radioresistant tumour cells.

Clinical application

Some tumours are highly radiosensitive and may be cured at dose levels easily tolerated by normal tissue. Others, are moderately radiosensitive, but in favourable locations where high tumour doses can be given with relatively little damage to surrounding structures, cures may be obtained. Radioresistant tumours are normally treated by surgery.

Radiosensitive tumours

As a sole curative measure, radiotherapy can be used to sterilize wide fields of involvement or potential involvement in the following malignancies: seminoma of the testis, dysgerminoma of the ovary, medulloblastoma and localized or regional Hodgkin's and non-Hodgkin's lymphoma. All these conditions progress in a reasonably steady and predictable manner, but they are so sensitive to irradiation that low or moderate doses are curative in 80 to 90 per cent of early cases. Even in the later stages of the disease, substantial salvage rates can be achieved by judiciously using external radiotherapy in conjunction with antitumour drugs.

Moderately radiosensitive tumours

This group of tumours requires high doses of radiation confined to a small area. Such treatment can be curative in a high proportion of early cases of basal-cell and squamous-cell carcinomas of the skin, carcinomas of the cervix and body of the uterus, transitional-cell and squamous-cell carcinomas of the urinary bladder, carcinoma of the nasopharynx, adenocarcinoma of the breast, carcinoma of the ovary and some carcinomas of the prostate. For cancer of the larynx, radiation is exceptionally suitable as recurrence is rare in this tumour and the patient's voice is retained.

Radioresistant tumours

Radiotherapy may improve the cure rate of other tumours if used intelligently in conjunction with surgery, cytotoxic therapy, hormones or immunotherapy. These include: Wilm's tumour, locally advanced carcinomas of the breast, bladder, prostate, bowel and thyroid gland, some gynaecological cancers, small cell carcinoma of the lung, acute lymphatic leukaemia and most cases of moderately advanced lymphoma. In this field, the major contributions of radiotherapy are in reducing the local bulk of the disease to make surgical operation easier and other forms of systemic therapy more effective. Postoperatively, it may eradicate residual malignant cells. Radiotherapy works best before surgery, but often renders surgery more difficult or delays wound healing if full dosage is used. A compromise of sandwiching the surgical operation between two half courses of radiation is used in some centres for carcinomas of the bladder, bowel, breast, testis and for gynaecological neoplasms.

Palliative radiotherapy

Radiation can be used as palliative therapy for the relief of both local symptoms and systemic effects with some measure of success and prolongation of useful life. Care must always be taken of course to treat the patient as a whole and not as a collection of symptoms. It could, for example, be a mistake to relieve the obstruction of a patient's ureter surrounded by incurable cancer when systemic spread is already apparent. Such treatment could deprive the patient of a comfortable uraemic death and leave him to die in pain and distress from the rest of his disease.

CHEMOTHERAPY

The more we know about the differences between normal and malignant cells, the easier it will be to find specific chemotherapeutic agents for the treatment of cancer. The ultimate aim is to develop new drugs which are cytotoxic only to malignant cells without damaging normal cells but, apart from the enzyme L-asparaginase (p. 34), this ideal has not yet been achieved. The antitumour drugs currently used are toxic to both neoplastic and normal cells, almost all have carcinogenic activity and most of them are immuno-suppressive. Their clinical use, therefore, is always associated with a considerable degree of toxicity to normal cells and with some risk of developing a second malignancy.

Classification of antitumour drugs

Like normal cells, tumour cells require DNA, RNA and protein for their continued growth. Because of this requirement, various blocking agents are being used for therapy which interfere with essential synthetic processes and metabolic pathways. Antitumour drugs, therefore, can be classified according to the specificity of their action in regard to the cell cycle (Fig. 10.2).

The antimetabolites (S-phase specific)

These drugs belong to various groups. Each one resembles a natural substance with which it competes in the enzymatic process. The more common analogues are:

1. *5-Fluoruracil (5-FU)* is a pyrimidine antagonist which inhibits the enzyme thymidylate synthetase involved in the synthesis of DNA. Since gastrointestinal tumours preferentially take up uracil, 5-FU is the standard drug therapy for adenocarcinoma of the gastrointestinal tract.

2. *6-Mercaptopurine (6-MP)* is a purine antagonist. It has little value in the treatment of solid tumours, but it is used in acute

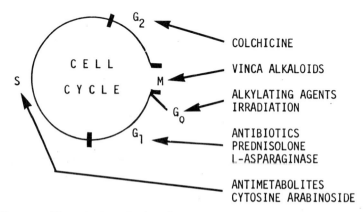

Fig. 10.2   The main sites of action of the antitumour drugs in relation to the cell cycle

leukaemias in children and is often combined with methotrexate and hormones. 6-Thioguanine has a similar effect.

3. *Methotrexate* is a folic acid antagonist. It competes with folic acid for the enzyme folic acid reductase and interferes with DNA synthesis. It is used in acute leukaemia in children and produces spectacular results in choriocarcinoma.

4. *Arabinosyl cytosine* (*ARA-C*) acts solely against cells actively synthesizing DNA.

5. *Procarbazine* probably exerts its effect in disrupting mitosis and depolymerizing DNA and is used in Hodgkin's disease.

Vinca alkaloids (*M-phase specific*)

These alkaloids are extracted from the *Vinca Rosea* plant (periwinkle). Two compounds are used, *vinblastine* and *vincristine*. Like colchicine, they inhibit spindle formation leading to arrest of mitosis in metaphase. They are rapidly cleared from the blood and are excreted almost entirely in the bile. They are useful in the treatment of lymphomas and in acute lymphatic leukaemia. Vincristine is particularly useful in Hodgkin's disease.

Alkylating agents (*non-cell cycle specific*)

The difunctional alkylating agents (p. 43) are highly reactive electrophilic compounds which react with neutrophilic groups in DNA, RNA and protein. They cross-link the strands in the double helix, preventing DNA replication. Alkylating agents kill cells in all phases of the cycle. Examples in current clinical use include:

1. *Nitrogen mustard* used in the treatment of chronic leukaemia and lymphomas.

2. *Cyclophosphamide* is activated by the enzyme phosphaminase. Theoretically, the drug was produced to exploit the high levels of the enzyme in tumour cells, but, in fact, it is predominantly activated in the liver. It is used in Hodgkin's disease, myeloma and carcinomas of the lung, breast and ovary.

3. *Phenylalinine mustard* (melphalan) used in myeloma, lymphomas, seminoma of the testis and Ewing's sarcoma of bone.

4. *Triethylene melamine* (TEM) is of value in the treatment of lymphomas and, in combination with radiotherapy, in retinoblastoma.

5. *Triethylenephosphorimide* (*thio*-TEPA) is more stable and less toxic than TEM. It is used in chronic lymphatic leukaemia and to a lesser extent in carcinoma of the bladder and seminoma of the testis.

Antibiotics (non-cycle specific)
The antibiotic groups of antitumour agents are derived from a species of *Streptomyces* and include *actinomycin-D, rabidomycin, adriamycin* and *bleomycin*. Of these, actinomycin-D is the most active and least toxic.

Actinomycin-D binds to guanine of DNA particularly in a double helix configuration to form a stable complex, and the degree of binding parallels the amount of guanine in the molecule. Single stranded DNA binds much less actinomycin-D. This binding occurs at the site of the DNA template where *RNA polymerase* normally functions and thus selectively inhibits RNA synthesis and hence protein synthesis. Because of its inhibitory effect on RNA synthesis, actinomycin-D exerts an influence in the action of hormones (growth hormone, ACTH, adrenal steriods, oestrogen, testosterone, insulin and thyroxine).

Actinomycin-D is a potent immunosuppressant and commonly used in patients with renal transplants. It is poorly absorbed from the gut and when given intravenously it is cleared from the blood within two minutes, approximately half being excreted in the bile and 10 per cent in the urine.

Therapeutic aspects
Our present concept of the cell cycle and the cell kinetics of tumour growth provides an insight into some of the problems encountered in the chemotherapy of tumours.

Growth fraction (GF)
In the initial stages of growth, all the tumour cells are undergoing division, so that the growth of the tumour is exponential due to successive doubling in cell numbers. As the tumour increases in size, the percentage of actively proliferating cells (GF) decreases, that is, it is high at the periphery of the tumour, but progressively decreases to zero towards the centre of the tumour. This decrease in the GF has been attributed to a corresponding decrease in the blood supply which carries oxygen and other nutrients to the cell. The cell cycle time remains constant throughout the tumour, suggesting that the GF is the major determinant of growth.

Large tumours may be regarded as consisting of three concentric compartments (peripheral, middle and central) each with a different GF and a different significance for chemotherapy (Fig. 10.3).

1. *The peripheral compartment* has a high GF and nearly all the cells are synthesizing DNA. It is in this compartment that therapy

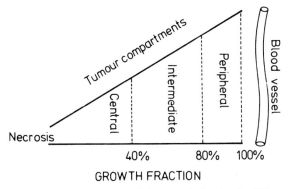

Fig. 10.3 The variation in the size of the growth fraction in different tumour compartments

with currently available drugs, particularly the cycle specific anti-metabolites can be directed most effectively.

2. *The intermediate compartment* has a low GF. Although it contains a large proportion of non-dividing cells (phases G_1 and G_0) the cells retain their capacity to re-enter the cycle. As the tumour increases in size, more cells move into this compartment, a phenomenon which is the major limitation of chemotherapy. Recognition of this compartment has led to the use of combinations of drugs that employ both cycle and non-cell cycle specific agents in an attempt to deal with both the dividing and non-dividing cell fractions.

3. *The central compartment* consists of cells that have lost their capacity to divide but they still occupy volume in the tumour mass. The importance of the concept of the GF in the effectiveness of chemotherapy is clear: antitumour drugs must be used in relation to the cell cycle in order to ensure maximum cytotoxicity and maximum therapeutic response, the actively proliferating cells being the most susceptible.

There are three obstacles in obtaining a complete chemotherapeutic cure. First, a given dose of a drug destroys a constant fraction of cells not a fixed number. This is the *fractional cell-kill hypothesis* which implies that a single treatment will not eliminate all the neoplastic cells in a tumour, it reduces the cell population by a constant percentage. Repeated doses of a drug are therefore necessary to kill all cells. Secondly, stable cells in the intermediate compartment which have retained their capacity to proliferate may start dividing and thus contribute to the growth fraction. For this reason, all regimes of combination chemotherapy incorporate the idea of intermittent courses of therapy. Thirdly, the amount of any antitumour drug that can be given depends on its toxicity. Virtually all chemotherapeutic agents exert some depressing effect on the bone marrow, but the degree of depression varies considerably from drug to drug. In addition, each agent may have its own specific adverse effects which preclude more of the drug being given but do not prevent another being used. For example, the amount of vincristine that can be administered is limited by its neurotoxicity, not by its effect on the marrow. It can, therefore, be used readily with an alkylating agent such as nitrogen mustard, which is not neurotoxic but has more effect on the marrow. In this way, a greater antitumour effect can be obtained without increasing toxicity.

Assessing response to therapy

A major problem in chemotherapy is the difficulty in estimating the *cell-kill fraction* and the remaining surviving cells after each course of treatment. In functioning tumours, the amount of specific product secreted is dependent on the residual mass of tumour cells and serves as an indirect index of the surviving tumour mass. For example:

Index substance	*Tumour*
Chorion gonadotrophin	Choriocarcinoma
Immunoglobulin	Myeloma
Alpha faetoprotein	Hepatoma
Carcinoembryonic antigen	Gastrointestinal carcinoma
Catacholamine	Phaeochromocytoma
Serotonin	Carcinoid

HORMONE THERAPY

Carcinoma of the prostate grows especially well in an environment where antigens predominate over oestrogens and some cases of carcinoma of the breast where oestrogens predominate over androgens. The mechanism of this hormone dependence (p. 31) has not yet been fully elucidated but the phenomenon has been exploited in the palliative treatment of carcinomas of the breast, prostate and uterus, and in the treatment of leukaemia.

Both naturally occurring and synthetic hormones are used.

1. *Corticosteroids* reduce the ability of lymphocytes to undergo mitosis and therefore, are of value in the treatment of leukaemia and the lymphomas. They may be used alone or in combination with other cytotoxic drugs. In children with leukaemia, corti-

costeroids have a direct effect on the malignant cells as well as being advantageous in the anaemia of malignancy by lessening the degree of haemolysis, decreasing the degree of haemorrhage in thrombocytopoenia and possibly in protecting the marrow against the toxic effects of other forms of chemotherapy or radiotherapy.

2. *Androgens* have two uses in the treatment of malignancy: (a) as a palliative agent in female breast cancer and (b) as an anabolic agent in the treatment of cachexia and in stimulating the bone marrow.

3. *Progestins* have recently been used in the treatment of carcinoma of the uterus, ovaries and kidney.

Clinical application

Alterations in the hormonal environment may be produced in two ways:

1. *Additive treatment*, by giving massive doses of hormones.

2. *Ablative or suppressive treatment*, by removing the physiological sources of hormone production, either surgically or by irradiation.

Carcinoma of the breast

Surgery and irradiation remain the best methods of treatment when the disease is localized. In advanced, inoperable carcinoma of the breast, whilst no cure can be claimed, hormone therapy offers considerable extension of useful life, alleviation of pain, especially in bone metastases, and improvement in the general condition of the patient through the anabolic effects of androgen.

For the purposes of hormone therapy, carcinoma of the breast may be subdivided into three groups:

1. *Oestrogen dependent* cancers occur mostly in the younger age group (premenopausal, up to five years post menopausal). Oophorectomy is the preferred treatment in this group. It indicates if the tumour is oestrogen dependent and, at the same time, removes the main source of oestrogen production. Approximately 50 per cent of selected patients respond to oophorectomy. When the condition relapses androgen therapy is commenced.

2. *Hypophyseal dependent and non-oestrogen dependent.* This group occurs in the older age group of patients (sixty years and over). Treatment is aimed at inhibiting anterior pituitary production of trophic hormones (medical hypophysectomy) with oestrogens.

3. *Hormone independent group.*

Carcinoma of the prostate
Surgical excision is possible only in approximately five per cent of patients. Oestrogen therapy is effective in over 90 per cent of cases. The oestrogen of choice is stilboestrol given orally, but it has a number of adverse effects such as gynaecomastia, atrophy of the testis, gastrointestinal disturbance and a risk of inducing carcinoma of the male breast. Cessation of androgen secretion can also be achieved by orchidectomy.

IMMUNOTHERAPY

Immunotherapy is the intentional manipulation of the host's immune response to enhance its effect in the prevention and treatment of cancer. The concept is not new, its history dates back to the beginning of the century. Cases of tumour regression associated with bacterial infection have been reported, and vaccines and bacterial products have been administered to patients with cancer to inhibit the growth of the tumour. In addition, the lymphocytic infiltrations in and around some primary tumours and sinus histiocytosis in regional lymph nodes also provide indirect evidence of a possible immunological host reaction.

Therapeutic aspects
Cancer immunity is a mixed response to the presence on the surface of tumour cells of *tumour transplantation antigens* (TSTA) which are foreign to the host (p. 58). Tumours induced by nonviral carcinogens contain individually different TSTAs, whereas all tumours induced by a given virus share the same TSTAs. The immune response to TSTAs is weak. Two types of response are recognized:

1. *Antibodies* (immunoglobulins) in the serum, which bind to TSTA on the cell surface.

2. *Small lymphocytes*, which react specifically with TSTAs and activate the complement system. In this type of cell-mediated immunity, the lymphocytes release a migration inhibiting factor which prevents migration of macrophages and enables them to accumulate at the site where lymphocytes have reacted.

Clinical application
Before immunotherapy can become a standard form of treatment for cancer it will be necessary to find ways and means of increasing the patient's immune response. This can be achieved, to a limited

extent, by specific and nonspecific approaches.

In the specific approach, patients with cancer are treated either by active or passive immunization, or by both methods.

1. *Active immunization* consists of stimulating the patient's immune system against the tumour by injecting (a) whole tumour cells inactivated by heat, chemicals or irradiation, or (b) subcellular fractions, especially tumour cell membranes.

2. *Passive immunization* consists of administering sensitized lymphocytes or antibodies obtained from an appropriately immunized donor to the patient with the tumour.

In the nonspecific approach, agents that cause a general increase in immunity are used. Such agents may be injected either directly into the tumour or at sites remote from the tumour. The commonly used nonspecific immunotherapeutic agents for the treatment of cancer are:

1. *BCG* (Bacillus Calmette-Guérin) for melanoma and acute leukaemia.

2. *DNCB* (dinetrochlorobenzene) for squamous-cell carcinoma of the skin.

3. *Levamisole* for most tumours.

There is evidence that BCG vaccination may produce remissions in patients with acute leukaemia and that intratumour injection in cutaneous metastases of malignant melanoma may cause regression in small tumours (less than 100 mg).

In acute leukaemia, once remission has been achieved by combination chemotherapy, it is possible to maintain the remission with immunotherapy, using nonspecific stimulation with BCG together with a specific stimulus such as irradiated leukaemic cells.

The value of immunotherapy has yet to be proven. There is no doubt that in experimental animals, immunological procedures can both prevent the induction of malignant disease and cause regression of small tumours. Animal experiments and results from patients with leukaemia indicate that the immune mechanism can only destroy small numbers (less than 10^5) of malignant cells. Thus, for immunotherapy to be successful, the main requirements are: (a) that the tumour is small and (b) that the host must be capable of mounting an immune response.

t present, immunotherapy holds promise for eliminating micrometastases in patients with an intact immune system. Its major value is to mop up and destroy residual cells after the main tumour has been removed by surgery or radiotherapy.

CONCLUSIONS

In the simplest terms, therefore, the strategy of treatment in malignant disease may be summarized as follows:

1. To reduce the population of malignant cells to the lowest possible number by surgery, radiotherapy or chemotherapy.

2. To give additional treatment to kill residual cells which may remain locally, in regional lymph nodes or at distant anatomical sites by radiotherapy, chemotherapy or immunotherapy.

3. To use techniques such as the secretion of hormones and other products to detect early relapse.

4. To maintain patients free from disease by further chemotherapy or immunotherapy, where this form of treatment has been shown to be effective.

FURTHER READING

Cline, M. J. & Haskell, C. M. (1975) *Cancer Chemotherapy.* Philadelphia: W. B. Saunders Co.

Humphrey, L. J., Jewell, W. R. & Murray, D. R. (1971) Immunotherapy for the patient with cancer. *Ann. Surg.,* **173**, 47.

Lawrence, W. & Terz, J. J. (1977) *Cancer Management.* New York: Grune & Stratton.

Murphy, W. T. (1967) *Radiation Therapy,* 2nd edn. Philadephia: W. B. Saunders Co.

Naib, Z. M. (1976) *Exfoliative Cytology,* 2nd edn. Boston: Little, Brown and Co.

Nealon, T. F. (1965) *Management of the Patient with Cancer.* Philadelphia: W. B. Saunders Co.

Sutton, D. (1975) *A Textbook of Radiology,* 2nd edn. Edinburgh: Churchill Livingstone.

II

Tumours of the skin

Skin tumours are situated in a particularly favourable position from the point of view of early diagnosis and treatment. As with tumours of other tissues, there are two main biological types of skin tumours – benign and malignant, of which the vast majority are primary. In addition, there is a group of premalignant lesions which occur in the skin, mucous membranes and mucocutaneous junctions and which probably represent a stage between normal cellular growth and overt malignant growth. It is not yet possible to detect these premalignant stages with any degree of certainty, but some skin lesions are known, from experience, to have a tendency to develop into cancer.

Primary tumours of the skin are divided broadly into those derived from the epidermis, those from melanocytes and those from skin appendages.

EPIDERMAL TUMOURS

Malignant
Squamous-cell carcinoma
Basal-cell carcinoma
Premalignant Lesions
Leukoplakia   Solar keratosis
Radiation dermatitis   Bowen's disease
Xeroderma pigmentosum
Tumour-like Lesions
Pseudo-epitheliomatous hyperplasia
Keratoacanthoma   Keratotic papilloma
Virus warts   Cysts

Squamous-cell carcinoma

Squamous-cell carcinoma usually occurs on exposed skin surfaces, mucous membranes and muco-cutaneous junctions. It tends to occur in people whose occupation entails prolonged exposure to sun (farmers, sailors and fishermen) or prolonged contact with tars, dyes, arsenic or other carcinogens. Skin cancer occurs more commonly in fair-skinned than in dark-skinned people. Coloured people are virtually immune because the melanin pigment in the skin acts as a protective barrier against the ultraviolet rays of the sun. Men are affected much more commonly than women and most patients are middle-aged or elderly, but the disease may appear in early adult life. In mucous membranes and muco-cutaneous junctions, *leukoplakia* may be a premalignant condition and in the skin solar keratosis, radiation dermatitis, Bowen's disease and xeroderma pigmentosum.

Macroscopic features

Squamous-cell carcinoma occurs mainly on the cheek, ear, tip of nose, forehead and dorsum of hands. It may present either as a small, hard, scaly nodule in the skin or as an ulcer. A typical ulcer is irregular in outline and its edges are often raised and everted. The base of the ulcer is indurated and may become attached to deeper structures. Regional nodes may be involved. A biopsy is always necessary for diagnosis.

Microscopic features

The tumour tissue is composed of irregular masses of squamous cells which show varying degrees of differentiation. In the well-differentiated tumours (Fig. 11.1a), the cells are large, pink-staining and polygonal in shape with well defined prickles and, in the centre of such masses of cells, whorls of flattened keratinized cells may occur (*keratin pearls*). Prolongations of tumour cells may extend into the dermis branching in all directions like the roots of a tree. In any section therefore, such roots appear as groups and strands of isolated cells, in which mitoses are frequent and irregular. The connective tissue stroma between the masses of tumour cells is often oedematous and infiltrated by a moderate number of lymphocytes and plasma cells.

Two uncommon variants of squamous-cell carcinoma are recognized:

1. The *adenomatoid (acantholytic) squamous-cell carcinoma*, which shows a glandular pattern and contains squamous cells.

2. The *spindle-cell type of squamous-cell carcinoma*, in which the cells resemble fibroblasts.

Course and prognosis

In general, all squamous-cell carcinomas progress. Some progress very slowly and years may pass before metastases occur, others spread rapidly. The outlook is good if the lesion is localized and operable, but poor if the lesions are multiple, as in xeroderma pigmentosum, or if metastases have developed. Prognosis, therefore, depends on the duration, extent and location of the growth.

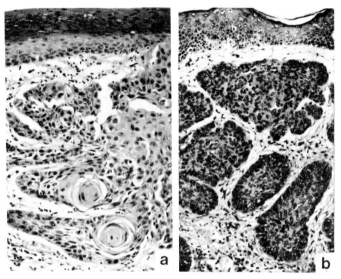

Fig. 11.1 Well differentiated squamous-cell carcinoma of the skin: (a) showing groups of large squamous cells with keratinization in the centre to form the *pearls* that are characteristic of this tumour; (b) basal-cell carcinoma composed of groups of small, dark-staining cells similar to the basal cells of the skin. The cells at the periphery of each group show palisading of the nuclei (× 200)

Basal-cell carcinoma (Rodent ulcer)

Basal-cell carcinoma occurs on hair-bearing skin and arises from basal cells of the epidermis. As in squamous-cell carcinoma, the main aetiological agents are sunlight, X-rays, arsenic and tar. It rarely occurs before middle-age and is commoner in males than in females. Approximately 60 per cent of malignant tumours of the skin are basal-cell carcinomas.

Macroscopic features

Over ninety per cent of basal-cell carcinomas occur on the face, especially in the region of the inner canthus of the eye. Initially, the growth appears as a pearly nodule with blood vessels on the surface. Eventually the overlying skin becomes eroded and an ulcer forms. The tumour is locally destructive and, as the ulcer extends, it destroys the surrounding skin and erodes through deeper tissues such as muscle, cartilage and even bone.

Microscopic features

The essential differences between squamous-cell carcinoma and basal-cell carcinoma are the characters of the cells. In basal-cell carcinoma, the tumour tissue is composed of irregular masses and strands of cells surrounded by a connective tissue stroma (Fig. 11.1b). The tumour cells are small, oval or round, tightly packed and have a round, dark-staining nucleus. The cells at the periphery of the masses of cells resemble those of the basal layer of the epidermis being arranged in a definite layer which frequently shows palisading of the nuclei. In haematoxylin and eosin stained sections, the deep blue masses of cells of basal-cell carcinoma are in contrast to the pink masses of cells of squamous-cell carcinoma. The tumour cells tend to spread in a lateral direction rather than downwards.

A variety of histological patterns occur in basal-cell carcinoma – solid, cystic or adenoid types and, in some, melanin pigment may be present.

Course and prognosis

The great majority of basal-cell carcinomas grow slowly, but even when the tumour grows rapidly, the prognosis is good. Basal-cell carcinomas rarely, if ever, metastasize.

Leukoplakia

The term leukoplakia is used to designate the presence of white plaques on the mucous membranes of the mouth, tongue, oesophagus and vulva. Two types are recognized which cannot be distinguished on clinical grounds:

1. *Simple hyperkeratotic leukoplakia*, in which the plaque is due to hyperkeratosis and parakeratosis resulting from chronic irritation. This type is not premalignant and disappears when the irritation is removed.

2. *Premalignant leukoplakia*, which, in addition to hyperkeratosis and parakeratosis, show acanthosis, cellular disarray and atypicality, and a lymphocytic infiltrate in the subjacent connective tissue. This type of leukoplakia is usually irreversible and may progress to invasive squamous-cell carcinoma.

Solar (senile) keratosis

Solar keratosis occurs principally on the face and backs of hands of fair-skinned, middle-aged or elderly people exposed to the sun for long periods of time. The senile skin undergoes degenerative changes characterized, either by areas of atrophy which are usually erythematous and covered by scales, or by raised hyperkeratotic areas which may be pigmented and form cutaneous horns. The lesions are usually multiple and a considerable proportion of patients (up to 20 per cent) may develop squamous-cell carcinoma in one or more areas.

Microscopically, three types of histological change may be seen: areas of epidermal hypertrophy, areas of epidermal atrophy and areas resembling Bowen's disease.

1. *The hypertrophic type* consists of alternating columns of para-keratosis and hyperkeratosis. The cells of the rete pegs show irregular, downward proliferation, hyperchromatic and pleo-morphic nuclei and many mitotic figures. The basal cells may show budding and whorl formation.

2. In *the atrophic type*, the epidermis is thin and devitalized, but there is basal cell atypia, the nuclei are hyperchromatic, pleo-morphic and, in places, crowded together.

3. *Bowen's disease* is characterized by the presence of scaly plaques in the skin and sometimes in the mucosa of the vulva. The plaques appear as reddish, crusted papules which may resemble psoriasis or eczema.

Histologically, the papules show thickening of the epidermis with crust formation, hyperkeratosis, acanthosis, elongation and broadening of the rete pegs and narrowing of the dermal papillae. There is disarray of the epidermal cells which vary in size and shape. The nuclei also vary in shape, they may be multiple or crowded together and mitotic figures may be present at all levels. Keratin pearls may be present in the acanthotic layer and, occasionally, individual cells may contain keratin inclusions.

Radiation dermatitis

Following repeated small doses of radiation, the skin may show areas of hyperkeratosis, hyperpigmentation and sometimes ulceration. Histologically, the epidermis is thin with loss of rete pegs and there is absence of hair follicles, sweat glands and sebaceous glands. The epidermal cells show degenerative changes and pyknosis of the nuclei. In the dermis, collagen bundles appear swollen and hyalinized, and an inflammatory infiltrate is present. The blood vessels are dilated in the superficial dermis, but in the deep dermis, the vessel walls are thickened with narrowing or occlusion of the lumen.

In long-standing cases, signs of cell proliferation appear with downgrowths of epidermal cells extending into the dermis. In these cases, squamous-cell or basal-cell carcinoma may develop.

Xeroderma pigmentosum

Xeroderma pigmentosum is a rare but strongly precancerous condition inherited via an autosomal recessive gene. It usually develops in childhood, sometimes in the first year of life, and is characterized by a hypersensitivity to sunlight (p. 75). The lesions may develop into basal-cell carcinoma, squamous-cell carcinoma or malignant melanoma.

Histologically, the patches show hyperkeratosis with atrophy of the rete pegs. There is increased melanin in the basal layer of the skin and many melanophores are present in the superficial dermis. Collagen destruction is a constant feature in the dermis.

Basal-cell papilloma (seborrhoeic keratosis)

This is a common lesion which occurs as a slightly raised, yellow to red nodule on the trunk and extremities of people with seborrhoea. The nodules are often covered with a greasy crust which can be scraped off.

Histologically, the nodule is composed of proliferating epidermal cells which form a thick network. The cells resemble basal cells and occasionally contain melanin pigment. Keratin cysts are a feature and represent horny invaginations.

Keratoacanthoma (molluscum pseudocarcinomatosum)

Keratoacanthoma is a relatively common, shell-like tumour which occurs on exposed skin surfaces, particularly the face and backs of hands. It usually starts off as a red pimple which grows to a diameter of 1 to 2 cm in a period of four to six weeks. During the next four weeks, it remains the same size, but the central part undergoes keratinization and may become umbilicated. The base is not fixed to underlying structures and moves freely with the epidermis. If untreated, the nodule shells out during the next three to six months.

Three histological features are characteristic of keratoacanthoma:

1. The nodule is elevated above the adjacent skin surface and is composed of a shell of squamous epithelium with keratin filling the crater.

2. Peripherally it is clearly demarcated from the adjacent epidermis.

3. On its deep aspect, the nodule has a broad base line by a

regular, intact layer of basal cells. Sweat glands are always present deep to the base.

These features indicate that keratoacanthoma grows by expansion, not by invasion.

Squamous (keratotic) papilloma

Although squamous papilloma is the most frequent and familiar tumour in animals, it is relatively uncommon in man. Cutaneous tags that commonly occur in the neck and other parts of the skin are a variant of squamous papilloma. The tumour is composed of a layer of hyperkeratosis overlying the hyperplastic prickle-cell layer (acanthosis). An inflammatory reaction is usually present in the underlying dermis.

Pseudocarcinomatous hyperplasia

Epidermal hyperplasia of the *irritated epithelium* type which is often seen at the edges of chronic varicose ulcers, burns, bromoderma and other chronic proliferative inflammations, may mimic or may even develop into squamous-cell carcinoma. Histologically, it shows downward proliferation of epidermal cells which is sometimes difficult to differentiate from carcinoma. However, the cells are usually regular in form, mitoses are not present in increased numbers, there is no intracellular keratinization and a leukocytic infiltrate may be present in the surrounding connective tissue stroma.

Virus warts

Warts are sessile or pedunculated horny growths of the epidermis caused by virus infections. Infection is usually by direct contact and the incubation period varies from one to nine months. The majority of virus warts are seen in young patients of both sexes.

Histologically, they show hyperkeratosis, an unusual form of parakeratosis in which the nuclei over the dermal papillae are retained, acanthosis and elongation of the rete pegs. Many of the cells are vacuolated. A number of distinct clinical varieties of virus warts occur.

1. *Verruca vulgaris* is the commonest type and is seen mostly in children, where they usually occur on the hands and fingers. They vary in size from 1 to 5 mm.

2. *Verruca plana* are also seen in young people, but they occur mainly on the face, neck and backs of hands.

3. *Verruca plantaris* occur on the soles of the feet and toes and they cause pain on walking.

4. *Verruca acuminata* occur in the genital regions, in moist areas.

5. *Molluscum contagiosum* is a contagious virus infection characterized by a small, pearly white nodule with a central punctum.
They occur mainly on the face, neck and genital region. The
prickly cells contain eosinophilic intracytoplasmic inclusion bodies,
but the cells of the basal layer are free of inclusions.

Cysts
The cystic lesions likely to be confused with tumours include:

1. *Dermoid cysts* which occur in the region of the facial clefts
are lined by well developed epidermis containing hair follicles and
sebaceous glands.

2. *Epidermal cysts* are lined by stratified squamous epithelium
and filled with keratin.

PIGMENTED SKIN TUMOURS

This group of tumours is derived from melanocytes which occur
in the basal layer of the epidermis, hair sheaths, sebaceous glands
and possibly sweat glands. The origin of melanocytes has not yet
been settled, but according to one theory, they migrate to the
epidermis from the neural crest of the embryo and are considered
neuroectodermal. Primary pigmented skin tumours may be benign
or malignant, the former are often called *naevi or moles* and the
latter *malignant melanomas.*

> *Benign lesions (naevi or moles)*
> Junctional naevus
> Compound naevus
> Intradermal naevus
> Blue naevus
> Juvenile melanoma
> Hutchinson's melanotic freckle
> *Malignant lesions*
> Malignant melanoma

Generally, the word naevus means a birthmark or blemish and
is basically a hamartoma. In oncology, the term is used to denote
a benign lesion derived from pigmented or dopa-positive cells.
Naevi should be distinguished from tumours containing non-
melanin pigment, particularly haemosiderin, which takes up iron
stains. They are extremely common lesions usually found on the
face, neck or mucous membranes. The vast majority are congenital,
being present at or appearing soon after birth, and exhibit a typical

clinical course which consists of a pre-pubertal phase of active growth, a quiescent post-pubertal phase and, later, a phase of atrophy. Often growth is reactivated during pregnancy but it subsides again postpartum.

Rarely, a malignant change may occur in a pre-existing naevus. Such a change cannot be diagnosed with certainty clinically, but the development of any of the following signs should be regarded with suspicion:

1. A recent increase in size.

2. A flat lesion which becomes raised and palpable.

3. Colour changes such as increase in pigmentation or the appearance of pale and non-pigmented areas.

4. Itching, weeping, bleeding, scaling or ulceration.

As the ultimate diagnosis rests on histological structure, suspicious nodules should be excised with a wide margin of normal tissue and the whole specimen sent to the laboratory for histological examination in order to make a diagnosis and to estimate the extent of invasion. When a histological structure indicates a malignant lesion, the full title *malignant melanoma* should be used to avoid confusion with benign naevi which are sometimes erroneously called melanomas.

Junctional naevus

Junctional naevi usually appear during the first few years of life, but they may occur at any age. Macroscopically, they vary in size from a few millimetres to several centimetres. They may be dark or light brown in colour and their surface is usually flat, smooth and hairless.

Microscopically, junctional naevi are composed of small clusters of proliferating naevus cells at the dermo-epidermal junction, hence the name (Fig. 11.2a). They may develop into compound or intradermal naevi, or they may remain inactive and even regress. Their most significant feature is that they may occasionally develop into a malignant melanoma.

Compound naevus

The great majority of naevi in children are compounded naevi, but they may occur at any age. Clinically, compound naevi are indistinguishable from intradermal naevi and may bear a superficial resemblance to malignant melanoma by virtue of their raised centre. Macroscopically, they present as brown to black elevated nodules of approximately 1 cm in diameter, but they may be larger. The

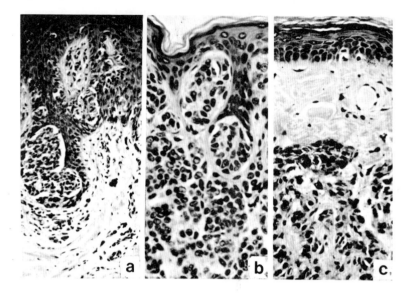

Fig. 11.2   The three main types of pigmented naevi shown together for comparison: (a) Junctional naevus composed of clusters of naevus cells confined to the dermo-epidermal junction; (c) Intradermal naevus in which there is no connection between the naevus cells and the overlying skin; (b) Compound naevus showing both junctional and intradermal patterns (× 160)

edge may be surrounded by a halo and hairs may be present on the surface.

Microscopically, a compound naevus possesses features of both a junctional and an intradermal naevus (Fig. 11.2b). Clusters of naevus cells similar to those described under junctional naevus are present in the junctional zone and in the dermis.

Intradermal naevus

This naevus is the common form in adults and usually occurs on the face and scalp. It develops from the compound naevus and represents the fully developed stage. The intradermal naevus is usually less than 1 cm in diameter, but occasionally, it may be huge, as, for example, the *bathing trunk naevus*. The surface is raised and may be flat and smooth, sessile or pedunculated. The edge is regular and coarse hairs are often present.

Microscopically, the naevus cells are confined entirely within the dermis (Fig. 11.2c). Giant multinucleated naevus cells are common, which are regarded as evidence of maturity and of the benign nature of the lesion.

Blue naevus

Blue naevi develop in the dermis from melanocytes which are believed to have failed to complete their migration from the neural crest to the epidermis. Their most distinguishing feature is the blue to blue-black colour. Blue naevi are usually less than 1 cm in diameter, they have a smooth hairless surface with a well defined regular edge. They are almost always benign.

Microscopically, they are composed of irregular collections of elongated melanocytes situated in the dermis and contain heavy accumulations of pigment. The pigment is melanin. The cells are often spindle-shaped and grouped in irregular bundles, sometimes they tend to form whorls and may extend into the subcutaneous fat. Blue naevi occur especially on the face, dorsum of hands and on the buttocks. Their blue colour is due to the refraction of light by the collagen layer superficial to the pigment cells.

Juvenile melanoma

This usually occurs as a solitary benign naevus on the face and limbs of young children. It is a reddish-brown, dome-shaped, small nodule less than 1 cm in diameter.

Microscopically, it is a variant of the compound naevus composed of nests of either spindle-shaped or epithelioid cells which may or may not contain melanin. The cells are irregular in form, the nuclei are hyperchromatic and there are usually many mitotic figures present. Because of these features, these naevi were once regarded as malignant melanomas.

Hutchinson's melanotic freckle (lentigo maligna)

Hutchinson's melanotic freckle usually starts as a brown macule on the face in middle-aged adults. Its rate of growth is unpredictable, but is usually very slow. The lesion varies in size, usually less than 1 cm in diameter, but occasionally it may cover almost the whole side of the face. The colour is typically uneven, brown with pale or black areas and the surface is flat and hairless. Development of papules, plaques or nodules suggest a malignant change.

Microscopically, there is linear proliferation of atypical melanocytes in the basal layer of the epidermis and sheaths of hair follicles. The cells are haphazardly arranged, but they tend to remain single without cluster formation. Many cells are elongated or spindle-shaped and may contain considerable amounts of pigment. The nuclei are pleomorphic. Severe solar degeneration is present in the dermis.

The lesions develop from melanocytes in the junctional zone and a significant proportion develop into frank malignant melanoma. Malignant melanomas developing from these lesions are said to have a better prognosis than those arising *de novo*.

Malignant melanoma

Malignant melanoma is the most malignant skin tumour and ranks among the most malignant of all tumours. Compared with the ubiquitous benign naevus, it is a rare condition accounting for approximately 1 in 1250 deaths and 1 in 250 tumours. Malignant melanoma is particularly rare before puberty, those cases in children diagnosed as juvenile melanomas are, in fact, variants of the compound naevus. Although most malignant melanomas arise *de novo*, a small but significant proportion (approximately 10 per cent) develop in a pre-existing naevus. They usually occur as solitary nodules, occasionally they may be multiple and, rarely, metastases may occur in the absence of a detectable primary tumour.

Macroscopic features
Malignant melanoma is a disease of exposed surfaces of the body and its highest incidence is in the head and neck. In females, the lower leg is a common site and, in males, the back of the trunk, but it can occur in any part of the skin, including the nailbeds where a subungual tumour may be mistaken for paronychia. The tumour varies in size from a few millimetres to several centimetres. It is usually black in colour but it may be tan, dark brown, grey, pink or show uneven speckling. In most cases the surface is hairless, raised and readily palpable and, in addition, it may be roughened, scaly, polypoidal or ulcerated. The edge of the tumour is often irregular with scalloped margins and may be surrounded by a zone of inflammation.

Histological features
Malignant melanoma arises at the dermo-epidermal junction and its development is determined by the presence of atypical melano-cytes invading the dermis. The tumour cells may be arranged in compact masses, cords, strands or single cells which may be polygonal, cuboidal or spindle-shaped with large, round nuclei containing nucleoli. The number of mitotic figures varies consider-ably from tumour to tumour and bears some relationship to the

degree of malignancy. Multinucleated giant cells may also occur. Melanin pigment may be present or absent, but has no prognostic significance (Fig. 11.3).

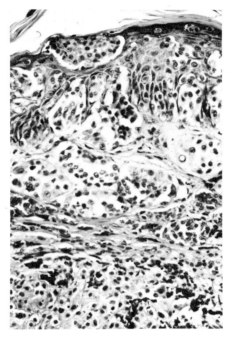

Fig. 11.3 Malignant melanoma showing extensive proliferation of melanocytes with deep and superficial invasion. The tumour cells are irregular in form, possess atypical nuclei and some contain melanin pigment (× 200)

According to McGovern, there are three major types of malignant melanoma. These differ in their mode of origin and prognosis and they can be distinguished histologically by the presence or absence of tumour cells within the epidermis.

1. *Malignant melanoma, invasive, with adjacent intra-epidermal component of Hutchinson's melanotic freckle type.* This type has the best prognosis, the five-year survival rate being approximately 90 per cent.

2. *Malignant melanoma, invasive, with adjacent intra-epidermal component of the Pagetoid type.* This type is characterized histologically by collections of cells resembling Paget's cells, which spread laterally along the dermo-epidermal junction. The tumour cells invade the dermal papillae in the superficial dermis or may

extend into the epidermis, hence the designation *superficial spreading malignant melanoma*. The five-year survival rate of this type is approximately 70 per cent.

_3. *Malignant melanoma, invasive, without adjacent intra-epidermal component*. This type has the least favourable prognosis, the five-year survival rate being approximately 50 per cent.

Course and prognosis
The behaviour of malignant melanomas is unpredictable. Some examples are highly malignant and have a very poor prognosis while others, with apparently similar histology, may behave in a relatively benign fashion. Lymphatic spread is indicated by the appearance of satellite nodules around the main tumour and by invasion of the regional lymph nodes. The lung is the most frequent site of blood spread although metastases may occur in other organs, brain, liver, heart, etc.

In addition to the histological types described above, the prognosis of malignant melanoma appears to be directly related to the depth of invasion, and the level of invasion of the tumour cell infiltrate is an important parameter in assessing the prognosis. Five levels have been described:

I.   Tumour cells are confined to the epidermis. There is no invasion of the dermis (malignant melanoma *in situ*).
II. Tumour cells invade the superficial or papillary layer of the dermis (superficial spreading malignant melanoma).
III. Tumour cells extend to, but do not invade the reticular dermis.
IV. Tumour cells invade the reticular layer of the dermis.
V.   Tumour cells invade through the dermis into the subcutaneous fat.

ADNEXAL TUMOURS OF THE SKIN

The adnexal tumours of the skin are an uncommon group of growths, in which the interrelationship between the epithelial components of the skin appendages and the subserving stroma are largely preserved. It is not known if all are true tumours, some are likely to be hamartomas in nature. Innumerable names have been given which merely describe the various histological patterns of these tumours. The prefix *tricho-* (trichos = hair) is used to denote a relationship to hair, *hidro-* to sweat glands, *spira-* to a coil-shaped pattern, *acro-* to extremities and *syringo-* to ductal origin. The following classification is based on the structural resemblance to hair follicles, sebaceous, apocrine and eccrine glands:

> *Hair follicles*
>> Trichoepithelioma
>> Calcifying epithelioma of Malherbe
>
> *Ductal tumours*
>> Syringoma
>> Syringocystadenoma
>
> *Glandular tumours*
>> Eccrine cystadenoma (trichadenoma)
>> Apocrine cystadenoma (trichadenoma)
>> Sebaceous adenoma

FURTHER READING

Clark, W. H. *et al.* (1969) The histogenesis and biologic behaviour of primary human malignant melanomas of the skin. *Cancer Res.*, **29**, 705.

Lever, W. F. (1975) *Histopathology of the Skin*, 5th edn. Philadelphia, Toronto: J. B. Lippincott Co.

Louis, C. J. (1958) Investigation of Tumours of the Skin (Epidermis) using a Histochemical Technique. *Surg. Gynec. Obstet.*, **107**, 317.

McGovern, V. J. *et al.* (1973) The classification of malignant melanoma and its histologic reporting. *Cancer*, **32**, 1446.

Ten Seldam, L. E. J. *et al.* (1974) *International Histological Classification of Tumours No. 12: Histological Typing of Skin Tumours.* Geneva: World Health Organization.

12

Tumours of the breast

Disorders of the breast are predominantly confined to females, and almost all present as localized swellings or lumps. The range of disorders that need be considered include:

> *Carcinoma of the breast*
>   (a) Noninfiltrating
>   (b) Infiltrating
> *Benign tumours*
>   (a) Fibroadenoma
>   (b) Duct papilloma
> *Non-neoplastic (tumour-like) lesions*
>   (a) Mammary dysplasia
>   (b) Duct ectasia
>   (c) Fat necrosis

It is not always possible to distinguish a cancerous growth from other benign tumours or non-neoplastic lesions. The age of the patient, the presence or absence of pain, the presence of a discharge from the nipple and a history of trauma to the breast may suggest certain conditions, but these symptoms do not provide the final answer. Even the clinical features of the mass itself, especially in the early stages of the disease, may not be sufficiently characteristic to enable a diagnosis to be made. The nature of the condition can only be evaluated by histological examination after excision of the mass. By use of the frozen section technique, an answer can usually be given in five to 10 minutes, while the patient is maintained under general anaesthesia. When there is a doubt about the diagnosis, it is in the patient's interest to limit surgery to local excision in the first instance and postpone any radical procedures for one to two days until a definite answer is available from paraffin section.

CARCINOMA OF THE BREAST

Aetiology

Carcinoma of the breast has now become the commonest form of cancer in women, accounting for approximately five per cent of all cancer deaths. Its cause is not known, but recent studies comparing patients with breast cancer with normal controls have revealed a number of factors which appear to influence the incidence of the disease.

Age

The incidence of breast cancer increases with age reaching a peak between 45 and 75 years. Although no age is exempt, the condition is rare before 25 years.

Racial factors

Different races living in different geographical areas show a significant variation in the incidence of breast cancer. The incidence is high in Denmark, Canada, England, United States of America and Australia and low in Japan. However, when different racial groups are exposed to the same environmental influences for a long period of time as, for example, Japanese migrants to Hawaii, the incidence of the disease gradually increases until it reaches that of the indigenous white population. These findings suggest that environmental rather than genetic factors are responsible.

Hereditary factors

The genetic effects of carcinoma of the breast have been investigated in families and twins. Identical (monozygous) twins with like genotypes show a greater incidence of the disease than do non-identical twins. Moreover, when the tumours develop, they commonly occur at the same age and in the same breast far more frequently in identical than non-identical twins. In various relatives of patients with breast cancer, there is at least a twofold increase in carcinoma of the breast among mothers and sisters of patients with the disease but not among grandmothers and aunts. It is not clear whether this relationship represents a genetic influence or whether it is a result of common environmental and social factors.

Initiating and promoting factors

In laboratory mice, the most important aetiological agents in the development of breast cancer are viruses (p. 63) and polycyclic hydrocarbons (7,12-dimethylbenz(a)anthracene). The carcinogenicity of both of these agents is only expressed in specific strains and is influenced by endocrine factors. Although it is dangerous at this stage of our knowledge to extrapolate in detail results obtained from experimental animals to the disease in man, it seems clear that there are two important prerequisites for the development of malignancy:

1. Some trigger mechanism must be responsible for initiating the malignant change within the cell.

2. The environment must be favourable for tumour growth.

It is not known which trigger mechanisms are applicable to man. At present, there is no conclusive evidence either for or against the existence of a viral agent comparable with the milk factor, chemical carcinogens or ionizing radiations.

A favourable hormonal environment has considerable significance in the development of breast cancer. As long as 200 years ago, Ramazzini noticed that in Padua there were more cases of breast cancer among nuns than among married women. This observation was later statistically substantiated and further clarified. For example: (a) it is known that the incidence of breast cancer is higher in single than in married women, (b) the high risk in affluent countries has been associated with women who marry late, who have a limited number of children and who, as a convenience, curtail the duration of lactation, (c) the risk is particularly high in those women who marry late and have no children, and (d) fertility and prolonged breast feeding appear to offer protection against the risk of developing the disease.

The manner in which hormones exert their effect in the development of breast cancer is not understood. In the case of oestrogens, tumour growth is related to the presence or absence of specific oestrogen-binding proteins in the cytoplasm of tumour cells (p. 31). More recent work indicates that specific binding of prolactin to the tumour cell membrane might also directly stimulate tumour growth. If prolactin should turn out to be the important endocrine factor in the aetiology of breast cancer, it is conceivable that control of the secretion of this hormone might have an important prophylactic value against the disease.

Classification
Virtually all carcinomas of the breast arise from ductal epithelium, only rarely from acinar epithelium (lobular carcinoma). The relationship of tumour cells to the ducts and acini has an important bearing on the prognosis of these tumours, the prognosis being

good in the absence of extraduct spread and less favourable when tumour cells have invaded through ducts. Thus when examining sections from these tumours histologically, it is important to determine whether the tumour cells are confined within the basement membrane of the ducts or lobules, or whether they have penetrated the basement membrane and infiltrated the surrounding connective tissue stroma. On this basis, two major histological groups of breast cancer are recognized: the non-infiltrating and the infiltrating carcinomas.

Non-infiltrating carcinoma

Neither the lobular nor the intraduct types of carcinoma form distinct masses in the breast; they merely give rise to an increased consistency of the affected region. The essential histological feature of this group of cancers is an atypical and irregular epitheliosis which shows loss of cell polarity, pleomorphism, hyperchromatic nuclei and increased mitotic activity. The pattern of cell proliferation may take on various forms which further sub-divides this group:

1. *In solid intraduct carcinoma*, the ducts are filled and distended with masses of tumour cells which are irregular in form. The cells are usually larger than those lining the ducts, polyhedral in shape and show numerous mitotic figures.

2. *In comedocarcinoma*, the central mass of cells within the ducts degenerates, leaving only a narrow cuff of cells at the periphery. The bulk of the lumen is filled with eosinophilic debris which can be easily expressed by slight pressure on the cut surface. The expressed material resembles that of blackheads or comedos, hence the name *comedocarcinoma*.

3. *Cribriform carcinoma* is an uncommon type in which the cells are arranged around clear spaces. It is sometimes referred to as *adenoid cystic carcinoma*.

4. *Papillary carcinoma* is the rarest type of intraduct group. Cell proliferation takes the form of papillary processes which often have a well developed core. The cells are pleomorphic with many mitotic figures and frequently infiltrate the stroma of the core.

5. *Lobular carcinoma*, presumably arising from breast lobules, is the rarest form of breast cancer. It is characterized by intralobular epithelial overgrowth in which there is cell irregularity and atypicality, and the cytoplasmic margins between the tumour cells are indistinct. Some workers consider this as a premalignant lesion (lobular carcinoma *in situ*). It has the most favourable prognosis.

Infiltrating carcinoma

All infiltrating carcinomas of the breast develop from the intraduct or intralobular variety. Infiltration implies extension of tumour cells beyond the limits of the basement membrane. As this process continues, distinct masses become palpable in the breast and the prognosis of the condition becomes progressively worse. Although any section of the breast may be involved, infiltrating carcinoma usually commences in the upper and outer quadrant. The approximate relationship of cancer to the anatomical regions of the breast is as follows:

Upper and outer quadrant – 60%
Subareolar area   – 20%
Upper and inner quadrant – 10%
Lower and inner quadrant – 5%
Lower and outer quadrant – 5%

Morphologically infiltrating carcinomas of the breast may take various forms: they are classified on the degree of fibrosis (scirrhous or medullary) or on metaplastic changes (mucoid or squamous).

Scirrhous carcinoma

Among the infiltrative forms of breast cancer, the scirrhous is the predominant type (90 per cent). On palpation, the mass feels stony hard, its outline is indistinct, and in the early stages of the disease, it may move freely, but it soon becomes adherent to the skin and pectoral muscles, causing shrinkage and retraction of the breast. When cut with a scalpel, it gives a gritty sensation which has been likened to that produced by cutting an unripe pear. Both cut surfaces appear concave, grey in colour, and may show small, yellow spots which represent elastic fibres. The periphery of the tumour is irregular in outline, with scalloped edges, from which claw-like extensions taper out and fix the mass to skin and muscle. Fixation and retraction of the nipple, and wrinkling of the overlying skin, are late signs caused by involvement of the main ducts and lymphatics (Fig. 12.1).

Scirrhous carcinoma is composed predominantly of fibrocollagenous tissue which is characteristically dense and hyaline, and contains isolated or small strands of epithelial cells. The individual cells are round or polygonal in shape, regular in form, with small, dark-staining nuclei and very few mitotic figures. Usually, the deeper part of the tumour tends to be acellular and fibrous, whereas

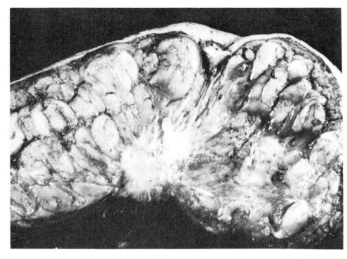

Fig. 12.1 Scirrhous carcinoma of the breast showing an irregular mass with scalloped edges, retraction of the nipple and invasion of the pectoral muscle

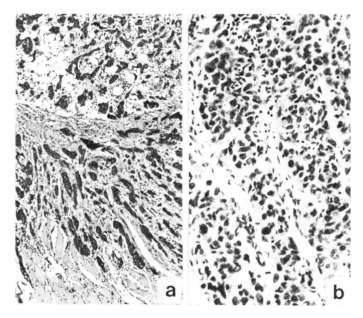

Fig. 12.2 Infiltrating carcinoma of the breast: (a) scirrhous carcinoma showing cords of tumour cells separated by fibrous tissue and invading the subcutaneous adipose tissue above and the pectoral muscle below (× 40); (b) medullary carcinoma showing densely packed cells (× 120)

the periphery of the tumour is more cellular. The tumour cells at the periphery infiltrate the adjacent adipose tissue and tend to invade blood vessels and lymphatics (Fig. 12.2).

Medullary (encephaloid) carcinoma

This is a less common variety of breast cancer which tends to occur in young women with well developed breasts. It is usually large (2 to 6 cm in diameter), round, bulky and well-circumscribed. Its soft consistency resembles bone marrow or brain tissue, and its cut surface, unlike that of scirrhous carcinoma, bulges and frequently shows areas of necrosis and haemorrhage.

Histologically, these tumours are highly cellular with very little stroma. The cells are arranged in large groups or sheets, sometimes separated by lymphocytic infiltrates. They are usually spheroidal in shape, with large vesicular nuclei and there are many mitotic figures. Those cases which show prominent lymphocytic infiltration indicate a host reaction against the tumour, but the presence of large collections of lymphocytes is not of any definite prognostic significance.

Mucoid carcinoma (colloid carcinoma, gelatinous carcinoma)

This is a rare tumour which tends to be bulky, fluctuant and well circumscribed. The cut surface shows a translucent, moist, gelatinous appearance often intersected by fine white strands of tissue.

Histologically, this is an adenocarcinoma composed of multilocular, cyst-like spaces, filled with pale blue, amorphous material containing small clusters of epithelial cells. The tumour cells are small; they have round, eccentrically located nuclei and the cytoplasm is vacuolated giving a *signet-ring* appearance. The material in the vacuoles takes up mucin stains.

Squamous-cell carcinoma

This also is a very rare tumour of the breast. It spreads very slowly in the epidermis around the nipple and, histologically, it shows typical features of a well differentiated squamous-cell carcinoma (p. 142).

Paget's disease of the nipple

This condition, first described by Sir James Paget in 1874, is one of the most interesting diseases affecting the breast. It is a rare disease occurring in women over the age of 40 years. The patient develops an acute eczema of the nipple which becomes erythematous, scaly and weepy, and later, the nipple becomes indurated and retracted or destroyed. A hard mass can often be felt deep to the nipple.

Histologically, the hallmark of this disease is the so-called *Paget-cell* which is a large, ovoid cell with clear cytoplasm and a vesicular nucleus; often it shows a positive PAS staining reaction. In the early stages of the disease, only a few Paget-cells are present scattered through the epidermis, but as the cells increase in number, they tend to compress the adjacent squamous cells and invade into the dermis (Fig. 12.3).

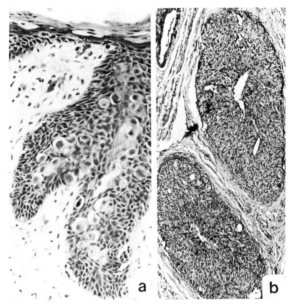

Fig. 12.3 Paget's disease of the nipple and associated intraduct carcinoma showing: (a) typical Paget's cells which are large with clear cytoplasm (× 120); (b) intraduct carcinoma in which the tumour cells are confined within the ducts (× 60)

Most authors now regard Paget's disease of the nipple as an infiltrating carcinoma of one of the main mammary ducts, not as a cancer of the skin. The lesion grows slowly, invades the stroma and eventually produces a scirrhous type carcinoma.

Modes of spread of breast cancer

Local spread
Breast cancer spreads radially, infiltrating through tissue spaces and invading adjacent lymphatic and blood vessels. When this

process is slow, the primary growth may acquire a pseudo-capsule, retain its mobility and be mistaken for an innocent tumour. More often, the tumour involves the main ducts of the breast, produces retraction of the nipple and becomes fixed to the skin.

Lymphatic spread

Permeation of the small lymphatic vessels interferes with the drainage of local areas of skin, causing lymphoedema and producing a typical orange peel appearance (*peau d'orange*). Lymphatic embolism involves the axillary glands, at first on the same side, and later, on the opposite side. The tumour may also spread to the internal mammary nodes in the second and third intercostal spaces, then to the mediastinal nodes in the thoracic cavity and to the deep lymphatic chain of the neck, involving the supraclavicular glands. During pregnancy, carcinoma of the breast tends to infiltrate extensively and may involve many lymphatics, producing acute swelling of the breast with redness and tenderness of the skin (*inflammatory carcinoma*).

Blood spread

Involvement of blood vessels results in metastatic deposits to any part of the body, particularly the lungs, liver, bone and adrenals. Metastases in bone are predominantly osteolytic (85 per cent), occasionally, osteoblastic (15 per cent).

Course and prognosis

Recurrence of breast cancer

Patients treated for breast cancer appear to run a greater risk of developing a second tumour in the other breast than the normal female population. In some cases, the second tumour is clearly a metastasis from the primary, but there is considerable evidence which shows that the risk of developing a second primary tumour might be as much as 10 times the risk of developing a single primary.

The prognosis and suitability for treatment of individual cases of carcinoma of the breast depend on the histological type of the tumour and on the extent of the disease. As a general rule, relatively better results are obtained in papillary, colloid and Paget's carcinomas than in scirrhous and medullary types. In cases where there is no microscopic evidence of metastases in the axillary nodes, the five-year survival rate is over 80 per cent, but the rate falls to 45 per cent when the axillary nodes are involved.

BENIGN TUMOURS

Fibroadenoma

Fibroadenoma is the commonest benign tumour of the female breast. It occurs in the age group 15 to 35 years, usually as a solitary nodule, but occasionally more than one tumour is present in the same breast. Rarely, the tumours may be bilateral. Fibroadenoma is rare in the male breast.

Some authors consider that fibroadenomas are not neoplasms, but localized hormonal hyperplasias representing focal areas of breast tissue which are more sensitive to oestrogens than the rest of the breast. In support of this view, they point out that the tumours increase in size during pregnancy and regress after lactation, both the epithelial and connective tissue components of the tumour respond to the action of hormone and that the surrounding breast tissue nearly always shows some degree of hyperplasia. Others maintain that fibroadenomas are true neoplasms, because on rare occasions, they undergo malignant change.

Fibroadenomas are round to oval tumours which vary in size from 1 cm to 4 cm in diameter, but may be much larger. They may be soft or hard in consistency. On gross section, the hard variety is uniformly grey-white in colour and the soft variety often contains small yellow foci of glandular tissue.

Microscopically, the tumours consist of both epithelial and connective tissue components. Two typical patterns are distinguished, pericanalicular and intracanalicular, although most tumours show a mixture of these two patterns.

1. *Pericanalicular fibroadenoma* is composed of proliferating ducts surrounded by concentric layers of cellular fibrous tissue. The ducts are lined by two or more layers of cells which may be cuboidal, columnar or spheroidal. This is the hard variety of fibroadenoma and commonly occurs in a young age group (15 to 25 years).

2. *Intracanalicular fibroadenoma* is composed predominantly of loose fibrous tissue which tends to grow against the ducts. Overgrowth of fibrous tissue disturbs and invaginates the ducts which become elongated and appear as slit-like branching structures lined by two layers of epithelium (Fig. 12.4). The loose areolar stroma often shows myxomatous and degenerative changes which give these tumours a soft consistency. They are uncommon tumours usually seen in a slightly older age group than the hard variety (25 to 35 years).

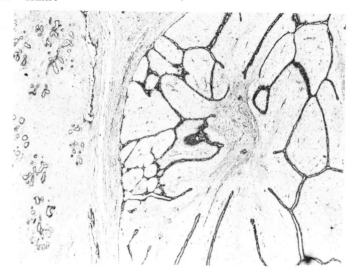

Fig. 12.4 Margin of an intracanalicular fibroadenoma of the breast showing stromal proliferation compressing the duct system and producing a pattern of elongated branched clefts (× 20)

Occasionally, a giant fibroadenoma occurs which may reach a weight of several kilograms. This tumour is a variant of the intra-canalicular fibroadenoma and appears in older women (40 to 60 years). Microscopically, there is a predominance of cellular con-nective tissue which show myxomatous change and may undergo malignant transformation (*cystosarcoma phylloides*).

Intraduct papilloma

The intraduct papilloma is usually a small, single tumour situated in one of the main breast ducts close to the nipple. It is a rare tumour, which occurs in middle-aged women and which is generally regarded as a benign lesion, but sometimes it may be difficult to differentiate from early cases of intraduct carcinoma. The cardinal symptom of duct papilloma is a bloodstained discharge from the nipple. No swelling can be felt in the breast, but by stroking different segments of the breast radially towards the nipple, it may be possible to show that the blood issues from a particular segment.

When the duct is opened longitudinally, the tumour is seen as a granular, raspberry-like nodule projecting into a dilated duct in the vicinity of the nipple. Microscopically, it consists of numerous delicate villi attached to the wall of the duct either by a narrow stalk or a broad base. The villous processes are composed of a core of loose connective tissue lined by a hyperplastic ductal epithelium which is regular in form. The connective tissue core contains thin-walled blood vessels which bleed easily, hence the bloodstained discharge.

TUMOUR-LIKE CONDITIONS

Mammary dysplasia

The mechanisms involved in the normal development, hormonal control and involution of the female breast are complex and do not always operate smoothly. Abnormalities arising from this system are grouped under the general heading of *mammary dysplasia* and are seen in the breasts of over 50 per cent of females between the ages of 30 and 50 years. The morphological features of mammary dysplasia include cystic disease, epithelial proliferation and metaplasia, fibrosis and infiltrations of lymphocytes and plasma cells. These components are seen in varying combinations, they vary in severity and their distribution may be diffuse or focal. Normally, the changes themselves do not require treatment, but biopsy of the lesions is frequently necessary to exclude the presence of malignant disease.

Cystic disease

Microcysts are found in over 50 per cent of post-menopausal women, so that their presence is considered normal. They form during normal involution of the breast ducts by the fusion of acini but the cysts retain their communication with the duct system and do not give rise to symptoms. When their communication is blocked either by fibrosis and kinking of the ducts or by intraductual epithelial proliferation, fluid secretion by the cells lining the cysts continues and gradually distends the small cysts into a palpable lump.

Palpable cysts are often found in the breasts of parous women nearing menopause. They may be single or multiple and usually contain clear or turbid fluid under tension. When the breast is incised, large solitary cysts with clear fluid appear blue, the blue-domed cyst of Bloodgood. In some cases, fluid may leak out from the cyst into the surrounding stroma causing a chronic inflammatory reaction with induration, giving the impression of malignant invasion.

Microscopically, two types of cyst occur in breasts showing mammary dysplasia:

1. *Simple cyst* lined by a single layer of flattened epithelium which shows no evidence of proliferative activity.

2. *Papillary cyst*, in which the lining epithelium is proliferating and tends to form papillary processes into the lumen. Sometimes apocrine metaplasia (pink epithelium) is also present (Fig. 12.5a).

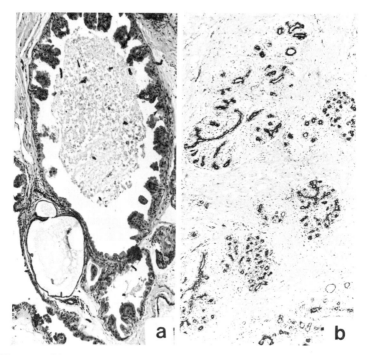

Fig. 12.5 Mammary dysplasia: (a) cystic hyperplasia showing dilation of ducts lined by hyperplastic epithelium, papillary processes and apocrine metaplasia (× 100); (b) lobular hyperplasia showing small ducts grouped into lobules (× 40)

Fibrosclerosis
Fibrosis of the breast, although an uncommon condition, is another variant of mammary dysplasia. It may occur before or after the menopause and usually presents as a hard, round lump in the upper and outer quadrant of the breast. The condition is probably due to hormonal imbalance; it is not a post-inflammatory fibrosis. The cut surface has a glistening white colour. Microscopically, it mainly consists of hyalinized fibro-collagenous tissue, very few atrophic epithelial structures and is devoid of adipose tissue.

Adenosis

Proliferation of ducts is the predominating feature in this form of mammary dysplasia, hence the name *adenosis*. Often it is accompanied by fibrosis and cystic change. The condition commonly occurs in women between the ages of 35 and 45 years and tends to affect the upper and outer quadrant of the breast. Macroscopically, the lesion is grey-white in colour, firm in consistency, and on the cut surface, small cystic spaces may be seen with the naked eye. Microscopically, the characteristic feature is an increase in the number of ducts. The arrangement of these ducts and the degree of intralobular fibrosis determine the type of adenosis.

1. When the ducts are grouped together into small lobules, the condition is referred to as *lobular hyperplasia*. These ducts are lined by two layers of cells, an inner layer composed of columnar cells which are regular in form, and an outer layer of proliferating myoepithelial cells. The connective tissue stroma within the lobules is loose areolar or myxomatous in type and devoid of fat (Fig. 12.5b).

2. In some cases, there is replacement of the loose intralobular connective tissue by dense hyaline fibrous tissue. This fibrous overgrowth compresses the ducts, obliterating the lumen and giving the appearance of solid cords of cells surrounded by collagen. This appearance, described as *sclerosing (fibrosing) adenosis*, gives rise to a hard lump which can be mistaken for infiltrating carcinoma. The presence of myoepithelial cells are an important aid in making a diagnosis; sometimes they proliferate and show palisading.

Epitheliosis

Proliferation of epithelial cells within existing small and large ducts is the histological hallmark of epitheliosis. Various patterns of proliferation may be seen within the duct system and sometimes in cysts. Three types are recognized:

1. In *solid epitheliosis*, the ducts are filled with a solid sheet of cells which are regular in form.

2. In *papillomatosis*, multiple minute papillary processes project into the lumen of the ducts or cysts.

3. *Cribriform epitheliosis* shows an acinar pattern without stroma formation.

Epithelial proliferation, *per se*, does not cause clinical symptoms unless it produces a nipple discharge. It is usually recognized by the pathologist in biopsy specimens and is an important change, because sometimes, it is difficult to differentiate from intraduct carcinoma. Normally, in epitheliosis, the cells are regular in form, mitotic figures are sparse and the peripheral layer of cells which show palisading of the nuclei is attached to the basement membrane. *Apocrine metaplasia*, characterized by large pink-staining cells, often accompanies epitheliosis. Sometimes cell proliferation may be of such a degree as to suggest a malignant change. Epitheliosis can progress to malignancy, so that any form of pleomorphism and excessive mitotic activity should be regarded with suspicion.

Duct ectasia

Ectasia means dilatation. Duct ectasia is seen in the breasts of parous women over the age of 40 years. As the ability of the ducts to absorb acinar secretion is impaired, the ducts become distended and a palpable mass may be felt in the region of the nipple. Mild degrees of distension are a common finding during the involutionary period and do not produce symptoms, but when distension is extensive, the ducts may rupture or leak fluid into the surrounding stroma and give rise to an inflammatory reaction. Occasionally, the inflammatory process leads to fibrosis of the ducts and retraction of the nipple which, in the presence of a palpable mass, causes alarm because of the possibility of malignancy.

The cut surface is grey and contains dilated ducts filled with a yellow cheesy material which can be easily squeezed out. Microscopically, the ducts are dilated and contain amorphous material and crystalline lipid bodies surrounded by macrophages and polymorphonuclear leucocytes. The lipid material dissolves out during processing and in haematoxylin and eosin sections appears as crystalline clefts. The surrounding stroma shows varying degrees of fibrosis and an infiltrate of plasma cells, polymorphonuclear leucocytes, large pale macrophages (epithelioid) and foreign body giant cells. Sometimes, plasma cells dominate the inflammatory exudate and, in those cases, the term *plasma-cell mastitis* is used by some pathologists.

Gynaecomastia

This refers to enlargement of the male breast. When unilateral, it often presents as a firm mass deep to the nipple and may be mistaken for carcinoma. Microscopically, there is hyperplasia of both ducts and stroma, but the cells lining the ducts are regular in form and clearly demarcated from the surrounding stroma.

Fat necrosis

The breasts, being superficial organs composed largely of fat, are particularly vulnerable to trauma and are occasionally the site of fat necrosis. The condition usually occurs in corpulent women with large breasts between the ages of 30 and 70 years, and approximately half of the patients cannot recall a definite injury to the breast. The lesion, which may occur in any part of the breast, is situated superficially, close to the skin. Its appearance varies according to its age. At approximately one month following the injury, a round mass forms in the subcutaneous fat. It feels firm on palpation, and its cut surface has an opaque yellow colour, areas of altered blood and foci of calcification. Microscopically, there are groups of necrotic fat cells, proliferation of fibroblasts and accumulation of epithelioid cells. Later, multinucleate foreign body giant cells form, especially around fatty acid crystals and blood pigment. Eventually, the necrotic area is replaced by fibrous tissue which contracts and causes skin dimpling. The importance of fat necrosis is that it gives rise to a palpable lesion which can either simulate a scirrhous carcinoma or obscure an underlying malignancy.

FURTHER READING

Antonius, J. I. & Jones, H. W. (1963) The significance of certain types of epithelial proliferation occurring in the female mammary gland. *Bull. Mason Clin.*, **17**, 17.

Helman, P. & Kilman, M. (1956) Paget's disease of the nipple: A clinical review of 27 cases. *Brit. J. Surg.*, **43**, 481.

Louis, C. J. (1958) Tumours of the Breast: A Study employing a histochemical technique. *Brit. J. Surg.*, **46**, 147.

McDivett, R. W. *et al.* (1967) *Tumours of the Breast*, Fascicle 2, second series. Washington, D.C.: Armed Forces Institute of Pathology.

Scarff, R. W. & Torloni, H. (1968) *International Classification of Tumours No. 2: Histological Typing of Breast Tumours.* Geneva: World Health Organization.

13

Tumours of lymphoid tissue

All primary tumours arising in lymphoid tissue are malignant and the whole group is collectively referred to as *malignant lymphomas*. Two major groups are recognized:

1. Non-Hodgkin's lymphoma.
2. Hodgkin's disease (HD).

They account for approximately 5 per cent of all cancers. Clinically, malignant lymphomas usually present as enlargement of a single node or a group of regional nodes, but occasionally, they may present as generalized lymph node enlargement associated with splenomegaly and hepatomegaly. Malignant lymphomas are not the only cause of lymph node enlargement, they must be distinguished from other causes, namely:

1. Reactive hyperplasia
2. Inflammations (acute and chronic)
3. Drugs (especially the antiepileptic drugs)
4. Infiltrations (lipids, amyloid)
5. Leukaemias
6. Neoplasms (secondary)

Diagnosis of the cause of enlargement of a lymph node can only be made by biopsy and histological examination, because the clinical features of each condition are not sufficiently distinctive to allow differentiation of the disease process. The lymph node to be removed for microscopic study should be carefully selected. When several lymph nodes are enlarged, the largest node in the cervical area should be taken, since axillary and particularly inguinal nodes are often the site of chronic inflammation. It should be excised with care, avoiding pressure on the node because it tends to distort the histological architecture, and the whole node should immediately be sent to the laboratory in a sterile container. This enables the pathologist to make imprints and to prepare cell cultures, frozen sections and paraffin sections. Knowledge of the histological structure of the lymphoma is essential before considering treatment and, to achieve this, a second biopsy may be necessary.

CLASSIFICATION OF NON-HODGKIN'S LYMPHOMAS

Until recently, malignant lymphomas were classified into four groups: follicular lymphoma, lymphosarcoma, reticulum-cell sarcoma and Hodgkin's disease. In 1956, Rappaport noted that follicular lymphoma was not a specific entity, but simply represented an expression of nodular deposition of tumour cells as compared with the more common, and prognostically worse, diffuse distribution. Later, doubt was cast on the nature of reticulum-cell sarcoma because its constituent cell resembled the histiocyte more than the reticular cell of lymphoid tissue. Rappaport, therefore, proposed a new classification for the non-Hodgkin's lymphomas based on these three histological criteria:

1. *The cell type* (lymphocytic, histiocytic or mixed lymphocytic-histiocytic). Identification of the cell type is made on routine haematoxylin and eosin stained sections. Imprints, histochemistry and electron microscopy do not appreciably contribute to the classification and are only used as diagnostic adjuvants in selected cases.

2. *The degree of cell differentiation* (well differentiated or poorly differentiated).

3. *The pattern of proliferation* (nodular or diffuse). A nodular pattern has a better prognosis because it is believed that it represents an early involvement of the node and that the pattern becomes diffuse as the disease progresses. Nodularity constituted the follicular lymphoma of the old classification. On this basis, Rappaport proposed the following classification:

Cell type	*Lymphoma*
Lymphocytic	Malignant lymphoma, lymphocytic type, well differentiated (diffuse or nodular)
	Malignant lymphoma, lymphocytic type, poorly differentiated (diffuse or nodular)
Mixed cell type (lymphocytic-histiocytic)	Malignant lymphoma, mixed cell type (usually nodular)
Histiocytic	Malignant lymphoma, histiocytic type.

In addition to Rappaport's classification, a further sub-division of the non-Hodgkin's lymphomas was put forward by Lukes and Buttler to indicate the functional potential of the cell type. The basis of their classification depends on histochemical and immunological identification of the cell types. For example:

1. *Histiocytes* contain a non-specific esterase which can be detected in tissue imprints or frozen sections.

2. *Lymphocytes* fall into two categories: (a) *T-cells* which are thymic dependent and can be identified by their ability to form rosettes with sheep red cells, and (b) *B-cells* which are thymic independent, but have receptors for heavy and light chains of immunoglobulin by which they can be identified. Both T and B lymphocytes, when exposed to foreign antigen transform into large forms which then undergo cell division. The small forms are the dormant cells, and the large forms, the metabolically active cells.

The fact that there are no firmly established T-cell lymphomas limits the value of Luke's classification. Most lymphomas arise from B-cells which develop in the centre of the lymphoid follicles. The follicular centre cell-types are classified as small cleaved, large cleaved, small non-cleaved and large non-cleaved. The last type resembles a fully transformed lymphocyte and is called an immunoblast when it leaves the follicles and enters the interfollicular tissue.

Incidence

Non-Hodgkin's lymphoma is not a common disease; it has a world-wide distribution and its incidence seems to be increasing. It occurs at any age, the incidence reaching a peak between the ages of 50 and 70 years and males are affected twice as frequently as females. Burkitt's lymphoma (p. 61) has a peak at five to six years and seldom occurs before the second and after the fifteenth year.

Aetiology

The aetiology of lymphoma is not known. Patients with certain long-standing autoimmune diseases such as systemic lupus erythematosis, Sjorgen's syndrome and rheumatoid arthritis, and those on immunosuppressants are more prone than the normal population to develop lymphoma. The aetiological implication of this association is not understood. Growing evidence appears to be implicating viruses as aetiological agents, but there is no definitive evidence for this view. Some forms of lymphoma in animals are caused by viruses and the diseases can be transmitted by cell-free extracts. In man, there is a strong suggestion that Burkitt's lymphoma might be caused by the E-B virus (p. 61).

Macroscopic appearance

The involved nodes are generally enlarged and discrete, but they may become matted together, especially in the latter stages of the disease. The cut surface shows a thick capsule and usually a homogeneous grey-white colour. Sometimes a nodular pattern is seen, the nodule being approximately 1 mm in diameter and occasionally foci of necrosis and haemorrhage are present. The spleen, bone marrow, liver, lung, tonsils and intestinal mucosa may also be involved.

Histological features

Microscopically, the normal pattern of the lymph node is partially or completely obliterated and replaced by closely packed cells arranged either diffusely or in nodules. The cell type is usually uniform in any given tumour (Fig. 13.1).

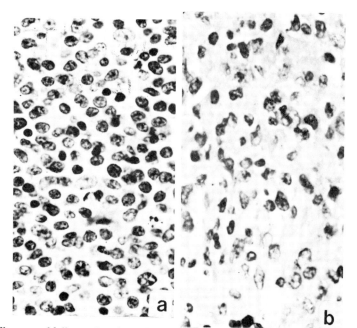

Fig. 13.1 Malignant lymphona: (a) lymphocytic type, well differentiated (× 160); (b) histiocytic type (× 160)

1. *Malignant lymphoma, lymphocytic type, well-differentiated.* The lymph node structure is replaced by sheets of small mature lymphocytes which are uniform in size and shape with very few mitotic figures present. A significant number of these lymphomas develop into chronic lymphatic leukaemia and, in the absence of a peripheral white cell count, it is not possible to distinguish between the two conditions. Occasionally, the lymphocytes in this type of lymphoma resemble plasma cells (*Waldenstrom's macroglobulinaemia*) in which the cytoplasm increases in amount due to production of immunoglobulin (IgM), becomes pyroninophilic and gives a positive PAS.

2. *Malignant lymphoma, lymphocytic type, poorly differentiated.* This lymphoma is characterized by cells larger than lymphocytes, but smaller than histiocytes. The cells show considerable variation in size and shape, the nuclei are cleaved (indented or twisted) and the chromatin is coarsely clumped. Prominent nucleoli are frequently present. Lymphoblasts which represent the extremes of immaturity are characterized by a fine chromatin mesh and prominent nucleoli.

3. *Malignant lymphoma, mixed-cell type.* In the mixed-cell type of lymphoma, there is proliferation of both lymphocytes and histiocytes in approximately equal numbers. The population of lymphocytes may also vary from small, mature cells to large immature cells or lymphoblasts.

4. *Malignant lymphoma, histiocytic type.* The lymph node architecture is replaced by proliferating neoplastic histiocytes. These mononuclear cells are large, with ill-defined cell outlines, oval vesicular nuclei and prominent nucleoli. The cytoplasm is pale pink in haematoxylin and eosin stains, but sometimes it is granular and may contain phagocytosed material. Mitoses are numerous and lymphocytes may be present. In doubtful cases, the esterase and reticulin stains might be helpful.

HODGKIN'S DISEASE

In 1832, Thomas Hodgkin described seven patients who had a disease characterized by generalized lymphadenopathy and splenomegaly. The condition subsequently became known as Hodgkin's disease and it is now the commonest member of the lymphoma group in Western countries. In China and Japan, malignant lymphoma histiocytic type is more common.

Incidence

HD may occur in children, but it is uncommon under the age of 15 years. The age-specific incidence is typically bimodal, the first peak occurring between 15 and 35 years, and the second, between 55 and 75 years. Although the overall sex incidence of HD is approximately 1.5 times more common in males than in females, it has been shown to vary according to the age group. The approximate frequencies are:

1. *Under 10 years of age*, 85 per cent of cases occur in boys.
2. *In the 15 to 35 year age group*, males and females are equally affected.
3. *In the 55 to 75 year age group*, males are affected twice as frequently as females.

Aetiology

The cause of the disease, like that of the other lymphomas, is not known; it is as obscure today as it was in 1832. There is no animal counterpart of HD. There are two opposing views concerning its aetiology:

1. It is an *infectious granuloma* similar to those of tuberculosis, sarcoidosis and brucellosis. Interest in a viral aetiology was aroused when cells indistinguishable from *Sternberg-Reed cells* were demonstrated in biopsies of lymph nodes from patients with infectious mononucleosis. The significance of this association has not been established.

2. It is a *true neoplasm* because of the infiltrating nature of the cells in the latter stages of the disease.

Pathologically, Hodgkin's disease occupies a mid-position between chronic inflammation and neoplasia. It has been suggested that the granulomatous reaction is an expression of the host's response to the disease.

Macroscopic appearances

Characteristically, the enlarged nodes are painless, smooth or nodular, discrete and rubbery in consistency. Late in the disease, invasion of the capsule occurs and they become matted together. The lymph nodes vary in size from 2 to 5 cm in diameter and their cut surface has a uniform grey-white appearance, although some lesions may show varying degrees of fibrosis and nodularity. The *spleen* is also frequently involved; commonly it weighs between 500 and 800 gm but occasionally it may reach a weight of 2 000 gm. The cut surface of the spleen often shows sharply outlined grey masses of tissue which are irregular in size and shape and which stand out against the pulp. This is the typical Hodgkin's tissue. The *liver* is usually large but rarely over 2 kg in weight and contains Hodgkin's tissue. The *bone marrow* may also contain nodules of Hodgkin's tissue and, when present, the nodules are indistinguishable from those of carcinomatosis.

Histological features

The microscopic diagnosis of Hodgkin's disease is based on two criteria: (a) the presence of typical Sternberg-Reed cells, and (b) a characteristic cellular environment (the *tissue reaction*). Both components are necessary for diagnosis because cells resembling SR cells can be found in many other conditions (metastatic carcinomas, infections, mononucleosis, sarcomas etc.) and the cellular environment characteristic of Hodgkin's disease can also be seen in other diseases.

1. *The SR cell* is regarded as the essential prerequisite for the diagnosis of Hodgkin's disease. Characteristically, it is a large (15 to 50 μm), well defined cell with abundant cytoplasm which shows variable staining affinities. There may be one single bilobed, or two vesicular nuclei with a thick, intensely stained nuclear membrane. At least one nuclear segment contains a large, smooth, spherical inclusion-like nucleolus which is attached to the nuclear membrane by strands of chromatin and surrounded by a clear halo (Fig. 13.2).

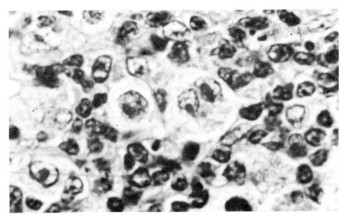

Fig. 13.2 Hodgkin's disease showing a Reed–Sternberg cell at the centre. The cell is binucleate, the nuclear membrane is coarse, each nucleolus has a clear halo and is attached to the nuclear membrane (× 350)

2. *The histiocytes* are the most characteristic cells. They are large cells (10 to 15 μm in diameter) with distinct cell outlines and pale, pink-staining, slightly granular cytoplasm. An oval or kidney-shaped nucleus with fine chromatin mesh uniformly distributed throughout is usually situated at one pole of the cell. The nucleolus is small and darkly stained.

3. In addition, there are *lymphocytes, plasma cells, neutrophils, eosinophils* and various degrees of *fibrosis*.

Classification

The histological pattern of Hodgkin's disease is complex. In all cases, the same cells are involved but various attempts to classify the disease and to correlate each type with length of survival have proved unsatisfactory. The sub-division into paragranuloma, granuloma and Hodgkin's sarcoma by Jackson and Parker that has been used for many years is unsatisfactory, because over 80 per cent of cases of HD fall into the granuloma group which shows variable survival times. The most recent acceptable classification is the *Rye Classification* proposed by Lukes and Buttler, in which four types are described:

	Relative frequency (%)	5-year survival (%)
Group I		
Lymphocytic predominance	10–15	55
Mixed-cell type	20–40	15
Lymphocytic depletion	5–15	5
Group II		
Nodular sclerosing	20–50	45

Lymphocytic predominance

Lymphocytes constitute the main component in this lymphoma. Other inflammatory cells such as plasma cells, neutrophils and eosinophils are scarce and necrosis and fibrosis are absent. SR cells are sparse and may have to be carefully searched for. The pattern may be diffuse or nodular. This type of HD corresponds to the paragranuloma of Jackson and Parker (Fig. 13.2).

Mixed-cell type

This type of HD is sometimes referred to as the fibrocellular variety. The cellular component is made up of a mixture of lymphocytes, histiocytes, fibroblasts, mature neutrophils, eosino-phils, plasma cells and SR cells. In addition, there are discrete areas of fibrosis; collagen deposition is not seen. The mixed-cell type of HD represents an intermediate phase in the progression from the early lymphocytic predominance stage to the late lymphocytic depletion stage. Because of its intermediate position, borderline cases may be difficult to classify and, in such cases, the interpretations of different pathologists will often vary.

Lymphocytic depletion
There are two types in this group – cellular and hypocellular. The hypocellular type shows a diffuse fibrosis made up of hyalinized collagen, few histiocytic cells and very few SR cells. The cellular type is a highly malignant form composed of pleomorphic histiocytes showing many mitoses and many bizarre SR cells. Necrosis is common in this type of HD which was originally called Hodgkin's sarcoma by Jackson and Parker.

Nodular sclerosing Hodgkin's disease
The criteria laid down for the diagnosis of nodular sclerosing Hodgkin's disease are:

1. *A thick capsule* surrounding the lymph node.

2. *Bands of birefringent collagen* surrounding irregular nodules containing lymphocytes, mature granulocytes, eosinophils, plasma cells and SR cells in varying proportions (Fig. 13.3).

3. The presence of *lacunar cells*. These are large cells (up to 40 μm in diameter) with abundant water-clear or pale eosoniphilic staining cytoplasm. The cell has a sharply defined peripheral margin which retracts away from adjacent cells during fixation giving the appearance of a large cell in a lacunar space. These cells are not peculiar to HD they are seen in reactive lymph nodes.

COURSE AND PROGNOSIS OF MALIGNANT LYMPHOMAS

Most patients who present with lymph node enlargements are otherwise healthy. As the disease progresses, certain systemic manifestations such as anaemia, fever, night sweats, weight loss and weakness gradually become apparent. These patients have a significantly greater tendency to succumb to certain types of infection, particularly fungal infections and tuberculosis, than other people. The most common fungal infection is torulosis (*Cryptococcus*

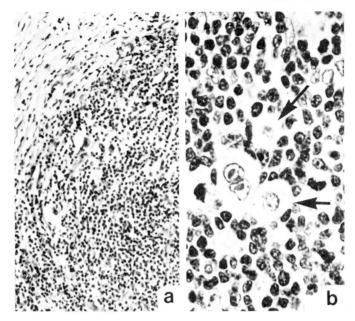

Fig. 13.3 Nodular sclerosing Hodgkin's disease showing: (a) fibrosis at the upper left corner (× 40); (b) lacunar cells indicated by arrows (× 160)

neoformans) which is found in approximately 15 per cent of patients with HD. Furthermore, treatment of these diseases with X-rays, hormones, immunosuppressants and cytotoxic drugs increases the chances of the patients developing tuberculosis and other opportunistic fungal infections.

The natural course of malignant lymphoma is one of progression until death. In the individual case, prognosis is difficult to estimate, but in general, it depends on two factors:

1. *The histological type* as determined by biopsy.

2. *The extent of involvement* (stage) as determined by lymphangiography and surgical exploration.

Histological classification and staging provide an indication of the prognosis of a given lymphoma and what form of therapy will be most effective. In the non-Hodgkin's lymphomas, the nodular and well differentiated types generally have a better prognosis than the diffuse and poorly differentiated varieties.

Four clinical stages are recognized and are shown below together with their relative survival rates. Each stage is further sub-divided into A or B depending on the absence or presence respectively of general symptoms.

Stage	Extent of Involvement
I	Limited to 1 anatomical region
II	2 or more anatomical regions involved but on the same side of the diaphragm.
III	Disease on both sides of diaphragm but limited to lymph nodes and spleen.
IV	Involvement of other tissues: bone marrow, lung, liver, gut etc.

The distribution of the histological types of HD correlates well with the clinical stages. The following figures, obtained from various sources, have been rounded off for simplicity:

	Clinical stages (%)		Symptoms (%)	
Histological type of HD	I and II	III and IV	Absent (A)	Present (B)
Lymphocytic predominance	90	10	100	0
Nodular sclerosing	70	30	70	30
Mixed-cell type	50	50	50	50
Lymphocytic depletion	30	70	30	70

FURTHER READING

Braylan, R. C. et al. (1975) Malignant lymphomas: Current classification and new observations, *Pathology Annual*, **10**, 213.

Gough, J. (1970) Hodgkin's disease: A correlation of histopathology with survival. *Int. J. Cancer*, **5**, 273.

Kaplan, H. S. (1972) *Hodgkin's Disease*. Cambridge, Massachusetts: Harvard University Press.

Lukes, R. J. & Collins, R. D. (1975) New approaches to the classification of the lymphomata. *Br. J. Cancer*, **31**, 1.

Rappaport, H. et al. (1956) Follicular lymphoma: A re-evaluation of its position in the scheme of malignant lymphomas, based on a survey of 253 cases. *Cancer*, **9**, 792.

14

Tumours of the salivary glands, mouth and pharynx

TUMOURS OF THE SALIVARY GLANDS

The salivary glands consist of the major salivary glands (parotid, submandibular and sublingual) and the minor salivary glands found throughout the oral cavity. Tumours arising in these glands are ten times more common in the parotid than in the submandibular gland, and rare in the sublingual glands. The classification and relative frequency of salivary gland tumours are as follows:

	Frequency (%)
Adenomas:	85
(a) Pleomorphic adenoma (mixed tumour) (75)	
(b) Adenolymphoma (9)	
(c) Oxyphilic adenoma (1)	
Acinic-cell tumour	1
Mucoepidermoid tumour	3
Carcinomas:	11
(a) Adenocystic carcinoma (3)	
(b) Adenocarcinoma (1)	
(c) Epidermoid carcinoma (1)	
(d) Undifferentiated carcinoma (3)	
(e) Malignant mixed tumour (3)	

Pleomorphic adenoma

Pleomorphic adenoma, or mixed salivary tumour, is the commonest tumour found in the salivary glands and is a well-known clinical entity. It is slightly more common in females than in males and the peak incidence appears to be between 30 to 50 years of age. Pleomorphic adenoma is of unusual interest for three reasons: its natural history, the question of its histogenesis and the nature of its mucoid substances.

At present, most authors support the epithelial theory of origin. This conclusion was arrived at from histological observations that all transitions from glandular tumour elements to spindle and stellate cells surrounded by mucoid and cartilaginous material often occur in a single tumour. Especially convincing is the occasional presence of squamous epithelium with its various forms of differentiation. Such squamous metaplasia is common in a wide variety of epithelial tissues. The chief obstacle to the epithelial theory is the frequent occurrence of connective tissue mucin and cartilage, and the occasional presence of bone.

A further difficulty encountered with these growths is the assessment of their degree of malignancy. Whilst the mixed tumour is regarded as benign, in that it rarely metastasizes, some workers consider it malignant because local recurrence is a predominant characteristic.

Macroscopic features

Pleomorphic adenoma is a hard, somewhat rounded, slowly growing tumour which frequently occurs in that part of the parotid gland overlying the angle of the jaw. It varies in size from 1 cm to 5 cm in diameter but occasionally it may be much larger. Its cut surface is solid and grey-white in colour, often with small bluish areas which represent cartilaginous foci, and soft moist areas which represent mucoid change. Occasionally, cystic spaces and areas of fibrosis, calcification and bone formation may be present.

Microscopic changes

Usually the nodules are separated from the surrounding glandular tissue by a well developed capsule of connective tissue. In places, the capsule is incomplete and minute excrescences from the main tumour mass jut out through these gaps. It is from these extra-capsular islands of tumour tissue that recurrence develops following enucleation. Histologically, the tumours show cellular and relatively acellular areas (Fig. 14.1a).

1. *The cellular areas* are composed of sheets or groups of polyhedral cells with basophilic, homogeneous cytoplasm containing large, ovoid, vesicular nuclei. The cell outlines are indistinct and often merge with the scanty intercellular stroma. Other areas are composed of tubular structures which vary in size and are lined by two layers of cells, an inner layer of epithelial and an outer layer of myoepithelial cells. The tubules differ from normal salivary gland ducts in that they lack a basement membrane, the lining cells are not in close contact with each other, but are often surrounded by a homogeneous mucoid material suggesting loss of polarity of secretion.

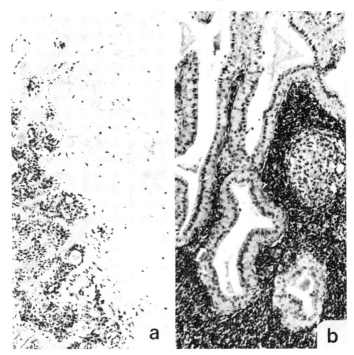

Fig. 14.1 Salivary gland tumours: (a) pleomorphic adenoma (mixed salivary tumour) showing cells forming ducts and containing mucin, and a hyaline area resembling cartilage (× 60); (b) adenolymphoma showing lymphoid follicles and spaces lined by characteristic tall epithelium with the nuclei situated near the free margin (× 200)

2. In the *relatively acellular areas*, the cells are usually scattered singly or in groups of two or three within a voluminous connective tissue stroma. The cells may be triangular or spindle-shaped, they possess darkly staining nuclei and their cytoplasm tapers out into fine processes which blend with the stroma. In some areas, circumscribed zones of fibromucoid material are seen, in other areas, the stroma is homogeneous in structure with cells embedded in lacunae giving the appearance of cartilage.

Adenolymphoma

This is a benign, slow growing, encapsulated tumour which arises in the ducts of the parotid gland. It seldom occurs in the other salivary glands. Histologically, it is composed of glandular and cystic structures lined by two layers of cells. The inner layer of cells is tall columnar with granular eosinophilic cytoplasm and

small nuclei, the deep layer consists of cuboidal cells. The stroma
is densely infiltrated with lymphocytes in which well-formed
germinal centres are prominent (Fig. 14.1b).

Oxyphilic adenoma (oncocytoma)

Oxyphilic adenoma is an uncommon benign tumour of glandular
origin and mainly occurs in the parotid gland in patients over 50
years of age. It is round or oval, firm, well encapsulated and freely
mobile; its cut surface is grey and lobulated. Histologically,
oxyphilic adenoma is composed of large cells with pink granular
cytoplasm (oncocytes). Electron microscopy shows they are rich
in mitochondria. These cells are also found in the thyroid gland
(Hürthle cells), parathyroid, pancreas and adrenal glands. The
cells are arranged in columns or irregular groups with very little
stroma between them. A few lymphocytes may be present, but they
are not a feature.

Acinic-cell tumour

The acinic-cell tumour is a well circumscribed slow growing lesion
with a cut surface which has a grey-white colour, but may show
areas of necrosis and haemorrhage. Most occur within the parotid
gland and are more common in females than in males. Histologically,
it is composed of solid sheets or groups of cells which resemble
the serous cells of the parotid gland, in that they have a basophilic
granular cytoplasm and a round nucleus. Sometimes, clear cells
may be present in variable proportions. Secretions may accumulate
within the tumour to form cystic spaces, and occasionally, small
infiltrates of lymphocytes may be present.

Acinic-cell tumours are benign in the early stages, but sooner
or later, they may invade locally and spread to regional lymph nodes.

Mucoepidermoid tumour

This tumour arises from the ducts of the major salivary glands,
usually the parotid. It may be solid or cystic. Histologically, it is
composed of epidermal or mucin-secreting cells, one of which
usually predominates. Solid tumours consist mainly of squamous
cells which are recognized by their eosinophilic cytoplasm, intercellular bridges and keratin formation. Cystic tumours contain
spaces lined by goblet cells and filled with mucin. The proportion
of epidermoid and mucoid components varies in each tumour.

Mucoepidermoid tumours vary in their degree of malignancy.
Generally, they are slow growing and well encapsulated but they
may infiltrate locally and occasionally metastasize to regional lymph
nodes.

Carcinoma

Carcinomas are uncommon tumours in the salivary glands. They arise in the ducts and occur in many different forms which vary in appearance and prognosis; many arise in a pre-existing mixed salivary tumour. Generally, they are more common in men and occur in the 50 to 70 year age group.

1. *Adenocystic carcinoma* differs from other salivary gland tumours in that it is common in the submandibular gland and may occur in the minor salivary glands. Histologically, it is a poorly encapsulated, infiltrating carcinoma in which the constituent cells show a characteristic cribriform pattern surrounding tubular or cystic spaces which may be empty or contain eosinophilic, PAS-positive material (Fig. 14.2). Two types of cells are present, those resembling cells lining the ducts and myoepithelial cells. Occasionally, the cells may be arranged in sheets or form trabeculae. This tumour grows typically by infiltration and has a tendency to infiltrate into perineural spaces. Facial paralysis is an unfavourable sign. Local recurrence and involvement of lymph nodes may occur following excision.

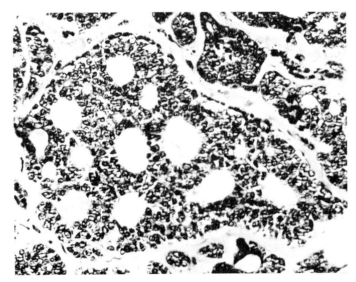

Fig. 14.2 Adenoid cystic carcinoma of the parotid gland showing groups of small cells set in a connective tissue stroma and arranged around cystic spaces (× 100)

2. *Adenocarcinoma* is an infiltrating tumour composed of a single cell type which tends to form glands or tubules, often with papillary projections. No *mixed tumour* components are present. Occasionally, mucus-secreting adenocarcinoma may occur but these must be distinguished from mucoepidermoid tumours by the presence of an epidermal component.

3. *Squamous-cell carcinoma* is composed of well differentiated squamous cells showing intercellular bridges and keratin formation. No mucus secretion is present. These tumours are rare and probably arise in areas of squamous metaplasia which occurs in ducts in association with chronic infections or calculi.

4. *Undifferentiated carcinoma* is an uncommon tumour which is often difficult to distinguish from sarcoma.

5. *Malignant mixed tumour* shows areas of malignant change in a mixed salivary tumour. The malignant change is usually an adenocarcinoma, but undifferentiated or squamous-cell carcinomas may develop.

Course and prognosis

Since tumours of the salivary glands are radioresistant, surgery is the usual form of treatment. In pleomorphic adenomas, the high rate of recurrence following surgical treatment appears to be due partly to the frequent presence of extracapsular tumour tissue and partly to spilling of tumour cells during the operation. For this reason, a preoperative biopsy is usually contraindicated. Benign tumours of the parotid gland are treated by removal of the tumour with a good margin of normal parotid tissue, after identification and preservation of the facial nerve. Malignant tumours require total parotidectomy with removal of the facial nerve and the involved surrounding tissues. Adjuvant chemotherapy might be helpful. The approximate five-year survival rate of malignant salivary tumours are:

Tumour	Five-year survival (%)
Malignant mixed tumours	40
Mucoepidermoid tumour:	
(a) Low grade malignancy	80
(b) High grade malignancy	20
Acinar tumour	80
Squamous-cell carcinoma	20
Undifferentiated carcinoma	20

TUMOURS OF THE MOUTH AND PHARYNX

Malignant	*Benign tumours*	*Tumour-like lesions*
Squamous-cell carcinoma	Papilloma	Dermoid cyst
Lymphoma	Angiofibroma	Mucous cyst
Transitional-cell carcinoma	Giant-cell epulis	Ranula
Sarcoma	Other soft tissue tumours	Thyroglossal cyst
Melanoma		Ectopic thyroid

The tumours that arise in the mouth and pharynx cover the whole spectrum of tumour pathology. The vast majority are derived from the lining mucous membrane and, microscopically, the vast majority (over 90 per cent) are well differentiated, keratinizing, squamous-cell carcinomas. It is with this tumour that the present discussion will be mainly concerned. Tumours other than squamous-cell carcinoma occasionally occur in this area, sometimes as localized tumours, sometimes as symptomatic manifestations of generalized disease such as lymphoma, leukaemia, plasmacytoma and other soft tissue tumours. These will not be discussed in this section. Benign tumours are many and varied and only three are worthy of mention, the papilloma, the juvenile angiofibroma and the giant-cell epulis, all of which are rare. Tumour-like lesions of the oral cavity are also common, but their recognition depends on histological diagnosis.

Malignant tumours

Carcinomas of the mouth and pharynx present as ulcers with raised edges, or as nodular infiltrating lesions and occur most commonly on the lip and tongue and less commonly in the pharynx. The degree of malignancy varies with the site, being lowest in the lip and highest in the tongue. These cancers are seen in patients with *unstable mucous membranes* and who show a tendency to have second and even third primaries in different areas. This emphasizes the need for critical initial evaluation and long-term follow-up. The established lesions are readily recognized but diagnosis should be aimed at the early stages of the disease because late signs, such as fixation and lymph node involvement, make treatment difficult and the prognosis correspondingly poor. The golden rule, therefore, is that when a small mucosal lesion is seen which cannot be pronounced benign with certainty, it should be immediately excised and biopsied.

Carcinoma of the lip

Carcinoma of the lip is the commonest form of oral cancer, being more prevalent in pipe smokers and workers in outdoor occupations such as farmers, seamen and fishermen. It is ten times more common in males than in females, the lower lip is most frequently affected and the peak incidence is between the ages of 50 and 70 years.

There is strong evidence that pipe smoking is an important predisposing factor. For example, carcinoma develops at the site where continual pressure from the pipe-stem has been exerted, and there is a high incidence of cancer of the lip in Irish peasant women and negro women who smoke clay pipes. The carcinogens in tobacco are probably the initiating factor and the irritating pressure from the pipe-stem the promoting factor. The role of actinic rays in the development of carcinoma of the lip is indicated by the disproportionate incidence of the condition in sunny countries, such as Australia. The preponderance of tumours of the lower lip may be explained by the constant exposure of the mucocutaneous junction to sunlight, whereas the corresponding part of the upper lip is relatively shaded. The lower lip drains to the submental, submandibular and upper deep cervical lymph nodes. Except in the midline tumours, there is seldom spread to the lymph nodes of the opposite side of the neck.

Carcinoma of the tongue and floor of the mouth

Squamous-cell carcinoma of the tongue and mouth is the second most common cancer of the oral cavity. It is substantially more frequent in men than in women, the peak incidence being in the age group between 50 and 70 years. Predisposing causes include smoking, tobacco chewing and chronic dental sepsis. It occurs predominantly on the lateral border and upper surface of the anterior two-thirds of the tongue; carcinoma of the posterior third of the tongue is rare. The ulcer is hard with raised indurated edges and must be distinguished from:

1. *Simple ulcers* which occur at the edge or tip. They are small, shallow, painful, inflamed and often associated with a sharp-edged tooth.

2. *Tuberculous ulcers* occur at the tip. They are indurated and associated with pulmonary tuberculosis.

3. *Syphilitic ulcers* occur on the dorsum of the tongue. They

have a serpiginous outline and are associated with tertiary syphilis. Because of the rich lymphatic drainage and constant muscular movement of the tongue, lymphatic spread to the cervical nodes occurs early and is frequently bilateral. The prognosis is generally poor, the five-year survival rate being less than 30 per cent.

Carcinoma of the pharynx
The pharynx extends from the base of the skull to the junction of the oesophagus in the neck and is divided into three regions, mainly on anatomical and pathological grounds.

1. *The nasopharynx* is the space below the base of the skull and above the soft palate, having the inner ear as its lateral border and the nasal cavity its anterior border. Tumours in this region are usually poorly differentiated squamous-cell carcinomas, sometimes associated with lymphocytic infiltration (*lympho-epithelioma*). They are rare except among Chinese, Korean and South East Asian people, in whom they have been associated with the Epstein–Barr virus (p. 62). They remain silent for a long period of time and often present as an enlarged lymph node in the neck. Because of their invasive potential, they spread widely to involve structures related to the boundaries of the nasopharynx and may cause: (a) deafness and otitis media by involving the Eustacian tube, (b) cranial nerve palsies and headache from involvement of the base of the skull, and (c) nasal obstruction and bleeding if spread is anterior. A change in the character of a chronic post-nasal discharge may be the only symptom related to the primary tumour.

2. *The oropharynx* includes the tonsil and its arches, the soft palate, the base of the tongue as far forward as the circumvallate papillae and the anterior surface of the epiglottis. Tumours here are rare and the symptoms they produce are minimal, for example, sore throat, a tickling sensation on swallowing or intermittent pain referred to the ear. Spread to cervical glands is common and early. Most tumours are squamous-cell carcinomas, occasionally a malignant lymphoma may develop submucosally.

3. *The hypopharynx* represents the rest of the pharynx and extends from the oropharynx to the oesophageal junction. It is subdivided into posterior wall, pyriform fossa and postcricoid region. Although squamous-cell carcinoma arising in the pharyngeal mucosa is commoner in men than in women, this sex incidence is reversed in carcinoma arising in the hypopharynx and upper end of the oesophagus. Cancer of the hypopharynx is, in fact, almost exclusively a disease of women and is preceded, in a large proportion of cases, by the *Plummer–Vinson syndrome*. Symptoms in

this region depend on the site of the primary tumour: (a) pyriform fossa tumours are often silent and an enlarged cervical node may be the first sign, and (b) tumours of the postcricoid region and posterior pharyngeal wall produce dysphagia. Approximately 90 per cent of these tumours are squamous-cell carcinomas, the rest are either transitional-cell carcinomas or lymphoepitheliomas.

Benign tumours

Juvenile angiofibroma
Angiofibroma is a rare tumour which occurs in the nasopharynx of adolescent boys. Although benign, it can be a major problem because of the risk of precipitous haemorrhage. Characteristically, these tumours grow to a large size before being recognized and frequently involve the paranasal sinuses.

Papilloma
This is a wart-like lesion occurring on the lips, tongue and palate. Papillomas may be flattened, mushroom-shaped or pedunculated and are composed of papillary processes of fibrovascular connective tissue lined by proliferating squamous epithelium. On the lip, papillomas should be regarded with suspicion because they are frequently malignant.

Giant-cell epulis
This lesion is more common in females than in males and occurs at all ages. It is a round, blue-red swelling arising from the gums and may be pedunculated or sessile. Histologically, it is composed of a fibrovascular stroma containing many monocytes and multi-nucleated giant cells of the foreign body type. The lesion is not neoplastic, it does not recur and is now considered to be a granuloma.

Cystic lesions

Mucous cyst
This is a rounded swelling usually less than 1 cm in diameter and covered by normal mucosa which is often thinned and translucent. Mucous cysts are retention cysts caused by obstruction of the gland orifice following trauma or inflammation. They occur on the inside of the lips, cheeks, floor of the mouth, and occasionally, the palate.

Ranula

This is a smooth, round, blue cyst situated beneath the front of the tongue to one side of the midline. It is caused by obstruction of a mucous gland and its wall is composed of fibrous tissue infiltrated by leukocytes and lined by epithelium. The cyst may reach a large size, compress the duct of the submandibular gland and cause secondary changes in the gland.

Thyroglossal cyst

Thyroglossal cysts arise in the thyroglossal duct which extends from the junction of the anterior two-thirds and posterior third of the tongue along the midline to the upper border of the thyroid cartilage. From these, it diverges slightly to one or other side of the midline and its course is represented after birth by the pyramidal lobe of the thyroid gland. Abnormalities of this duct which may be mistaken for tumours are:

1. *Thyroglossal cysts* which occur anywhere along the line of the duct and are connected to the foramen caecum of the tongue by the remainder of the duct. Cysts above the thyroid cartilage are central, those below slightly to one side. Removal of the cysts entails removal of the attachment to the foramen caecum. The cyst is lined by squamous or ciliated columnar epithelium and foci of thyroid gland tissue may be seen in the wall.

2. *Ectopic thyroid*. Thyroid gland tissue also may occur anywhere along the line of the duct. Sometimes it is found on the back of the tongue (*lingual thyroid*). Carcinoma may develop in these aberrant thyroids.

FURTHER READING

Beckman, J. S., Westbrook, K. C & Thompson, B. W. (1974) Lip cancer: surgical management. *Am. J. Surg.*, **128**, 732.

Louis, C. J. & Bremner, D. A. (1962) Mixed salivary tumours. *Aust. & N.Z. J. Surg.*, **31**, 254.

Thackaray, A. C. (1972) *International Histological Classification of Tumours No. 7: Histological Typing of Salivary Gland Tumours*. Geneva: World Health Organization.

Thackaray, A. G. & Lucas, R. B. (1974) *Tumours of the Salivary Glands*, Fascicle 10, Second Series, Washington D.C.: Armed Forces Institute of Pathology.

Wahi, P. N. (1971) *International Histological Classification of Tumours No. 4: Histological Typing of Oral and Oropharyngeal Tumours*. Geneva: World Health Organization.

15

Tumours of the gastrointestinal tract

TUMOURS OF THE OESOPHAGUS

Carcinoma is the most important tumour affecting the oesophagus. Other tumours such as leiomyoma, squamous papilloma and sarcoma occasionally occur, but are extremely rare.

Carcinoma

Oesophageal cancer accounts for approximately 2 per cent of all cancer deaths and shows great variation in geographical distribution. In America, Canada and Australia the incidence is approximately 2 to 3 per 100 000 population, in England, 5 to 6 per 100 000 and in France, Puerto Rico and Switzerland, 10 to 15 per 100 000. Generally, it is more common in men than in women (4:1) but the post-cricoid carcinoma, which is frequently superimposed on a long-standing *Plummer–Vinson syndrome*, is much more common in women (20:1). Most of the patients are between 50 and 70 years of age.

Aetiology

The aetiology of oesophageal cancer is obscure. In many high risk countries, low socio-economic standards, inadequate diet and a heavy intake of alcohol and tobacco are considered significant. Recent studies have implicated carcinogenic food contaminants, particularly high concentrations of nitrosamines in certain alcohols and foods. For example, in Zambia, a dramatic rise in the incidence of carcinoma of the oesophagus was recently reported in men who consumed large quantities of locally brewed spirit (*kashasu*), and in France, where wine is the national drink, the incidence is twice that in England and America. Middle-aged women with Plummer–Vinson syndrome are more prone to develop carcinoma of the upper part of the oesophagus and hypopharynx. The incidence is also higher in patients with achalasia of the oesophagus.

Macroscopic features

Carcinoma may arise in any part of the oesophagus. The approximate distribution is:

(a)	Middle third	50%
(b)	Lower third	30%
(c)	Upper third	20%

The majority are solid or fungating tumours which project into the lumen. Less frequently, they are ulcerating lesions with rolled up edges, and least frequently, infiltrating or stenosing carcinomas are seen.

Microscopic features

Most carcinomas of the oesophagus are squamous-cell carcinomas which show varying degrees of differentiation, ranging from keratinizing carcinomas with well developed keratin pearls to completely undifferentiated and unrecognizable types. Sometimes, an adenocarcinoma involves the lower end of the oesophagus. This type may either represent an upward extension from a carcinoma of the stomach, or it may arise from ectopic gastric mucosa.

Course and prognosis

Carcinoma of the oesophagus is highly malignant and tends to spread early. Direct spread may involve the lung, trachea, bronchus or great vessels in the vicinity. Fistulae may also form with the air passages producing pulmonary complications. The left recurrent laryngeal nerve may be involved, either directly by the growth or by secondary tumour in lymph nodes. Lymphatic spread from the upper part of the oesophagus goes to the lymph nodes in the cervical region, from the middle of the oesophagus, to the root of the lung, while that from the lower part of the oesophagus, to the nodes along the lesser curvature of the stomach, coeliac axis and then to the liver.

Dysphagia, first for solids and later for liquids, is the first symptom, but this symptom only appears after the disease has involved at least half the circumference of the oesophagus and occluded three quarters of its lumen.

The prognosis of oesophageal cancer is generally poor, the survival rates being related to the site and stage of the disease. In tumours of the middle third of the oesophagus, the five-year survival rate is only 5 per cent, whereas in those of the lower third, 15 per cent.

TUMOURS OF THE STOMACH

Benign tumours of the stomach are rare; fibromas, myomas, lipomas and single adenomas are occasionally found. Lymphomas are also rare. By far the most common and most important tumour affecting the stomach is carcinoma.

Carcinoma of the stomach

Carcinoma of the stomach is prevalent in all civilized communities, although statistics show variations between and within countries. It is particularly common in Japan, Iceland, Sweden, Finland and Russia where the incidence is approximately 50 cases per 100 000 population. In England, Canada, America and Australia the disease is less frequent (10 to 15 cases per 100 000) and, in some parts of South Africa, it is uncommon (2 to 5 cases per 100 000). Within countries, carcinoma of the stomach shows a distinct socio-economic distribution related to habits and standards of living.

Social class	Incidence ratio
Professional classes	2
Skilled labourers	3
Unskilled labourers	5

Carcinoma of the stomach occurs predominantly in the sixth decade of life and is twice as common in males as in females.

Aetiology

The pattern of distribution of gastric cancer among certain populations indicates that environmental factors, genetic predisposition and certain pathological conditions are important in the development of the disease.

   1. *Environmental factors.* Different dietary habits and methods in food preparation appear to play an important role in the incidence of gastric cancer. For example: (a) fish is the staple diet in Iceland. In the coastal areas, where fresh fish is readily available, the incidence of gastric cancer is low, but in the inland areas, where smoked fish is mainly consumed, the incidence is high; (b) smoked and barbecued food contains high concentrations of carcinogenic hydrocarbons, particularly benzo(a)pyrene, which if ingested continuously over many years, may constitute an important cause of gastric cancer; (c) fat used repeatedly for frying and brought to high temperatures, is also an important source of carcinogens; (d)

in Japan, where the incidence of carcinoma of the stomach is the highest in the world, asbestos has been implicated as an aetiological factor. Japanese people consume large quantities of raw fish coated with a dressing of starch and talc which is nearly always contaminated with asbestos fibres.

2. *Hereditary factors.* A familial tendency towards gastric cancer is well established. Whether this tendency is due to hereditary or to some common environmental factor is not yet known, but family histories of high incidence of carcinoma of the stomach are occasionally recorded. The medical history of the Bonaparte family, for example, is of historical interest. Napoleon's father, three brothers and three sisters died from gastric cancer, and Napoleon himself, is reputed to have had carcinoma of the lesser curvature of the stomach. More convincing evidence of a hereditary pre-disposition is shown by the fact that gastric cancer is more common in individuals with blood group A than in those with other blood groups.

3. *Precancerous conditions.* Certain pathological conditions of the gastric mucosa are well known to carry a high risk of malignancy: (a) conditions associated with intestinal metaplasia of the mucosa, namely, atrophic gastritis, achlohydria and pernicious anaemia carry a 40 to 50 per cent risk. It is doubtful whether people with peptic ulcer run a significant risk of developing carcinoma of the stomach. Most authorities would place the risk at one per cent or less, and this is understandable, since both carcinoma and peptic ulcer are common conditions and both occur predominantly at the same sites in the stomach.

Macroscopic features

The anatomical distribution of gastric cancer in the stomach is similar to that of peptic ulcers. Approximately 50 per cent occur in the pyloric antrum, 2·5 per cent along the lesser curvature, 15 per cent at the cardia and 10 per cent in the rest of the stomach. In common with cancer of the gastrointestinal tract, carcinoma of the stomach may take one of three forms:

1. *Ulcerating carcinoma* is the commonest type and is character-ized by its raised edges, a rough necrotic floor and by its size which is usually greater than 3 cm in diameter. This is the commonest type.

2. *Fungating carcinoma* appears as a large cauliflower-like mass which is usually attached to the mucosa by a broad base and fills the lumen of the stomach. Often ischaemic necrosis occurs at its centre and when the necrotic tissue sloughs off, it becomes an ulcerating carcinoma.

3. *Infiltrating carcinoma* is the least common type and may take on two forms depending on its mode of growth: (a) it may spread superficially over the surface of the mucosa to give rise to a flat plaque-like lesion, or (b) it may infiltrate diffusely through the wall of the stomach, which becomes thick and rigid (*linitis plastica* or *leather-bottle* stomach). Section of the stomach shows white tumour tissue permeating the wall, particularly along the submucosa and subserosa (Fig. 15.1a).

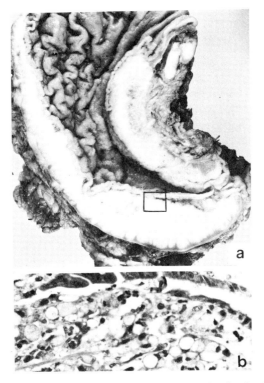

Fig. 15.1 Diffuse infiltrating carcinoma of the stomach ('leather bottle stomach', 'linitis plastica') showing: (a) diffuse thickening of the wall of the stomach by white tissue which mainly involves the submucosa but also penetrates the muscle coat; (b) the area shown in the square in (a) showing the 'signet ring' type cells of the tumour (× 200)

Microscopic appearances

Most carcinomas of the stomach are well-differentiated adeno-carcinomas, some are poorly differentiated or undifferentiated. In the ulcerating type, tumour tissue is present both at the periphery and base of the ulcer and, in this respect, it differs from peptic ulcer which contains granulation tissue at the base. Fungating tumours show a glandular and papillary pattern, whereas the infiltrating carcinomas are usually undifferentiated and associated with varying degrees of fibrosis. Often, a mucin stain is necessary to identify the undifferentiated tumour cells. All types of gastric cancer secrete mucin. Sometimes, the mucin remains within the cells pushing the nucleus to the periphery and giving rise to *signet ring* cells. At other times, it is located extracellularly either within the lumina of glands or in the interstitial tissue (Fig. 15.1b).

Spread
Direct spread may occur along the submucosa towards the oesophagus or duodenum, along perforating vessels to the serosa, through the serosa to the liver and pancreas, portal vein or common bile duct, or to the spleen and transverse colon. Transperitoneal spread may involve the ovaries giving rise to a Krukenberg tumour, or the mesentery and bowel causing a sero-sanguinous ascites. Lymphatic spread occurs early and frequently. The regional nodes are involved in approximately 80 per cent of operated specimens. Spread occurs to the epigastric and coeliac nodes first, and later along the thoracic duct to the left supraclavicular nodes (*Troisier's sign* or *Virchow's node*). Blood spread may occur via the portal vein or thoracic duct and metastases may develop anywhere in the body, especially in the lungs, brain, bone, liver and suprarenal glands.

Prognosis
The outlook of patients with carcinoma of the stomach is poor; less than 10 per cent survive five years. The prognosis in individual cases depends on the type of the tumour (fungating tumours have the best and infiltrating the worst prognosis), on the extent of invasion and on the degree of differentiation.

Leiomyoma
In the stomach, smooth muscle tumours are as common as epithelial polyps. Generally they are small, firm subserosal nodules which often project into the lumen of the stomach, but sometimes they may be intramural or subserosal in position. These small tumours are covered by intact mucosa, produce no symptoms and are discovered incidentally at necropsy or operation. Occasionally, when the tumours are greater than 5 cm in diameter, the overlying mucosa ulcerates and may be responsible for recurrent haemorrhage, anaemia and even pyloric obstruction.

Microscopic appearances

Leiomyomas are well-demarcated from the surrounding tissue but have no capsule. They are composed of spindle-shaped cells arranged in bundles and whorls, intermingled with bundles of fibrocollagenous tissue. It is often difficult to differentiate the muscle cells from fibroblasts, because both stain pink with haematoxylin and eosin. The nuclei of smooth muscle cells are long, thin, blunt-edged and often show palisading, whereas those of fibroblasts are thicker and taper at the ends. Reliable differentiation is possible with special tissue stains such as the van Gieson which stains muscle yellow and collagen red. Distinction between leiomyoma and leiomyosarcoma is not clearcut. The presence of pleomorphic nuclei and increased numbers of mitotic figures indicates a malignant change.

A variant of leiomyoma is composed of bizarre cells which are round or polygonal rather than spindle-shaped. These cells resemble epithelioid cells in that they have pink cytoplasm in haematoxylin and eosin stained sections and are characterized by clear spaces which partially or completely surround the nucleus. Foci showing transitions to typical spindle-shaped smooth muscle cells are frequently present and areas of haemorrhage, necrosis and mucoid change are common. These *bizarre leiomyomas* (epithelioid leiomyomas) are frequently found in the wall of the stomach, but occasionally they occur in the intestine, mesentery or omentum. They vary in size from 1 to 10 cm in diameter and they are usually benign.

TUMOURS OF THE SMALL INTESTINE

Tumours are uncommon in the small bowel; less than 5 per cent of tumours of the gastrointestinal tract occur in this area.

Adenomatous polyp

Pedunculated or sessile polyps occasionally occur in the small intestine but they are rare. More often they are seen in persons with the *Peutz–Jegher's syndrome*, a disease inherited as a Mendelian dominant and characterized by: (a) polyposis of the alimentary tract, particularly the small intestine and (b) melanin pigmentation of the lips, buccal mucosa and digits. The polyps rarely become malignant but they may cause recurrent bleeding or intussusception. They are regarded as hamartomas, not as neoplasms.

Lymphoma

Over 50 per cent of primary malignant tumours in the small intestine are lymphomas. Most of them are single; multiple tumours, when they occur, are often part of a generalized disease. The tumour appears as a grey-white, localized thickening of the bowel wall which causes narrowing of the lumen and may even perforate. All types of malignant lymphomas are seen from the well-differentiated lymphocytic type to the histiocytic and undifferentiated types. Occasionally, Hodgkin's disease involves the small bowel.

Carcinoid tumour

Carcinoid tumours or argentaffinomas may occur anywhere along the gastrointestinal tract from the stomach to the rectum. Their approximate anatomical distribution is as follows:

Site	Frequency (%)
Appendix	65
Ileum	25
Colon	5
Rest	5

They arise from argentaffin cells in the base of the crypts of Lieberkühn and develop in the sub-mucosa. Carcinoids have also been reported in the lungs, gall bladder, Meckel's diverticulum and in teratomas of the ovary.

Macroscopic features
Carcinoids arising in the appendix are usually single and occur near the tip, where they present as a yellow thickening which encircles the lumen. Those arising in the intestines are usually multiple and occur predominantly in the terminal part of the ileum and less frequently in the rectum, colon, stomach and duodenum. Characteristically, they are small, well-circumscribed tumours situated in the submucosa with the overlying mucosa usually intact. Tumour cells tend to infiltrate the muscle coat of the bowel and may involve nearby lymph nodes which are larger than the primary growth. The tumour tissue is firm and turns a bright yellow colour a few minutes after fixation in formalin.

Microscopic features
Typically, carcinoid tumours are composed of solid clumps of

small, closely packed cells. The nuclei are uniform in size, shape and staining affinities with very few mitotic figures present. Often, the peripheral layer of cells in the clumps is palisaded as in the basal cell carcinoma of the skin. The cytoplasm contains numerous granules which have an affinity for silver stains and contain serotonin (5-hydroxytryptamine). Serotonin, in the presence of formaldehyde, is converted to a cyclic compound (β-carbaline) which has a characteristic fluorescence in ultraviolet light and which probably accounts for the yellow colouration of the tumours that develops after formalin fixation.

Course and prognosis

Tumours in the appendix rarely spread, probably because they cause acute appendicitis and are detected early. Intestinal carcinoids, on the other hand, commonly spread to the regional lymph nodes and may invade the blood vessels to metastasize to the liver. Rarely, metastases may be seen in the lungs, brain, skin and bones.

Carcinoid tumours secrete 5-hydroxytryptamine (5-HT). 5-HT secreted by tumours confined to the intestines enters the portal blood and reaches the liver, where it is broken down by the enzyme *monoamine oxidase* to 5-hydroxyindoleaceticacid (5-HIAA), which is excreted in the urine. The estimation of urinary 5-HIAA is used both as a diagnostic test for the detection of carcinoids and as an estimate of the mass of tumour tissue present. The normal rate of excretion of 5-HIAA is 10 to 30 μmols/24 h.

5-HT secreted by liver metastases enters the systemic circulation via the right side of the heart and is responsible for the carcinoid syndrome (headaches, flushing, diarrhoea and a pulmonary stenosis murmur). The most entertaining description of the syndrome was given by Bean and Funk in 1959;

> This man was addicted to moanin',
> Confusion, oedema and groanin',
> Intestinal rushes,
> Great tricoloured blushes,
> And died from too much serotonin.

Carcinoma

Carcinoma of the small bowel is similar to that in the large bowel, except that its incidence is less than one per cent of all malignant tumours in the gastrointestinal tract. Approximately half of these occur in the duodenum where they may obstruct the common bile and pancreatic ducts. The rest occur in the proximal part of the jejunum and distal parts of the ileum where they tend to encircle the bowel producing constriction or obstruction of the lumen. In these cases, the portion of the bowel proximal to the tumour is frequently dilated and hypertrophied.

All carcinomas of the small bowel are moderately well-differentiated adenocarcinomas. They tend to spread early through all layers of the bowel wall to involve the regional lymph nodes. The prognosis, therefore, is usually poor.

TUMOURS OF THE LARGE INTESTINE

Benign tumours	*Malignant tumours*
Adenomatous polyp	Carcinoma
Villous adenoma	Lymphoma
Mixed adenoma	Carcinoid tumour
Juvenile polyp	
Hereditary polyposis	

Benign tumours

Polyps are common tumours in the colon; their incidence increases with age reaching a peak at 60 years, when they are found in approximately 20 per cent of the population. Occasionally, they are found in children (juvenile polyps) and may cause bleeding. Most of them occur in the rectum with the sigmoid colon, descending colon, transverse colon and caecum in descending order of frequency. Three main morphological types are recognized:

1. *Adenomatous polyp (Tubular adenoma)*. This is the commonest type of benign tumour. Macroscopically, it resembles a raspberry being approximately 1 cm in diameter, soft, red and attached to the colonic mucosa by a stalk of variable length. The stalk is composed of a central core of connective tissue which is an extension of the muscularis mucosa and submucosa of the colon and which is lined by normal or hyperplastic mucosa. The head of the polyp is also lined by normal or hyperplastic mucosa which branches out and forms deep crypts (Fig. 15.2).

2. *Villous adenoma (Villous papilloma)* is a sessile papillary tumour attached to the colonic mucosa by a broad base. It is less frequent than the pedunculated adenoma but larger, ranging from 4 to 6 cm in diameter. Microscopically, it is composed of elongated villi which are individually attached to the mucosa of the colon and lined by tall, mucus-secreting columnar cells. The epithelial cells rest on the muscularis mucosa and secrete copious amounts of mucin rich in potassium.

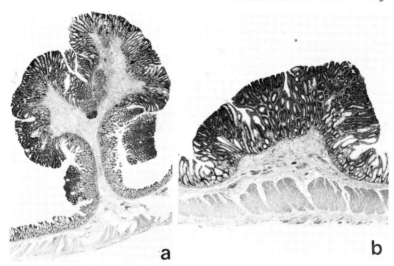

Fig. 15.2 Polyps of the large intestine showing: (a) benign pedunculated polyp attached to the wall of the colon by a stalk or pedicle; (b) benign sessile polyp attached by a broad base. Both polyps are lined by a regular form of epithelium which is clearly demarcated from the submucosa by a well-defined muscularis mucosa (× 5)

3. *Mixed adenoma (Tubulo-villous)*. This variety of polyp is intermediate in frequency and in histological features between the adenomatous polyp and the villous adenoma. It is composed of both tubular and papillary structures, hence the term *mixed*.

4. *Hereditary polyposis coli* is a well-established precursor of carcinoma. It is a rare autosomal disease carried by either parent and transmitted as a Mendelian dominant. Both sexes are equally affected. When one parent carries the defect, half the children will inherit and transmit the disease, the other half cannot transmit it. Tumours develop in postnatal life and symptoms appear before the age of 20 years. The polyps are common in the rectum and colon, but occasionally, they may extend to the small intestine, and even to the stomach. Macroscopically, the mucosa is studded with small pedunculated polyps. If polyps have not appeared by the age of 40 years, it is unlikely that they will develop. However, when present, malignancy invariably supervenes.

Carcinoma of the colon and rectum
Carcinoma of the colon and rectum is one of the major cancers in industrialized communities. Statistical studies show a steady

increase in frequency, the incidence approaching that of carcinoma of the lung. Every nation, race and social class is affected by this disease; the English-speaking countries, Denmark and Belgium have a particularly high incidence (40 to 50 per 100 000 population), whereas in Japan the incidence is low (5 per 100 000). In the rectum, carcinoma is twice as common in males as in females, but in the rest of the colon, the sexes are equally affected. The peak incidence of carcinoma of the colon lies between 50 and 80 years.

Aetiology
Several studies on the causation of carcinoma of the colon are being conducted, but the variables involved are many and complex. So far, dietary factors appear to play a predominant role and certain high risk factors have been established.

1. *Dietary factors.* The large intestine contains an enormous population of metabolically active bacteria which have the capacity to produce carcinogens from food residues or from intestinal secretions that reach the colon. For example, the incidence of colorectal cancer is higher in those countries where the diet has a high content of fat, or fat combined with protein, than in those where the fat intake is low. High-fat/low-residue diets, common in affluent societies, prolong the transit time of food through the gastrointestinal tract and increase the contact time of faecal products with the mucosa. Fat in the diet also stimulates the secretion of bile, and the bile acids have a chemical structure resembling that of the polycyclic aromatic hydrocarbons which are well known to produce cancer in many sites. The likely steps by which intestinal bacteria can change bile salts to partially degraded polycyclic hydrocarbons have been elucidated. Comparison of faeces from people living in different countries has shown a striking correlation between the concentration of partially degraded bile acids and the reported incidence of colorectal cancer. Patients with colonic cancer have high concentrations of bile acid degradation products and high concentrations of *clostridium paraputrificum* which are responsible for the breakdown of bile acids.

2. *Polyps.* Most carcinomas of the colon are malignant from the start. Some, however, arise in pre-existing polyps. According to Morson, the three types of colonic polyps vary in both their frequency and their relationship to cancer. Polyposis coli is included in the list.

	Frequency (%)	Malignant potential (%)
Adenomatous polyp	75	15
Villous adenoma	10	40
Mixed type adenoma	15	20
Hereditary polyposis coli	rare	100

Apart from histological type, the malignant potential of a polyp varies with size and epithelial atypia. The risk of cancer being present in a given polyp rises significantly with increasing size over 1 cm, polyps less than 1 cm in diameter being rarely malignant. The degree of epithelial atypia may be graded into mild, moderate or severe. Mild atypia is common and frequently seen in adenomatous polyps, which have a low malignant potential, whereas severe atypia is uncommon, often seen in villous adenomas and probably accounts for the higher malignant potential of these

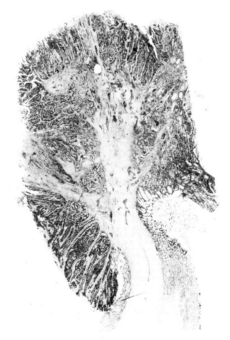

Fig. 15.3 Malignant pedunculated polyp of the colon showing early invasion of the stalk ($\times 5$)

tumours. Malignancy is determined only when there is unequivocal evidence of invasion across the line of the muscularis mucosa (Fig. 15.3).

3. *Ulcerative colitis* may also be of aetiological significance in carcinoma of the colon. There is general agreement that the overall risk of developing cancer is approximately 10 times greater in patients with ulcerative colitis than in the general population. This increased risk depends on three major factors: (a) the duration of the disease (after 10.years the risk progressively increases), (b) the extent of the disease (patients with pancolitis are at greater risk), and (c) the severity of the disease (patients that respond well to treatment and have long periods of remission are less likely to develop cancer than those that do not respond).

Macroscopic features
As in the stomach, carcinoma of the colon may assume three forms:

1. Fungating or polypoid
2. Ulcerating
3. Infiltrating or stenosing

Approximately 50 per cent of cancers occur in the rectum where they are equally divided between upper, middle and lower thirds, 25 per cent occur in the sigmoid colon and the rest are equally distributed in the ascending, transverse and descending colon. This anatomical distribution is statistically important, since 50 per cent of colorectal cancers can be reached with the examining finger and 75 per cent with the sigmoidoscope. In the rectum, the majority of cancers are of the ulcerating type. The stenosing type is more common in the descending colon, where it usually produces obstruction early because of the narrowing of the lumen and the solid consistency of the faeces at this site. Proximal to the obstruction, the pressure of inspissated faeces may cause ulceration of the mucosa (*stercoral ulcer*). The fungating variety which is more common in the caecum and ascending colon tends to cause recurrent occult bleeding and often presents late as an iron deficiency anaemia.

Microscopic features
The vast majority of carcinomas of the colon are well-differentiated adenocarcinomas. Occasionally, undifferentiated mucus-secreting carcinomas may occur in which the mucin may be intracellular (signet ring type) or extracellular and copious giving rise to a mucoid carcinoma.

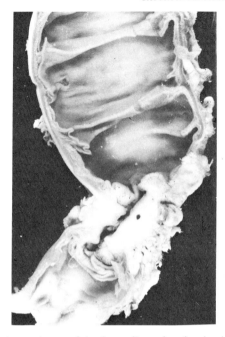

Fig. 15.4 Annular carcinoma of the descending colon showing invasion through the wall. The bowel above the growth is dilated and the wall thickened

Spread

Spread in carcinoma of the colon is generally slow, so that the tumour is confined to the bowel wall for a long time. Initially, spread is direct through the submucosa, muscle coat and serosa to involve the pericolic fat and adjacent organs (Fig. 15.5). Direct spread may lead to fistula or abscess formation. Lymphatic spread first occurs at the regional nodes and later to the aortic and caeliac nodes. The extent of lymphatic spread is important to the surgeon in planning surgical procedures. In carcinoma of the rectum, lymphatic spread is proximally along the superior rectal vessels which drain near the bifurcation of the common iliac arteries. When the superior rectal lymph nodes are blocked, downward or retrograde spread to the middle and inferior rectal lymphatics may occur and may involve the inguinal nodes. Blood spread to the liver via the portal vein is usually a late event. Occasionally, metastases to the ovaries may occur in females.

Course and prognosis

The tumour is resectable in over 80 per cent of patients, but the

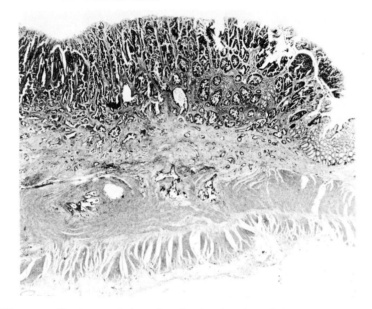

Fig. 15.5 Carcinoma of the colon showing invasion of the submucosa and infiltration of the muscle coat (× 5)

prognosis is dependent on the extent of local and lymphatic spread. Cuthbert Dukes has classified operative specimens of carcinoma of the colon into three major types according to pathological findings and the five-year survival rate. This is a convenient and accurate method of assessing the prognosis of individual cases:

		Operated Cases (%)	Five-year survival rate (%)
Type A	Spread confined to wall; not beyond the muscularis; no lymphatic spread.	15	95
Type B	Spread beyond muscle coat to pericolic and perirectal tissues. No lymphatic node spread	35	70
Type C	Lymphatic node spread	50	30

FURTHER READING

Lane, M. & Savage, H. (1975) Clinical application of the carcinoembryonic antigen (CEA) test. *Methods in Cancer Research*, **11**, 267.
Louis, C. J. (1957) A study of carcinoma of the colon, using an histochemical technique. *Aust. & N.Z. J. Surg.*, **27**, 146.

Martinez, I. (1969) Factors associated with cancer of the oesophagus, mouth and pharynx in Puerto Rico. *J. Nat. Cancer Inst.*, **42**, 1069.

Merlis, R. R. (1971) Talc-treated rice and Japanese stomach cancer. *Science*, **173**, 1141.

Ming, Si-Chun (1973) *Tumours of the Oesophagus and Stomach*, Fascicle 7, Second Series, Washington D.C.: Armed Forces Institute of Pathology.

Morson, B. C. (1974) Evolution of cancer of the colon and rectum. *Cancer*, **34**, 845.

Morson, B. C. (1976) *International Histological Classification of Tumours No. 15: Histological Typing of Intestinal Tumours*. Geneva: World Health Organization.

Morson, B. C. & Dawson, I. M. P. (1972) *Gastrointestinal Pathology*. Oxford: Blackwell Scientific Publications.

Overholt, B. F. (1975) Progress in gastroenterology: Colonoscopy. *Gastroenterology*, **68**, 1308.

Silberman, H. *et al.* (1974) Neoplasms of the small bowel. *Ann. Surg.*, **180**, 157.

16

Tumours of the liver, gall bladder and pancreas

TUMOURS OF THE LIVER

Benign tumours

Benign tumours of the liver are rare. They have no clinical significance because they are symptomless and only found incidentally at post mortem examination: most are developmental in origin or hamartomas and not true tumours. Recent studies indicate that liver-cell adenomas are becoming more common in females and have been associated with taking oral contraceptive hormones.

1. *Cavernous haemangioma* is the most common benign tumour in the liver. It is small (1 to 2 cm in diameter), well circumscribed, dark purple in colour and usually found just below the capsule near the anterior margin of the liver. It is really a localized telangiectasis consisting of a mesh of spaces lined by endothelium and filled with blood.

2. *Benign adenomas* may be single or multiple. They may arise either from the parenchymal cells of the liver (*hepatocellular adenoma*) or from the cells lining the intrahepatic bile ducts (*bile-duct adenomas*). The bile duct adenomas are usually multiple, well defined, grey-white nodules and consist of small, well differentiated bile ducts supported on a fibrous connective tissue stroma.

Primary carcinoma

Carcinoma is the most important primary tumour of the liver. It shows extreme variation in frequency in different countries and different races. For example, in the Bantu race in South Africa, liver cancer is the commonest form of malignancy and is found in 15 per cent to 20 per cent of all necropsies; Philipinos, Chinese and Javanese also show a very high frequency; the European countries, North America, Australia and New Zealand have the lowest incidence (0.1 per cent to 0.6 per cent of all necropsies).

In the liver, carcinoma may arise either from the hepatocytes or the cells lining the bile ducts. Thus two main types are recognized:

1. *Hepatocellular or liver-cell carcinoma.* This is the more common type, it accounts for over 80 per cent of all primary liver tumours, occurs predominantly in the male and is frequently associated with cirrhosis.

2. *Bile-duct or cholangiocarcinoma* is uncommon, it affects older people, occurs with equal frequency in the two sexes and is rarely associated with cirrhosis.

Aetiology

Surveys amongst some of the indigenous population of South Africa have shown that the most common form of malignancy is carcinoma of the liver, whereas in the white population living in the same geographical and climatic environment, the most common sites of malignancy are the stomach and colon. It is generally believed that these differences are basically due to diet, habits and customs. However, other factors such as exposure to carcinogens, cirrhosis, hepatitis B infection and parasitic infections also contribute to the development of this malignancy.

1. *Exposure to carcinogens.* Several naturally occurring compounds such as cycasin, senecio, pyrolyzodine alkaloids and the mycotoxins (p. 49), are known to be potent hepatocarcinogens in animals. These compounds may also have some relevance in the production of liver cancer in man. Aflatoxin exposure undoubtedly occurs, and the high incidence of liver cancer in some African countries is compatible with the consumption of food contaminated with this fungus. The extensive use of oral contraceptives is becoming more and more implicated in the induction of hepatic adenoma, but not in the induction of carcinoma. Ionizing radiations are a rare cause nowadays, since the withdrawal of thorotrast as a contrast medium for cholangiography.

2. *Relation to cirrhosis.* A distinct association has been established between cirrhosis and primary hepatocellular carcinoma. This association is mainly with macronodular cirrhosis (postnecrotic cirrhosis and the cirrhosis of haemochromatosis), and represents over 80 per cent of hepatocellular cancers. The fatty type of micronodular cirrhosis found in chronic alcoholics is not associated with a high incidence of liver cancer. No relationship exists between cirrhosis and bile-duct cancer. The nature of the relationship between cirrhosis and liver cancer is not clear. In experimental animals, it has been shown that the same agents are capable of

causing both disease processes, and it is possible that the same sequence of events occur in man. Carcinogens, being toxic substances, would first give rise to cirrhosis, and much later, to malignancy, which requires a long latent period.

Cirrhotic patients carry a significantly high risk of developing primary liver cancer. This risk is dependent partly on the morphological type of cirrhosis and partly on the country where the patient is residing. For example, a European with cirrhosis residing in Europe runs a 10 per cent risk of developing liver cancer whereas a Bantu residing in South Africa may run a risk of over 40 per cent.

3. *Relation to hepatitis B virus.* Hepatitis B has a long incubation period. Hepatitis B antigen (HBAg) can be readily detected in the serum of carriers, and it is generally accepted that this antigen is a marker for the presence of the virus. Field studies in Uganda, for example, where there is a high incidence of liver cancer, have shown that HBAg is present in 3 per cent of the normal population (young males are more commonly positive), in 30 per cent of patients with cirrhosis and in over 40 per cent of patients with primary liver cancer. Although these figures are significant and appear to implicate hepatitis B virus in the aetiology of hepatocellular carcinoma, the evidence is only circumstantial.

4. *Parasitic infection.* The Chinese liver fluke, *Clonorchis sinensis*, is associated with a very high incidence of cholangiocarcinoma in certain endemic areas. The parasite resides in the medium-sized intrahepatic bile ducts and induces epithelial proliferation, mucin secretion, and eventually a mucin-secreting adenocarcinoma develops. It is interesting that a high incidence of cholangiocarcinoma is also found in the domestic cat in endemic areas. Like the human, the cat is a definitive host for the parasite.

Macroscopic appearances
Primary carcinomas of the liver, both hepatocellular and bile-duct varieties, may assume one of three macroscopic types:

1. *Multinodular carcinoma* is the most common type. It consists of numerous nodules which may be difficult to distinguish from secondary deposits. The nodules vary in size from 0.5 to 4 cm in diameter and often project above the capsular surface. Their multiplicity suggests a multifocal origin of the tumour.

2. *Solitary massive carcinoma* is an expanding, large, soft tumour with areas of necrosis and haemorrhage. It is usually found in the right lobe of the liver, and is often accompanied by small, peripheral, satellite nodules.

3. *Diffuse carcinoma* is the least common type. It is an infiltrating growth, indistinguishable macroscopically from cirrhosis, and can only be recognized histologically.

In general, the hepatocellular carcinomas are soft haemorrhagic masses which may or may not be bile-stained. They tend to invade veins and cause thrombosis of the portal and hepatic veins. Bile duct carcinoma, on the other hand, is a tough, scirrhous type of growth. It spreads mainly by lymphatics and death usually results from carcinomatosis.

Histological features

1. *Hepatocellular carcinoma* is composed of hepatocytes of varying degrees of differentiation. In the well differentiated variety, the cells resemble normal liver cells and tend to be arranged in a trabecular pattern, simulating normal liver architecture. Intracellular and intracannalicular bile pigment may be present. The stroma consists of blood capillaries and is usually sparse. In the less differentiated type, the cells vary considerably in size and shape; they may be small, spindle-shaped, large or they may form giant cells. Venous invasion is common. The adjacent liver is frequently cirrhotic (Fig. 16.1a).

2. *Bile-duct carcinoma* is a mucus-secreting adenocarcinoma. It is composed of irregular-shaped glands separated by a fibrous connective tissue stroma which tends to form collagen bundles. The glands contain mucin, but no bile, and they cannot be distinguished from metastatic mucin-secreting adenocarcinomas. The adjacent liver is rarely cirrhotic (Fig. 16.1b).

Course and prognosis

Primary carcinoma of the liver has no characteristic symptomatology to enable early diagnosis. Most cases are associated with cirrhosis, which gives rise to clinical and biochemical findings of underlying liver disease. Other manifestations of carcinoma of the liver are hypoglycaemia and bleeding disorders. The antigen a_1-foetoprotein (p. 91) is present in approximately 75 per cent of cases.

The prognosis of adult patients with hepatocellular cancer is generally poor, the overall five-year survival rate being less than five per cent. In children with hepatoblastoma, the prognosis is good because these tumours are resectable. In cholangiocarcinoma, survival beyond one year after diagnosis is rare. Most patients die of widespread metastases and superimposed infections such as cholangitis, liver abscesses and bronchopneumonia; some die of portal hypertension and hepatic failure.

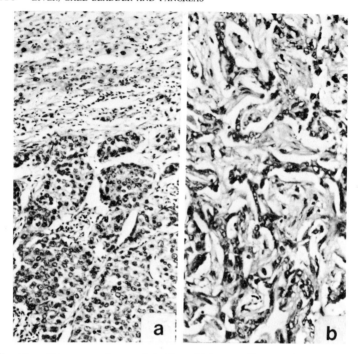

Fig. 16.1   Primary carcinoma of the liver: (a) hepatocellular carcinoma showing differentiation into liver cords (× 120); (b) cholangiocarcinoma showing differentiation towards bile duct type of adenocarcinoma (× 120)

TUMOURS OF THE GALL BLADDER AND MAJOR BILE DUCTS

Benign tumours

Benign tumours are rare in both the gall bladder and main bile ducts. The most common are:

1. *Adenoma*, which is a flat tumour composed of well differentiated biliary epithelium.

2. *Papilloma* which is a pedunculated polypoid growth made up of fronds or papillae consisting of a fibrovascular core covered by biliary epithelium.

Both adenoma and papilloma are commoner in the gall bladder than in the ducts. In the gall bladder, they are usually found in the fundus as small nodules approximately 1 cm in diameter. The adenoma is usually single, but the papilloma can be multiple. Although they are not precursors of malignancy, they should be distinguished from the following more common conditions: (a) *adenomyoma* of the gall bladder which is not a true neoplasm but a malformation composed of a mixture of glands and smooth muscle; it occurs in the fundus of the gall bladder as a small thickening which may simulate an adenoma, and (b) *pseudopolyp,* which is composed of granulation tissue or cholesterol accumulation; epithelial proliferation is absent.

Carcinoma

The most common malignant tumour of the gall bladder and major bile ducts is carcinoma. Soft tissue sarcoma, lymphoma and melanoma are extremely rare and will not be discussed. Carcinoma occurs mainly in the gall bladder and its incidence varies in different reports: in Britain and the U.S.A., carcinoma of the gall bladder accounts for less than one per cent of all cancer deaths and is three times more frequent in women than men, whereas duct carcinoma is less frequent (0.5 per cent of all cancer deaths) and affects the sexes equally. Biliary tract carcinoma is predominantly a disease of elderly people, the peak incidence being in the sixth and seventh decades.

Aetiology

Gall stones have been implicated, by association, as aetiological factors in the development of carcinoma of the gall bladder, and the male/female ratio of gall stones is compatible with the incidence of cancer of the gall bladder in the two sexes. The significance of this relationship is not clear and attempts to induce cancer in animals by implanting gall stones in the gall bladder have not been successful. Implants of pellets of 20-methylcholanthrene do give rise to carcinoma, and it is possible that cholesterol might be converted to 20-methylcholanthrene as a result of abnormal metabolism.

Macroscopic appearance

Most carcinomas of the gall bladder occur in the fundus, either as papillary growths or as scirrhous, infiltrating tumours. They usually invade the liver and neighbouring structures very early, and often infiltrate the cystic or common bile duct, resulting in cholecystitis and cholangitis. Very few carcinomas of the gall bladder are discovered in their preinvasive stage. In practice, therefore, it is more common to see advanced gall bladder cancers in which the whole organ is infiltrated by tumour tissue, and when this occurs, the site of origin of the tumour is difficult to determine.

Duct carcinomas are more common in the distal part of the

common bile duct and in the common hepatic duct, and are mostly of infiltrating type. Unlike carcinoma of the gall bladder, duct carcinomas produce early and progressive obstructive jaundice, so that extensive infiltration of the surrounding structures is not a common finding at operation. These tumours are easily confused with carcinoma of the head of the pancreas because of their close anatomical relationship (Fig. 16.2).

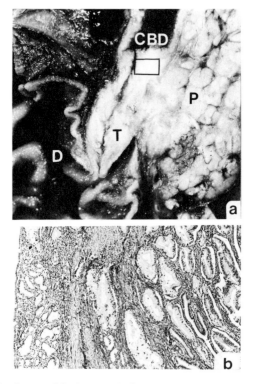

Fig. 16.2 Carcinoma of the lower end of the common bile duct showing: (a) the relationship of the tumour (T) to the common bile duct (CBD), duodenum (D) and pancreas (P); (b) the area in the square in (a) showing the lining of the duct and normal submucous glands on the left, and well-differentiated adenocarcinoma on the right (× 40)

Tumours arising in the large hepatic ducts, near the hilum, tend to infiltrate the undersurface of the liver. Those originating in the medium-sized ducts, along the course of portal tracts, are usually multicentric, appearing as whitish nodules which simulate metastatic carcinoma.

Histological features

Most carcinomas of the biliary tract are mucin-secreting adeno-carcinomas showing various degrees of differentiation. The following histological types are seen:

1. *Mucus-secreting adenocarcinoma* is the most common type. The tumour cells arrange to form well-differentiated glands containing mucin and surrounded by moderate amounts of fibrous stroma. Rarely, tumour cells may undergo squamous metaplasia with keratin production, a characteristic often retained in the metastatic lesions (*adenoacanthoma*).

2. *Signet-ring carcinoma* consists of cells distended with mucin, and the nucleus is pushed to the periphery of the cell giving the appearance of signet-rings.

3. *Mucoid carcinoma* produces a lot of mucin. It consists of single cells or cords of tumour cells which appear to be floating in a lake of mucin.

4. *Undifferentiated carcinoma* shows no specific pattern. It is commonly seen in the small diffuse cholangiocarcinomas, especially those associated with liver fluke infestation.

5. *Squamous-cell carcinoma* may also occur, but it is exclusive to the gall bladder. It accounts for two to three per cent of all biliary tract cancers.

Spread

Biliary tract carcinomas spread in a characteristic way; they rapidly invade adjacent structures, and metastasize to regional lymph nodes early and frequently. Gall bladder carcinomas often infiltrate the wall diffusely, resulting in contraction and induration of the organ. The regional lymph nodes are often involved and peritoneal seedings are common, but visceral metastases are infrequent. Duct carcinomas metastasize less frequently. Because of their strategic location, they give rise to obstructive jaundice enabling early diagnosis and treatment.

Course and prognosis

The most common presenting complaints of biliary tract cancers are epigastric pain, progressive jaundice, and often, considerable loss in body weight. Carcinoma of the gall bladder may produce symptoms indistinguishable from those of gall stones. Duct carcinomas often cause acute obstructive jaundice, and the gall bladder may become distended and palpable (*Courvoisier's law*). This is in contrast to jaundice produced by stones in the common bile duct, in which the gall bladder is small and contracted due to associated chronic inflammation. A correct diagnosis of duct carcinoma can only be made at operation because pancreatic tumours also give rise to similar signs and symptoms.

Gall bladder and duct carcinomas have a better prognosis than cholangiocarcinomas, but five year survivals are still rare. Occasionally, a patient with early cancer in the gall bladder may be cured when the lesion is incidentally removed in conjunction with gall stones.

TUMOURS OF THE PANCREAS

Tissue	Tumour
Exocrine	Cystadenoma
	Carcinoma
Endocrine	α-cell tumour
(Islet-cell tumours)	β-cell tumour
	δ-cell tumour

Tumours of the pancreas can be either of exocrine or endocrine origin. Exocrine tumours are far more common and account for approximately 10 per cent of all abdominal malignancies. Interestingly enough, all arise from the ductal epithelium; the acini do not appear to undergo malignant change.

Cystadenoma

This is a rare benign tumour, usually cystic and commonly occurring in the tail of the pancreas. It is made up of multilocular spaces filled with clear or gelatinous fluid. Microscopically, the spaces are lined by simple cuboidal or flattened epithelium which may form papillary projections. Rarely, a malignant cystadeno-carcinoma may occur.

Carcinoma

Carcinoma is the most common tumour of the pancreas. The highest incidence occurs between the ages of 50 and 70 years. It is more common in males than in females and it is extremely rare before the age of 40 years. Over 70 per cent of these tumours occur in the head of the pancreas, since the head represents the bulk of the organ. The remainder are equally distributed in the body and tail. Because of the close anatomical relationship of these tumours to the common bile duct, painless and progressively obstructive jaundice is an early and characteristic symptom. In carcinomas arising in the body and tail, symptoms of pain and wasting appear rather late in the disease, and the tumours are usually inoperable when diagnosed.

Macroscopic features
Characteristically, pancreatic carcinoma is firm with ill-defined borders and the cut surface usually shows haemorrhagic and necrotic foci. Tumours arising in the head of the pancreas may be very small (1 cm in diameter), while those arising in the body and tail are usually larger (10 to 15 cm in diameter). Since these tumours, especially those in the head, often impinge upon the common bile duct and large pancreatic ducts, secondary changes such as biliary ectasia and pancreatic acinar atrophy are common. Microscopically, they are all adenocarcinomas, some of which are scirrhous. Perineural invasion, and metastases to regional lymph nodes and liver are common.

The prognosis of pancreatic adenocarcinomas is extremely poor, because early diagnosis is difficult. Most patients die within one year and about 50 per cent of them die within six months. Surgically, the most hopeful tumour is one arising at the *ampulla of vater*.

Islet-cell tumours
All three types of cells (a-, β- and δ-cells) found in the islets of Langerhans are capable of giving rise to tumours, but such tumours are rare. In general, islet cell tumours may be single or multiple, and are usually small, spherical and encapsulated. They are more common in the body and tail than in the head of the pancreas, and occasionally, are found in aberrant locations (ectopic pancreas). The colour of the tumours varies from pinkish-red to yellow, depending on the amount of stromal fibrosis and hyalinization. In approximately 30 per cent of cases, multiple lesions are present and are associated with tumours in other endocrine organs (pituitary, parathyroid, adrenal and thyroid glands). Islet cell tumours may be functional or non-functional; the hormones they secrete are not controlled by the normal regulatory mechanism.

Histologically, they are composed of ribbons or cords of rather uniform cells. The precise identification of the cell type requires a combination of light microscopy, electron microscopy, immuno-fluorescence and hormone assay techniques. Both benign and malignant forms of islet cell tumours exist, but as with most other endocrine tumours, the usual cytological criteria for malignancy are not adequate to establish a diagnosis.

1. *β-Cell tumour* is the most common benign islet-cell tumour of the pancreas. It affects both sexes of all ages, from infancy to old age. Functional β-cell tumours release insulin at an uncontrolled rate resulting in severe hypoglycaemia which characteristically occurs in the morning, before breakfast. Whipple, in 1937, described three salient features in the manifestation of this tumour and considered that all three should be present in order to make a diagnosis. These features are: (a) an attack of hypoglycaemia should be precipitated by fasting and exercise, (b) during an attack, the blood sugar level should drop to 2.5 m mol/l or below, and (c) there should be prompt relief of symptoms by ingestion of glucose. Special cytoplasmic granules can be demonstrated in the β-cells with aldehyde-fuchsin stains. Approximately 10 per cent of β-cell tumours are malignant.

2. *a-Cell tumour* is very rare. It produces large amounts of glucagon which is responsible for the *hyperglucagon syndrome* (diabetes mellitus, anaemia and a skin rash).

3. *δ-Cell tumour* secretes excessive amounts of gastrin and is sometimes called a *gastrinoma*. High levels of blood gastrin cause increase in the parietal-cell mass which, in turn, is responsible for hypersecretion of hydrochloric acid, recurrent peptic ulceration in unusual locations, and frequently, diarrhoea and steatorrhoea. This complex is known as the *Zollinger–Ellison syndrome*. The tumours are often multiple, they may occur in aberrant locations such as the duodenum. Over 50 per cent of them are malignant and have metastases in the regional lymph nodes.

FURTHER READING

Becker, W. F. (1965) Cystadenoma and cystadenocarcinoma of the pancreas. *Ann. Surg.*, **161**, 845.

Beltz, W. R. & Gordon, R. E. (1974) Primary carcinoma of the gall bladder. *Ann. Surg.*, **180**, 180.

Douglas, H. D. & Holyoke, E. D. (1974) Pancreatic cancer. *J.A.M.A.*, **229**, 793.

Fechner, R. E. (1977) Benign hepatic lesions and orally administered contraceptives: A report on seven cases and a critical analysis of the literature. *Human Pathology*, **8**, 255.

Henson, S. W. et al. (1956) Benign tumours of the liver: I. Adenomas. *Surg. Gynecol. Obstet.*, **103**, 23.

Linder, G. T. et al. (1974) Primary liver carcinoma. *Cancer*, **33**, 1624.

Makk, L. et al. (1974) Liver damage and angiosarcoma in vinyl chloride workers. *J.A.M.A.*, **230**, 64.

Nevin, J. E. *et al.* (1976) Carcinoma of the gall bladder – staging, treatment and prognosis. *Cancer.*, **37**, 141.

Van Heerden, J. A. *et al.* (1967) Carcinoma of the extrahepatic ducts. *Am. J. Surg.*, **113**, 49.

Vogel, C. L. *et al.* (1974) Serum alpha-foetoprotein in 184 Ugandan patients with hepatocellular carcinoma. *Cancer*, **33**, 959.

17

Tumours of the lung

Most primary tumours of the lung arise from bronchial epithelium, and of these, the overwhelming majority are bronchogenic carcinomas. Other tumours, such as chondromas, fibromas, haemangiomas and hamartomas also occur, but they are rare and will not be discussed. Metastatic deposits are very common, and in fact, are the commonest malignant tumours in the lungs. The following classification lists the variety of primary lung tumours and the approximate frequency of each type:

Tumour	*Frequency* (%)
Bronchogenic carcinoma	
1. Squamous-cell carcinoma	65
(a) Well differentiated	
(b) Poorly differentiated	
2. Undifferentiated carcinoma	18
(a) Small-cell type (*oat-cell*)	
(b) Large-cell type	
(c) Giant-cell type	
3. Adenocarcinoma	8
(a) Acinar	
(b) Papillary	
Bronchiolar (bronchoalveolar) carcinoma	2
Bronchial adenoma (carcinoid tumour)	5
Mesothelioma	1
Others	1

Bronchogenic carcinoma
Early in this century, lung cancer was regarded as a rarity, but during the last 50 years, there has been such an alarming increase in the incidence of the disease that it is now the leading form of cancer affecting man. Indeed, the challenge of lung cancer to preventive medicine still remains unabated and the disease continues to increase annually. The highest mortality figures (40 to

70 per 100 000) have been recorded in the United Kingdom, Finland, Austria and Belgium, the lowest (5 to 10 per 100 000) in Japan, Portugal and Yugoslavia. Both morbidity and mortality of lung cancer are five times more common in males than in females, with a peak in the 50 to 70 year age group.

Aetiology

There appears to be no single aetiological agent responsible for bronchogenic carcinoma. The increase in mortality that has been demonstrated in various parts of the world has been associated with the introduction of carcinogenic agents in the respiratory environment. A careful study of the environment has revealed three major groups of factors in connection with the aetiology of lung cancer. In order of importance these are: cigarette smoking, atmospheric pollution and industrial hazards.

1. *Cigarette smoking.* Prospective studies following cohorts of individuals with different smoking habits and observing the causes of their deaths, have demonstrated that the risk of dying from lung cancer was closely related to the amount of smoking. The results of these studies showed that: (a) lung cancer is rare among non-smokers, (b) the risk among those who continued smoking was proportional to the number of cigarettes smoked daily, (c) the risk among cigar and pipe smokers was less than that of cigarette smokers but greater than that of non-smokers, and (d) those who inhale, those who smoke each cigarette to the very end and those who commence smoking at an early age are at greatest risk.

Apart from statistical evidence, the association between smoking and lung cancer rests on the identification of carcinogens such as benzo(a)pyrene in cigarette smoke, and on the demonstration that smoking induces high levels of aryl hydrocarbon hydroxylase (AHH) activity in some human tissues. AHH metabolizes benzo(a)-pyrene to an ultimate carcinogen, and this has led to the proposal that smoking causes high concentrations of active carcinogenic metabolites in target cells which subsequently give rise to cancer. However, benzo(a)pyrene is present only in trace amounts in cigarette smoke, and the possible importance of raised AHH levels in bronchogenic carcinogenesis in man is somewhat weakened by the failure to demonstrate AHH in bronchial epithelium. Furthermore, no one has been able to induce convincing invasive carcinoma in experimental animals by inhalation of cigarette smoke alone. There is probably no single aetiological agent in cigarette smoke responsible for bronchogenic carcinoma. Rather, the causation is most likely multifactorial.

2. *Atmospheric pollution* from industrial and motor car exhausts has long been considered significant in the development of lung cancer. The air in large cities contains many carcinogens, such as benzo(a)pyrene, arsenious oxide, coal tar fumes, petroleum oil mists and traces of radioactive substances. There is a fairly close relationship between the number of registered road vehicles and the incidence of lung cancer. Indeed, urban residents have a greater liability to the development of lung cancer than rural residents, even after correction for smoking.

3. *Occupational hazards* are responsible for a small but important subgroup of lung cancers. Once the association is recognized the carcinogens can be identified and adequate measures can be instituted to protect the worker. A variety of occupational hazards are known: radioactive dust in uranium and cobalt mines, asbestos, nickel, chromate, arsenic, beryllium and various tar compounds.

Macroscopic appearances
Lung cancer may arise in the central (perihilar region) or peripheral parts of the lung (Fig. 17.1).

1. Approximately 80 per cent are located centrally in a main bonchus or one of its branches, more commonly on the right lung. The majority of tumours arise as warty or ulcerating mucosal outgrowths, and at an early stage, tend to obstruct the bronchial lumen and invade the bronchial wall and surrounding lung tissue. The hilar nodes are often involved. When the tumour obstructs a major bronchus the lung distal to the obstruction collapses, and infection may set in, causing pneumonia, suppuration, fibrosis or bronchiectasis. Extension of the infection may cause pleurisy or empyema.

2. Peripheral lung cancers arise in small bronci or bronchioles, often in relation to scars. The centre of the mass may contain a dark anthracotic scar while the periphery of the tumour grows out into the surrounding lung presenting an irregular edge. Peripheral tumours may attain a very large size without producing a significant degree of atelectasis. Necrosis in these tumours may give rise to carcinomatous lung abscess.

Microscopic appearances
From a practical standpoint, three main histological types of bronchogenic carcinoma, which vary in frequency and sex incidence, are recognized. These are as follows:

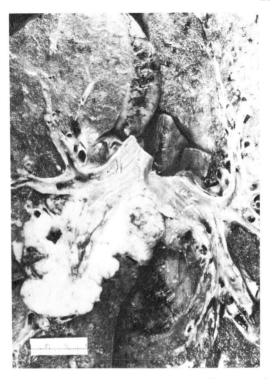

Fig. 17.1 Primary carcinoma of the lung arising centrally, obstructing the main bronchus and invading the wall and peribronchial tissues. There is spread to the hilar nodes

	Frequency (%)	Male/Female ratio
Squamous-cell carcinoma	70	6:1
Undifferentiated carcinoma	20	6:1
Adenocarcinoma	10	1.5:1

1. *Squamous-cell carcinoma* of the lung shows the complete range of appearances that are seen in squamous-cell carcinomas of other organs. Some are well differentiated and show intercellular prickles and keratin formation, others are poorly differentiated and may be difficult to recognize because they tend to merge with the undifferentiated large-cell type. Squamous-cell carcinomas are frequently associated with squamous metaplasia of the adjacent bronchial mucosa and it is probable that most of them arise in these areas. Approximately 90 per cent of squamous-cell carcinomas

of the lung are attributable to cigarette smoking (Fig. 17.2).

2. *Undifferentiated carcinoma* is one in which no squamous epi-thelium or glandular structures can be demonstrated. Three sub-types are recognized: (a) Small-cell type (oat-cell carcinoma) which is the second most common type of lung cancer and which is attributed to smoking and to individuals exposed to large doses of carcinogens. Histologically, it is composed of sheets of closely packed cells of the size of small lymphocytes with hyperchromatic nuclei, very little cytoplasm and indistinct cell outlines. The nuclei may be round, oval or spindle-shaped. Areas of necrosis are common within these tumours; (b) large-cell type, which is

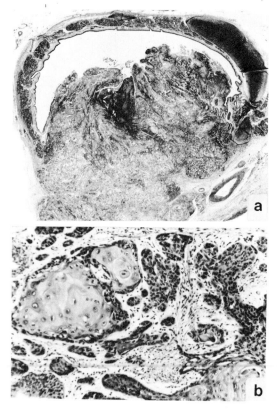

Fig. 17.2 Bronchogenic carcinoma showing: (a) invasion through bronchial wall and obstruction of lumen (× 5); (b) photomicrograph of the tumour in (a) showing a well-differentiated, keratinizing squamous-cell carcinoma

composed of pleomorphic undifferentiated cells arranged in irregular groups and trabeculae. The nuclei are large, hyperchromatic and there are many mitotic figures; and (c) giant-cell type, which is a variant of the large-cell type. It consists of large cells scattered in a loose connective tissue stroma and contains many bizarre tumour giant cells with several nuclei.

3. *Adenocarcinoma* is frequently associated with pulmonary scarring and is often located at the periphery of the lung. It is more common in smokers, even though the increase is not as great as in squamous-cell and oat-cell carcinomas. Histologically, adenocarcinoma is characterized by the presence of tubular and glandular structures which may or may not secrete mucin. Sometimes, a papillary pattern is present. Apart from smoking, it is not clear which aetiological factors give rise to adenocarcinoma. Asbestos-induced carcinoma is predominantly adenocarcinoma or bronchiolar carcinoma. Among carcinogenic metals, chromium appears to produce adenocarcinoma most often just as it produces adenocarcinoma of the nose and sinuses.

Bronchiolar (bronchoalveolar) carcinoma

This is an uncommon variety of lung cancer representing approximately two per cent of primary lung tumours. It arises from small bronchi and is located at the periphery of the lung. It may be diffuse, resembling the grey hepatization stage of lobar pneumonia, or nodular, which may be mistaken for multiple metastases or miliary tuberculosis. The cut surface shows a glossy, mucoid appearance due to the presence of mucin. Microscopically, the alveoli are filled with mucin and are lined by tall, mucous secreting columnar cells which commonly form papillary processes. Bronchiolar carcinoma is identified by its growth pattern rather than its cytological features. It has a tendency to grow along the alveolar walls, preserving the basic pattern of the bronchioles and alveoli, forming small papillary processes and secreting mucin. This type of growth pattern indicates a good prognosis and explains why the condition was called bronchial adenomatosis. A small proportion of bronchiolar carcinomas may metastasize to regional lymph nodes (Fig. 17.3).

Bronchial adenoma (carcinoid tumour)

These tumours occur in a younger age group than do other lung tumours, and no environmental factors have been shown to be responsible for their production. They are equally frequent in both sexes and represent approximately five per cent of lung tumours.

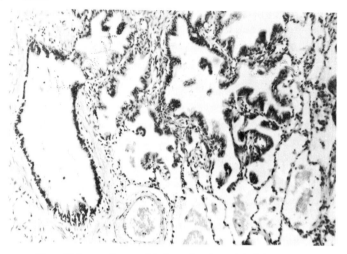

Fig. 17.3 Bronchiolar carcinoma of the lung showing origin from a small bronchiole (arrow) and growing along the interalveolar septa as a well-differentiated papillary adenocarcinoma (× 120)

They arise in a main bronchus as polypoid or sessile nodules and are responsible for early obstruction (Fig. 17.4). Their cut surface usually shows a yellow colour and a well circumscribed nodule. Microscopically, they resemble carcinoids of the intestine (p. 202). Occasionally, malignancy is difficult to determine with routine haematoxylin and eosin stains and some undifferentiated tumours may be mistaken for oat-cell carcinomas. Argentaffin stains or examination of fresh, paraformaldehyde-treated sections under ultraviolet light may reveal serotonin-containing granules.

Mesothelioma

Asbestos induces two types of lung cancer, bronchogenic carcinoma and pleural mesothelioma (p. 52). The causal relationship between asbestos exposure and mesothelioma was first suggested by Wagner in 1960 and evidence of this relationship is based on studies of human populations and animal experiments. The serous surfaces appear particularly vulnerable to asbestos, which causes pleural and peritoneal mesotheliomata.

Macroscopic appearances

The tumour spreads over the pleural surfaces, encasing and compressing the lung. This appearance is not specific, occasionally it is produced by metastatic carcinoma from the lung or from other

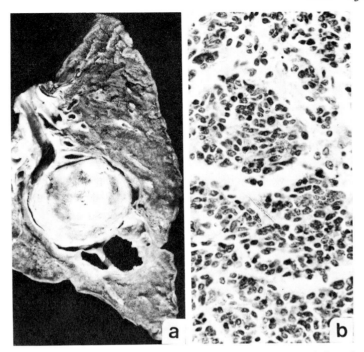

Fig. 17.4 Bronchial adenoma (carcinoid tumour): (a) situated in a main bronchus and expanding the bronchus; (b) the histological pattern of the tumour resembles that of a carcinoid (× 160)

organs. It is for this reason that some authorities question the existence of mesothelioma as a specific entity. Mesothelioma often invades the underlying lung but usually to a limited depth. Occasionally, it may metastasize to regional nodes, to the opposite lung, or to other organs. Pleural effusion, rich in mucopolysaccharides and pleural plaques which may be recognized on X-rays, are common manifestations.

Microscopic appearances
A variety of histological appearances occur. Tumour cells may resemble epithelial cells or spindle-shaped connective tissue cells:

1. *The epithelial type* represents the vast majority (75 per cent) of mesotheliomas. The cells of these tumours may be arranged into trabecular, tubular, glandular or papillary patterns. These patterns may be confused with those of metastatic carcinoma. Mesothelial cells normally elaborate mucins (acid mucopolysaccharides) which lubricate the sliding surfaces of the visceral and parietal pleura so

that increased amounts of these substances can be demonstrated in the tumour cells and in the pleural effusion.

2. *The spindle-cell type* ranges from the well differentiated to the poorly differentiated fibrosarcoma pattern.

3. *Mixed types*, in which both epithelioid and connective tissue components are present.

Course and prognosis

As with tumours of other organs, spread of carcinoma of the lung is by local infiltration through preformed pathways, and then by invasion of vessels and adjacent tissues. Lymphatic spread occurs (a) centripetally towards the hilar nodes; first to the mediastinal, peritracheal and pericardial nodes, and later, through the diaphragm to the aortic lymph nodes, and (b) centrifugally to the subpleural lymphatic plexus. Blood spread occurs by invasion of the pulmonary veins, bronchial veins or vertebral plexus. Metastases predominantly occur in the brain, bones, liver and adrenal glands.

The prognosis of lung cancer is generally poor because the disease is well advanced by the time diagnosis is made. Only 25 per cent of patients with centrally located tumours are suitable for surgery at the time of diagnosis, and the five-year survival rate following pneumonectomy is approximately five per cent. In patients with peripheral tumours, the five-year survival rate is 30 per cent.

FURTHER READING

Churg, J. & Kannerstein, M. (1970) Occupation exposure and its relation to type of lung cancer. In *Morphology of experimental respiratory carcinogenesis*, p. 105. A.E.C. Symp. Ser. vol. 21.

David, J. B. *et al.* (1967) Cancer of the lung: histology and biological behaviour. *Cancer*, **20**, 165.

Doll, R. *et al.* (1957) The significance of the cell-type in relation to the aetiology of lung cancer. *Brit. J. Cancer*, **11**, 43.

Kreyberg, L. (1967) *International Histological Classification of Tumours No. 1: Histological Typing of Lung Tumours*. Geneva: World Health Organization.

Lorenz. E. (1944) Radioactivity and lung cancer: A critical review of lung cancer in the mines of Schneeberg and Joachimsthal. *J. Natl. Cancer Inst.*, **5**, 1.

Louis, C. J. & Kushinsky, R. (1976) The effect of cigarette smoke on aryl hydrocarbon hydroxylase activity and cytochrome P450 content in rat liver and lung microsomes. *Oncology*, **33**, 197.

Royal College of Physicians of London: *Smoking and Health* (Pitman, London, 1962).

Spencer, H. (1977) *Pathology of the Lung*, 3rd edn. Oxford: Pergamon Press.

Wagner, J. C. (1970) The pathogenesis of tumours following the intrapleural injection of asbestos and silica, in *Morphology of Experimental Respiratory Carcinogenesis*, p. 347. A.E.C. Symp. Ser. vol. 21.

Willis, R. A. (1967) *Pathology of Tumours*, 4th edn. London: Butterworths.

Wynder, E. L. & Hoffmann, D. (1969) Bioassays in tobacco carcinogenesis. *Progr. exp. Tumor Res.*, **11**, 163.

18

Tumours of the thyroid, parathyroid and adrenal glands

TUMOURS OF THE THYROID GLAND

Benign	*Malignant*
Follicular adenoma	Papillary carcinoma
(a) Toxic	Follicular carcinoma
(b) Colloid (macrofollicular)	(a) Encapsulated
(c) Foetal (microfollicular)	(b) Non-encapsulated
(d) Hürthle-cell (oxyphil)	Undifferentiated carcinoma
(e) Embryonal (trabecular)	(a) Spindle-cell type
(f) Atypical	(b) Small-cell type
	(c) Giant-cell type
	Medullary carcinoma

Nodules are common in the thyroid gland; they may be solitary or multiple. At first, all thyroid nodules were regarded as neoplasms, but gradually, it was appreciated that the multiple nodules did not fall into this class. Their multiplicity, course, relation to ordinary functional variations of the gland and their histological features are now recognized and accepted as non-neoplastic localized hyperplasias.

Solitary nodules in the thyroid gland present a more difficult clinical problem. One important feature of solitary nodules is that they can be sub-divided into functional and non-functional by use of radioactive isotopes of iodine (^{131}I or ^{125}I).

1. *Functional nodules* can synthesize thyroid hormone and concentrate ^{131}I to an equal or greater extent than the surrounding glandular tissue. Such nodules are designated *hot* nodules because they emit radioactivity, and can be detected clinically.

2. *Non-functional nodules* are *cold* nodules because they do not take up ^{131}I and do not emit radioactivity.

Evaluation of the nature of a thyroid nodule is a very difficult clinical problem. Carcinomas are rarely functional, so that a *hot* nodule is nearly always regarded as benign. Since the incidence of malignancy in *cold* nodules is estimated at 15 per cent to 30 per cent, they are justifiably regarded with suspicion. Diagnosis of the nature of thyroid nodules is made by microscopic examination, after excision of the whole tumour. The normal criteria of malignancy, such as cellular atypia and increase in the number of mitotic figures, may not be present in well differentiated tumours of the thyroid gland. In such cases, diagnosis of carcinoma can only be made either by demonstrating capsular penetration or by invasion of capsular vessels.

Follicular adenoma

Adenomas are benign tumours which arise from the cells lining the thyroid follicles; they commonly occur in young adults. Since all adenomas of the thyroid gland possess more or less well defined follicles, they are collectively referred to as follicular adenomas. They are classified according to their histological structure.

Macroscopic features

Follicular adenomas are usually solitary, and vary considerably in size from 1 to 10 cm in diameter. The cut surface shows that they are clearly demarcated from the surrounding gland by a well-defined and sometimes thick fibrous capsule. The tumour tissue has grey-white colour, and often a mucoid appearance. In addition, it may show degenerative changes, haemorrhage, fibrosis, calcification, ossification and cystic spaces.

Microscopic features

The tumours are composed of thyroid follicles which range in size from very large (*macrofollicular*) to very small (*microfollicular*), and are lined by cuboidal to columnar epithelium. In places, they may show tubular or trabecular patterns. At the periphery of the tumour, the follicles are usually closely packed together and contain little colloid material, but in the centre, the follicles are larger, full of colloid and are often separated by an amorphous stroma. Areas of necrosis, haemorrhage and cystic spaces may be present. Various types of follicular adenoma are described depending on the different growth patterns (Fig. 18.1).

    1. *Toxic adenoma* is a relatively common nodule which is well demarcated from the surrounding gland. It consists of follicles which show all the features of hyperplasia, that is: (a) the follicles are small and free of colloid, (b) they are lined by tall columnar

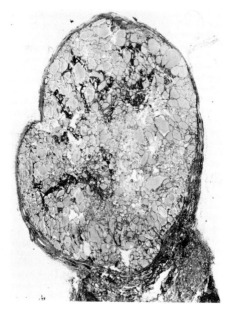

Fig. 18.1 Follicular adenoma of the thyroid gland showing considerable variation in the size of follicles, areas of haemorrhage and a well formed capsule

papillary processes which project into the lumen, and (c) there are numerous mitotic figures. A lymphocytic infiltrate may be present in the stroma.

2. *Colloid (macrofollicular) adenoma* is composed of follicles which resemble those of the adjacent thyroid gland, but they are usually dilated and filled with colloid material. The epithelial cells lining these follicles are regular in form and strictly comparable with those of the surrounding gland.

3. *Foetal (microfollicular) adenoma* is an encapsulated mass of homogeneous tissue with a glassy appearance, differing from colloid. Haemorrhages and cysts are common. Microscopically, there are numerous small follicles, arranged in strands resembling beads on a string, and separated by a homogeneous acellular material. Such an arrangement of cells and follicles with extra-follicular secretion is found in the thyroid gland of the foetus; in the adult, it merely indicates that the structure grows by budding of acini, it does not imply that there is reversion to a foetal form.

4. *Hürthle adenoma (oxyphilic adenoma)* is composed of large, granular, oxyphilic cells known as *Hürthle* or *Askanazy* cells, such

as those seen in chronic thyroiditis and other conditions of the thyroid gland.

5. *Embryonal adenoma* has a homogeneous structure which is more solid in appearance than the foetal type. It is composed of closely packed masses of cells in which an arrangement is not easy to discern. The cells are usually closely packed, forming solid trabeculae, but sometimes, small rudimentary follicles are scattered throughout the tissue. This nodule presents the greatest problem in prognosis.

6. *Atypical adenoma* is also encapsulated. It differs from the other types in that it is composed predominantly of proliferating cells, without any discernible pattern. Some areas are composed of islands of closely-packed cells, others of small trabeculae. The cells are small and uniform in appearance, with very few mitotic figures present. A vascular network is often present and conspicuous. It is important, in these cases, to exclude capsular penetration and invasion of capsular vessels to rule out malignancy.

Carcinoma of the thyroid gland

Cancer of the thyroid gland accounts for approximately 0.5 per cent of all cancer deaths. Although it is an infrequent form of cancer, the actual incidence of the disease is higher than that indicated by mortality figures, because many of these tumours are curable. The disease is more frequent in the endemic goitre areas of the world, but this cause is gradually being eradicated by dietary iodine. Thyroid cancer is twice as common in females as in males, and its peak incidence is between 40 and 60 years of age. The four main types of carcinoma, their incidence, age distribution and prognosis are as follows:

Type	Incidence (%)	Age in years	Prognosis
Papillary carcinoma	60	20–30	Very good
Follicular carcinoma	20	30–50	Good/fair
Undifferentiated carcinoma	10	50–80	Poor
Medullary carcinoma	5	20–40	Good/fair

Aetiology

1. *Experimental evidence.* The induction of carcinoma of the thyroid gland in experimental animals requires: (a) an initiator such as a chemical carcinogen (2-acetylaminofluorene, urethane or dibenzanthracene) which produces an irreversible and heritable effect on the epithelial cells lining the follicles and (b) a promotor, such as iodine-deficient diet, antithyroid drugs or a combination of the two, for the long-continued stimulation of these cells. Initiators

are not always necessary; thyroid tumours have been produced in some strains of rats by iodine-deficient diets alone. Similar factors appear to be responsible for the development of thyroid cancer in man.

2. *Irradiation.* Radiation exposures of 350 r carry a 30 per cent risk of developing thyroid nodules and a four per cent risk of developing cancer. The overall evidence suggests that the risk factor for doses greater than 20 r is linear; it is of the order of approximately 10 cases of malignancy per 100 000 subjects per rad. The latent period is approximately 20 years.

Whole body irradiation also appears to increase the incidence of carcinoma of the thyroid gland. Following the Hiroshima and Nagasaki atomic bomb detonations, thyroid nodules were more prevalent in those who received heavy doses of irradiation. In these patients, the incidence of malignancy in biopsy specimens of the nodules was 25 per cent, and of these, the vast majority (97 per cent in one series) were papillary carcinomas.

The role of clinically administered radioactive iodine in the aetiology of thyroid cancer in man is not established. Approximately 30 years have now elapsed since ^{131}I was introduced for the treatment of thyrotoxicosis, and many thousands of patients have been treated. On the basis of information available, it is doubtful whether millicurie doses of ^{131}I, used in the treatment of thyrotoxicosis in adults, carry any significant risk of inducing cancer. In children, however, there may be a risk. In a series of nine patients with thyroid cancer, six had received ^{131}I as children, and of these, three cases were follicular, two papillary and one undifferentiated carcinomas.

3. *Dietary iodine and geographical location.* The relationship between endemic goitre, caused by lack of iodine, and thyroid cancer is still debatable. On the one hand, mortality studies show that the highest incidence of thyroid cancer occurs in mountainous countries, such as Austria, Switzerland, the Himalayas and New Guinea. In these areas, there is a lack of iodine in the diet and a high incidence of hyperplastic goitre and carcinoma of the thyroid gland. On the other hand, in some parts of Japan and Iceland, where the mean daily iodine intake is very high, the incidence of thyroid cancer is also high. The possible relationship, therefore, between alterations in iodine levels, histological changes in thyroid epithelium and malignancy requires further study.

Papillary carcinoma

Macroscopic features
This is the commonest form of carcinoma in the thyroid gland, and affects particularly the younger age group (20 to 30 years). It varies in size from one millimetre up to 10 cm in diameter, and may replace the entire gland. The small type, is sometimes described as occult or *non-encapsulated sclerosing carcinoma*, because it appears as a tiny scar, and can only be recognized microscopically. The larger type has ill-defined edges, and its cut surface shows solid areas and cystic spaces filled with fluid, and myriads of minute papillae. Areas of fibrosis are often present, and there may be foci of calcium deposition which may be recognized radiologically.

Microscopic features
The tumour is made up of papillary processes, consisting of a well-defined core of vascular connective tissue, lined by cuboidal cells which are usually regular in form. The nuclei of these cells have a characteristic clear watery appearance which is unique to papillary carcinoma. Mitotic figures are sparse. Within the stroma there may be basophilic, laminated, calcified nodules, called *psammoma bodies*. Psammoma bodies are found in approximately 50 percent of papillary carcinomas of the thyroid gland, but they are rarely seen in benign tumours; their presence is very suggestive

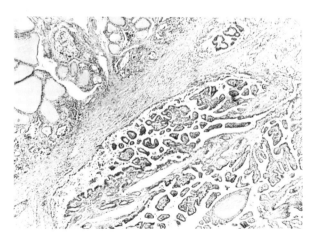

Fig. 18.2 Papillary carcinoma of the thyroid gland showing the margin of the tumour. Note invasion of a capsular vessel (× 40)

of malignancy. Thyroid follicles, many of which contain colloid, are almost always present, even in the metastases, and indicate origin from the thyroid gland (Fig. 18.2).

Some papillary tumours, show no histological evidence of malignancy, and are erroneously called *papillomas*. Careful examination of the capsule of these tumours, in sections prepared from several blocks, invariably reveals either penetration of the capsule or invasion of the capsular vessels. It is a good general rule to regard all papillary tumours in the thyroid gland as malignant.

Follicular carcinoma

Macroscopic features
Follicular carcinoma may be single or multiple and may vary in size from 1 to 10 cm in diameter. Two types are recognized:

1. *Encapsulated carcinoma*, which is difficult to differentiate macroscopically, and sometimes microscopically, from adenoma.

2. *Invasive carcinoma* is one in which local invasion of the thyroid gland, or beyond, can be demonstrated. The cut surface is grey-white in colour, firm in consistency and often shows central fibrosis and calcification. In addition, areas of haemorrhage, necrosis and cystic change may be present. Careful inspection of the capsule may show small almond-shaped islands of tumour tissue suggestive of capsular invasion.

Microscopic features
These are all adenocarcinomas composed entirely of follicles which vary in size and in their content of colloid material. The follicles are lined by a single layer of cells which resemble those of the adjacent thyroid gland. The nuclei are uniformly hyperchromatic, but very few mitotic figures are present. Oxyphilic or *Hürthle cells* may be present in varying proportions. In well-differentiated tumours, the demonstration of capsular invasion may be the only indication of malignancy (Fig. 18.3).

Undifferentiated carcinoma

Macroscopic features
The undifferentiated type of carcinoma of the thyroid gland differs from the preceding two types in that it is uncommon, affects an older age group, and is a highly malignant tumour which invariably causes death within six months. It presents as a bulky, poorly

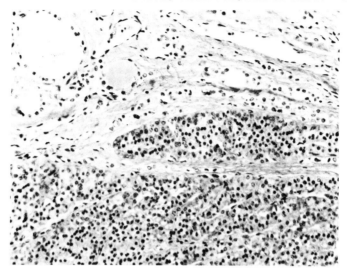

Fig. 18.3 Follicular carcinoma of the thyroid gland showing capsular invasion

defined mass which invades through the thyroid gland to encircle cervical structures and extend down into the mediastinum.

Microscopic features
These tumours are composed of proliferating cells which are totally undifferentiated and vary in shape and size. Three major histological types are recognized:

   1. *The spindle-cell type* in which the predominant cell is spindle-shaped, and the tumour may be confused with undifferentiated sarcoma.

   2. *The small-cell type* is composed predominantly of sheets of small, round, fairly uniform cells with little cytoplasm, and which may be mistaken for a lymphocytic lymphoma.

   3. *The giant-cell type* contains a great proportion of large, pleomorphic and multinucleate giant cells.

Medullary carcinoma

Macroscopic features
Medullary carcinoma occurs as a grey-white, usually well demarcated, but non-encapsulated tumour which varies considerably in size. It develops in the 40 to 50 year age group and is more common in females.

Microscopic features

The basic structure consists of groups of epithelial cells supported by an irregular stroma. The cells may be arranged in cords, trabeculae, festoons, whorls and nests of varying sizes, and may be round, polygonal or spindle-shaped. They have a pink, granular cytoplasm, with indistinct cell membranes and uniformly hyper-chromatic nuclei. There is no follicular or papillary pattern. The stroma nearly always contains a hyaline, amorphous and refractile substance which has all the properties of amyloid. Sometimes, amyloid is the predominating feature, at other times, it is inconspicuous.

Course and prognosis

Papillary carcinoma frequently spreads by lymphatics to regional nodes on both sides of the neck, but distant metastases are un-common. Often, cervical lymphadenopathy is the only sign, and diagnosis of a papillary carcinoma of the thyroid gland is made on a cervical lymph node biopsy.

The prognosis of carcinoma of the thyroid gland varies according to the histological type, and according to the stage.

1. Papillary carcinomas are, in fact, chronic cancers and their prognosis is generally very good. If left alone, even with lymph node involvement, 90 per cent of these patients can survive for 10 years, and with treatment, 95 per cent are alive after 20 years.

2. Follicular carcinoma can also have a good prognosis. The outlook of the encapsulated type is almost as good as that of the papillary carcinoma, but this does not apply to the invasive type. Invasive follicular carcinoma usually does not spread to cervical lymph nodes, it tends to invade blood vessels easily and metastasize to flat bones, lung and liver. Its prognosis is poor.

3. In contrast to the papillary and follicular carcinoma, undiffer-entiated carcinoma of the thyroid gland has an extraordinarily poor prognosis. Most patients with this tumour survive only a few weeks, over 95 per cent die within six months. The giant-cell type has the worst prognosis.

4. Medullary carcinomas are derived from C or parafollicular cells of the thyroid gland, and represent a distinct clinico-pathological entity. They synthesize calcitonin, prostaglandin, serotonin and histaminase. In addition, some tumours secrete immunoreactive ACTH in sufficient quantities to produce a Cushing's syndrome. Hypocalcaemia is not a feature of the disease, probably because parathyroid hyperplasia is associated with it and

maintains calcium homeostasis. Approximately 50 per cent of patients with medullary carcinoma of the thyroid gland may also have parathyroid adenomas, as well as a phaeochromocytoma and neuromas. The prognosis is relatively good, the 10-year survival rate being approximately 60 per cent.

TUMOURS OF THE PARATHYROID GLANDS

Most parathyroid tumours are adenomas, carcinomas being extremely rare, and in the absence of invasion or metastases, a distinction between the two is not possible. Adenomas occur more frequently in the inferior than in the superior glands, and they may be functional or nonfunctional. Functional adenomas are responsible for approximately 90 per cent of all cases of hyperparathyroidism, and in the vast majority of these cases, a solitary tumour is involved.

Parathyroid tumours vary considerably in size from minute nodules, barely visible macroscopically, to large growths which may be easily palpable and may resemble thyroid nodules. The cut surface has a variegated yellow to brown colour in which there may be areas of haemorrhage, cystic spaces, and occasionally,

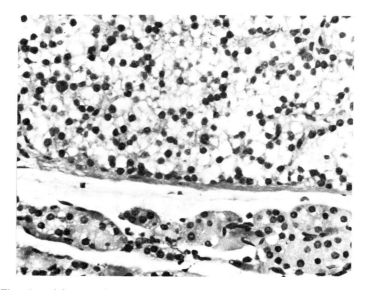

Fig. 18.4   Adenoma of the parathyroid gland showing a rim of parathyroid tissue below, a thin capsule of fibrous tissue, and above, the adenoma consisting of clear cells (wasserhelle cells) which are now thought to be active chief cells (× 100)

foci of calcification. The histological structure closely resembles that of the parathyroid gland. Functioning tumours are composed of chief cells, *water-cells (wasserheller)* or a mixture of the two in varying proportions. Among the chief cells, there may be considerable variation in nuclear size and shape, with giant nuclei and multinucleate cells often present. Mitotic figures are rare. In addition, there may be islands of oxyphilic cells (Fig. 18.4).

A histological distinction between hyperplasia and neoplasia cannot be made. In hyperplasia, all the glands are enlarged, though the enlargement may be unequal. A typical adenoma, on the other hand, has a compressed rim of normal parathyroid tissue at the periphery of the tumour, but serial sections may be required to identify this rim. If only one gland is enlarged, it is regarded as an adenoma, even if the rim of compressed parathyroid tissue is not identified. There are no other specific features by which an adenoma may be distinguished from a hyperplasia.

TUMOURS OF THE ADRENAL GLANDS

Metastases are the most frequent tumours in the adrenal glands. Primary tumours are not common, most of them are benign, and often small and difficult to explore clinically. Many of them are functional, and despite their small size, they give rise to serious clinical symptoms which need to be recognized.

Although the adrenal gland is an anatomical entity, it is made up of two distinct glands which differ from each other in origin, structure and function.

1. *The adrenal cortex* is derived from embryonic coelomic epithelium, and its development is controlled by ACTH. It consists of three layers of cells, the middle of which is the broadest and contains cells rich in lipid droplets and ascorbic acid. The principal cortical hormones are as follows:

Zone	Main hormone
Glomerulosa (outer)	Aldosterone
	Glucocorticoids (cortical)
Fasciculata (middle)	Sex hormones:
and	(a) Androgenic
Reticularis (inner)	(b) Oestrogenic
	(c) Progestogenic

2. *The adrenal medulla* develops from neural ectoderm and is

a specialized part of the sympathetic nervous system. It is composed of chromaffin cells and sympathetic ganglion cells. The medulla secretes two principal catecholamines (adrenaline and noradrenaline) together with traces of dopamine.

Structurally and functionally, therefore, two groups of primary tumours of the adrenal glands are recognized, one arising from cells in the cortex and the other from cells in the medulla.

Tissue	*Tumour*
Adrenal cortex	Adenoma
	Carcinoma
Adrenal medulla	Neuroblastoma
	Phaeochromocytoma

Adenoma

Adenomas of the adrenal cortex may be functional or nonfunctional. Functional adenomas are rare, whereas nonfunctional nodules are a common incidental finding at necropsy, the frequency increasing

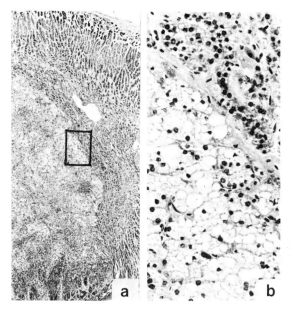

Fig. 18.5 Cortical adenoma of the adrenal gland showing: (a) the relationship of the nodule to the adrenal cortex (× 40); (b) the histological appearance of the area in the square in (a) showing the large clear cells of the tumour, the capsule of fibrous tissue and the adrenal cortex above (× 240)

with age. The tumours are usually small, round, well encapsulated nodules which vary in size from 0.5 to 5 cm in diameter, and may weight between 5 and 200 g. The cut surface is yellow to red-brown in colour, and in large tumours, there may be areas of haemorrhage and necrosis. The histological appearances resemble those of the adrenal cortex. The cells are large with a vesicular nucleus and granular, vacuolated or clear cytoplasm, and they may be arranged in small nests or tortuous columns (Fig. 18.5).

Carcinoma
Carcinomas may arise either in a pre-existing adenoma or *de novo*. They are three to four times more common in females than in males, and occur mainly between 25 and 50 years of age. Carcinomas are generally larger than adenomas, otherwise they have similar morphological features. Microscopically, it is not possible to distinguish between a benign and a well differentiated malignant tumour. In poorly differentiated carcinomas, the cells are spindle-shaped and pleomorphic, giant-cell forms are present and there is invasion of vessels and adjacent tissues. Malignant tumours are less likely to be functional and as a result, they are discovered late, the five-year survival rate being less than 10 per cent.

Clinical implications
Attempts to distinguish between functional and nonfunctional tumours of the adrenal cortex on the basis of histological structure have not been successful. Generally, three syndromes are recognized:

1. *Cushing's syndrome* results from excessive production of cortisol, and approximately 30 per cent of patients with this syndrome have a cortisol secreting tumour. Cortisol suppresses ACTH which, in turn, causes atrophy of the remaining normal adrenal cortex. Estimation of the plasma cortisol is of value in recognizing the condition. Normal values are: a.m.: 200–280 nmol/l; p.m.: 100–400 nmol/l.

2. *Conn's syndrome, or primary aldosteronism* is caused by hypersecretion of aldosterone, the major cause of which is a small functioning adrenocortical adenoma. The clinical features are due to: (a) low serum potassium, causing episodes of muscular weakness, (b) retention of sodium, which is the probable cause of hypertension, and (c) metabolic alkalosis, causing reduction in the ionized calcium and tetany. The excretion of aldosterone in the urine is high.

3. *Adrenogenital syndrome* results from excess adrenal androgens.

It causes virilism in women and girls, precocious sexual development in boys, but has no effect in adult males.

Phaeochromocytoma

This is an uncommon tumour found in less than 0.1 per cent of necropsies; it is more common in diabetics and hypertensives. It is responsible for approximately 0.5 per cent of all cases of hypertension, and because of the dramatic relief afforded by surgical removal, this tumour has attracted much attention.

Most phaeochromocytomas (90 per cent) occur in the adrenal medulla, more often on the right side than on the left. The remaining 10 per cent arise from the extra-adrenal chromaffin cells along the parasympathetic chain, namely to the coeliac and mesenteric arteries, the hila of the kidneys, the ganglion impar (organ of Zuckerkandl), neck of the bladder, and rarely, they occur in the mediastinum. The tumours are usually benign and functional. They form large quantities of catecholamines (mainly noradrenaline, in many cases adrenaline, and occasionally dopamine) which are released into the circulation. The release may be intermittent, producing *paroxysmal hypertension* (headaches, palpitation, sweating etc.), or continuous, producing *sustained hypertension*.

Diagnosis depends on finding excessive amounts of noradrenaline or adrenaline in the urine and plasma, especially during attacks. The site of the tumour can be localized by obtaining samples of blood from different levels of the inferior vena cava and superior vena cava. Samples should not be taken from the adrenal veins because they can give false high data. Differential assay of noradrenaline and adrenaline in the urine are also of value in predicting the site of the tumour. Almost all tumours which produce both adrenaline and noradrenaline are in the adrenal gland. Of those that produce only noradrenaline, 56 per cent are in the adrenal, the remainder are extra-adrenal. The upper limits of normal catecholamine levels are:

	Urine	Serum
Noradrenaline	100 μg/day	0.8 μg/l
Adrenaline	40 μg/day	0.3 μg/l

Macroscopic features
The tumour is usually round, smooth, well encapsulated and weighs approximately 100 g (5 cm in diameter). Much smaller and much greater sizes have been recorded. The cut surface is lobulated, and in the fresh state, has a grey-brown colour, but the

colour turns rusty-brown after the tumour has been standing in formalin solution.

Microscopic appearances
The tumour consists of a vascular connective tissue stroma supporting a variety of cells (Fig. 18.6).

1. Polygonal cells with granular or vacuolated eosinophilic cytoplasm resembling those of the adrenal medulla, but generally larger. The cytoplasmic granules take up chromaffin stains. The cells may be arranged in nests, whorls or trabeculae, and are intimately related to thin-walled blood vessels.

2. Larger cells with large hyperchromatic nuclei, sometimes multinucleate.

3. Small, round to oval cells with pale cytoplasm, resembling lymphocytes, may represent immature neural cells.

4. Ganglion-like cells in various stages of maturity, satellite cells, and Schwann cells with palisading nuclei.

Phaeochromocytomas generally behave as benign tumours. They metastasize only occasionally, and when they do, there are no distinctive histological features. The presence of atypical cells, such as spindle cells, large pleomorphic cells and giant cells, do not indicate malignancy.

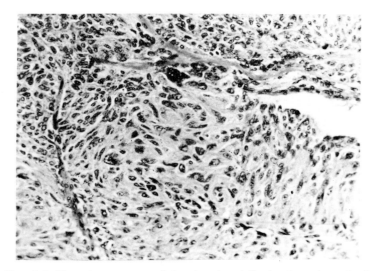

Fig. 18.6 Phaeochromocytoma of the adrenal medulla showing polygonal cells and cells with hyperchromatic nuclei (× 240)

Neuroblastoma

This is a highly malignant tumour which is common in young children, but rare in adults. It is more common in males than in females, especially under 10 years of age, with a peak incidence in the first two to three years of life. Over 50 per cent of tumours occur in the adrenal medulla, most of the others, along the sympathetic chain and in the retina (retinoblastoma). The provisional diagnosis of neuroblastoma can, in most cases, be confirmed by demonstrating abnormal quantities of catacholamines and their metabolites in the urine.

The tumours are large, round and lobulated. They are soft in consistency and their cut surface is usually grey with yellow flecks. Histologically, they are composed of large numbers of scattered and streaked cells, poorly supported by stroma. The cells have a dark, coarsely clumped nucleus, no obvious nucleolus and very little cytoplasm. In places, the cells tend to form *rosettes* which, with special stain, show fine neurofibrils. The PAS stain is negative, which helps to distinguish these tumours from Ewing's tumour, in which the stain is positive.

FURTHER READING

Dunegan, L. J. *et al.* (1974) Primary hyperparathyroidism. Preoperative evaluation and correlation with surgical findings. *Am. J. Surg.*, **128**, 471.

Franssila, K. O. (1973) Is the differentiation between papillary and follicular thyroid carcinoma valid?. *Cancer*, **32**, 853.

Glenner, G. G. & Grimley, P. M. (1974) *Tumors of the Extra-adrenal Paraganglion System*, Fascicle 9, Second Series, Washington D.C.: Armed Forces Institute of Pathology.

Hedinger, C. (1974) *International Histological Classification of Tumours No. 11: Histological Typing of Thyroid Tumours*. Geneva: World Health Organization.

Huvos, A. G. *et al.* (1970) Adrenal cortical carcinoma. Clinicopathologic study of 34 cases. *Cancer*, **25**, 354.

Louis, C. J. & Varasdi, D. (1960) Fluorescein-protein affinities of tumours of the thyroid gland. *Ann. Surg.*, **152**, 795.

Meissner, W. A. & Warren S. (1969) *Tumors of the Thyroid Gland*, Fascicle 4, Second series, Washington D.C.: Armed Forces Institute of Pathology.

Sjoerdsma, A. *et al.* (1966) Phaeochromocytoma: current concepts of diagnosis and treatment. *Ann. Int. Med.*, **65**, 1302.

19

Tumours of the urinary system

Tumours of the urinary system are divided into tumours of the kidneys and tumours of the urinary passages. Malignant tumours of the kidneys are uncommon, accounting for approximately 1 per cent of all primary cancers, whereas benign tumours are very common, but they are small and of little clinical significance. In the lower urinary tract, malignant tumours are twice as frequent as in the kidneys.

TUMOURS OF THE KIDNEYS

Benign	*Malignant*
Adenoma	Carcinoma
Fibroma	Nephroblastoma
Haemangioma	
Leiomyoma	

Adenoma (cortical adenoma)
In adult kidneys, small adenomas are found in over 20 per cent of routine post mortem examinations; their incidence appears to increase with age. Many pathologists regard them as forerunners of carcinoma, and indeed, the larger tumours may be difficult to distinguish from renal adenocarcinoma.

Macroscopic appearance
Adenomas are most commonly seen in scarred kidneys as greyish-yellow tumours situated just under the capsule in the outer part .of the renal cortex. They may be single or multiple, solid or cystic, and may vary in size from 2 mm to 2 cm in diameter. A nodule greater than 2 cm in diameter is likely to be a carcinoma.

Histological features
Microscopically, two patterns may be seen:

1. *Tubular adenoma* is composed of tubules lined by a single or several rows of cuboidal to columnar cells. The tubules may be convoluted and branched indicating their origin from renal tubules.

2. *Papillary adenoma* consists of small irregular cavities containing papillary processes. The papillae have a connective tissue core lined by cuboidal epithelium, and within the core there are foam cells in which lipid can be demonstrated and iron-containing macrophages.

Fibroma (medullary fibroma)
Fibromas are more common than adenomas. They occur as small, firm white nodules in the pyramids, and consist of closely packed fibrous tissue. It is not known whether they are true neoplasms or hamartomas.

Haemangioma
This is a rare tumour, which appears as a small, red, encapsulated nodule situated either under the capsule or in contact with the calyces. They are cavernous haemangiomas consisting of large vascular spaces, separated by connective tissue partitions, and lined by endothelium. When present in the renal cortex, they produce no symptoms, but when near the calyces, they may cause serious haematuria often necessitating nephrectomy. Diagnosis is made post-operatively. Renal haemangiomas may be associated with haemangiomatosis of the skin and other organs.

Leiomyoma
Renal leiomyomas probably arise from the smooth muscle cells of the renal capsule, or from perivascular mesenchymal cells. They are rare tumours found incidentally at post mortem examination, just under the capsule. They vary in size and are well circumscribed.

Renal adenocarcinoma
This is the most important kidney tumour in adults. Grawitz, in 1883, taught that it arose from misplaced adrenal rests, and the tumour became known as a *hypernephroma* or a *Grawitz tumour*. It is now generally accepted that this tumour arises from the epithelial cells lining the proximal convoluted tubules and should be referred to as *renal adenocarcinoma*. Adenocarcinoma represents approximately 80 per cent of malignant tumours of the kidney. It occurs in individuals past the age of 50 years, its peak incidence lies between 50 and 70 years of age and it is twice as common in males as in females.

Macroscopic appearance

Characteristically, the tumour arises in the cortex of the upper pole of the kidney, less commonly, it occupies the lower pole, and least commonly, the central part of the kidney. The two sides are equally affected. Sooner or later, the contour of the kidney is altered as the tumour grows and reaches the surface, and by the time the tumour is diagnosed, it is usually large (5 to 15 cm in diameter). On section, the cut surface shows a variegated colour pattern consisting of yellow zones, red haemorrhagic zones, foci of calcification and cyst formation. Glistening white bands of fibrous tissue intersect through the mass, giving it a lobular appearance, and similar fibrous tissue bands at the periphery of the tumour give a false impression of encapsulation. Frequently, small satellite nodules of tumour tissue are found outside the main mass, and cast-like cords of tumour within the renal vein, often extending to the inferior vena cava (Fig. 19.1).

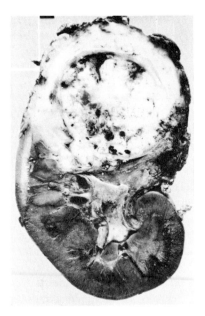

Fig. 19.1 Carcinoma of the kidney involving the upper half of the kidney. Translucent viable tumour tissue is present at the periphery, but centrally, the tumour is necrotic and haemorrhagic

Histological features

Two types of parenchymal cells are found in renal adenocarcinoma:

1. *Clear cells* are the most common type. Characteristically, they are large cells with clear cytoplasm which owes its appearance to the high content of lipid, cholesterol esters and glycogen. They have a small, round, dark-staining nucleus and a well defined cytoplasmic membrane. Mitotic figures are sparse (Fig. 19.2).

2. *Dark cells* are much less common than clear cells. They resemble the cells lining the renal tubules in having pink, granular cytoplasm, a distinct cell membrane and a small dark nucleus.

Clear and dark cells may co-exist in the same tumour, and they may be arranged in various patterns: (a) solid cords or nests, (b) cystic spaces into which papillary processes project, and (c) tubular pattern, suggesting that these tumours arise from renal tubules. The stroma is scanty, but rich in thin-walled blood vessels which are often invaded by tumour cells. Haemorrhages, areas of necrosis, foci of calcification and collections of iron-containing macrophages are frequent in the stroma.

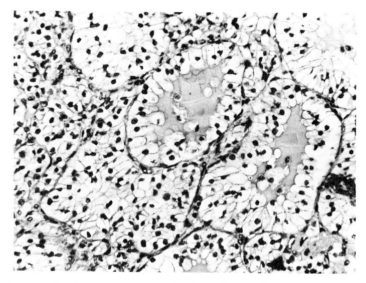

Fig. 19.2 Renal adenocarcinoma of the clear cell type. The cells form solid and tubular structures (× 200)

Course and prognosis
Carcinoma of the kidney generally presents late; three main symptoms may attract attention to the disease:

1. *Haematuria* is usually the first sign. It occurs in over 50 per cent of patients and is due to rupture of the thin-walled blood vessels in the stroma. Typically, it is painless, profuse and intermittent and occasionally it may be followed by clot colic.

2. *Pain* is present in half the patients. It indicates growth of tumour outside the capsule, and is usually a late symptom.

3. *A palpable mass* is also present in half of the patients, especially those with lower pole tumours.

In addition, (a) a *varicocoele* may develop when the left renal vein becomes involved and obstructs the entry of the left spermatic vein, (b) *polycythaemia* occurs in approximately 5 per cent of patients, due to production of erythropoietin by the tumour cells, and (c) *hypercalcaemia* may occur due to a vitamin D-like substance which increases absorption of calcium from the intestine.

Carcinoma of the kidney has a tendency to invade the veins. Blood spread, therefore, is a common and early complication and is directed particularly to the lungs, bones and brain. Lymphatic spread initially goes to the regional lymph nodes around the renal pedicle.

The prognosis of renal adenocarcinoma is unpredictable. Invasion of the renal vein is the most important single factor, the five-year survival rate being 60 per cent when there is no renal invasion, and 30 per cent when there is invasion of the renal vein.

Nephroblastoma (Wilms' tumour)
In children, especially infants, the commonest renal tumour is a mixed tumour, the nephroblastoma, often known as Wilms' tumour. It represents approximately 20 per cent of malignant tumours in children, the peak incidence being at three years; it is extremely rare after the age of 10 years. Clinically, it always presents as an abdominal mass, which increases rapidly in size, while the general health of the infant deteriorates. Haematuria does not occur until the late stages.

Macroscopic appearance
The tumour arises in any part of the kidney, and when discovered, it is large and tends to compress and destroy the infant organ. The cut surface is white and firm with cystic areas and small

patches of haemorrhage. While still small, it has a fibrous capsule, but as it grows, the capsule ruptures and the tumour becomes invasive, frequently involving the renal vein.

Histological features

The histological appearances vary from area to area. There are two main types of cells:

1. Epithelial cells arranged into rosettes and tubules.
2. Mesenchymal stromal cells which are spindle-shaped, with dark nuclei and scanty cytoplasm, and which Willis regards as the embryonic element.

Sometimes, the stromal cells form clumps which invaginate the tubular structures and resemble primitive glomeruli with poorly formed Bowman's spaces. Among the stromal cells, are thin-walled blood vessels, smooth and striated muscle cells, cartilage and fat. Tubules, primitive glomeruli and striated muscle fibres are the main histological criteria for diagnosis (Fig. 19.3).

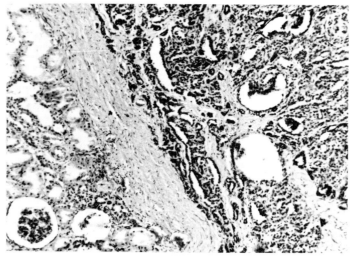

Fig. 19.3 Margin of a nephroblastoma (Wilm's tumour) showing normal kidney on left, tumour capsule and tumour tissue on right. The tumour cells tend to form tubular and glomerular structures (× 60)

Course and prognosis

Typically, the tumour spreads by direct invasion through the capsule, by the lymphatics to the local lymph nodes, and by the blood to the lungs, liver and bones. The younger the age at which diagnosis is made, the better the prognosis. In this regard, tumours at the lower pole of the kidney have a better prognosis, only because they are detected earlier. Nephrectomy and post-operative radiotherapy combined with actinomycin D give the best results, especially when the infant is less than one year old. Treatment at this stage gives a 95 per cent cure rate.

TUMOURS OF THE URINARY PASSAGES

Tumours of the renal pelvis, ureter and bladder are considered together, because they have certain features in common. In the first place, all these areas are lined by transitional epithelium which gives rise to tumours of similar morphological appearances, the majority of which are transitional-cell carcinomas; secondly, the tumours arising in these sites are probably all due to the same carcinogens present in the urine; and thirdly, painless, profuse haematuria is the presenting symptom in most patients.

In the majority of cases of tumours of the urinary passages, no cause is known. Among workers in the analine industry (dyeing, rubber, printing), who are exposed to β-naphthylamine, the incidence of carcinoma of the bladder is approximately 50 times greater than in the normal population. There is also a higher risk of bladder cancer among cigar and cigarette smokers, and in tropical countries, such as Egypt, there is a close association with schistosomiasis.

Tumours of the urinary passages generally appear late in life, 90 per cent occurring after the age of 50 years. They are three times more common in males than in females. The distribution in various organs appears to be related to the area of mucosa at risk, the commonest being the bladder, then the renal pelvis, and least common, the ureter. In the ureter, the lower third is the commonest site, whereas in the bladder, the area adjacent to the ureteric orifices and the trigone. Sometimes, tumours are seen in more than one site in a given patient, and occasionally, they are bilateral. In the past, the presence of multiple tumours was explained by the concept of spread by implantation, but the general feeling now is that multiple tumours are due to a multifocal origin in a field which is prepared by carcinogens in the urine.

As with other organs, tumours of the urinary passages may be benign (*papillomas*) or malignant (*carcinomas*). Other tumours such as fibromas, myomas, lipomas and haemangiomas occur occasionally, but they are discussed elsewhere.

Benign papilloma

This is a small, fragile, frond-like nodule which varies in size from 2 mm to 2 cm in diameter. It is usually attached to the mucosa by a narrow base and its structure and behaviour appear to be related to its size.

1. Small tumours, less than 1 cm in diameter, are characterized by masses of long, delicate branching, villous processes which, when seen through a cystoscope, resemble floating seaweed. Microscopically, the villous processes consist of a scanty, though highly vascular connective tissue core, covered by one or more layers of well differentiated transitional epithelium. The epithelial cells are arranged with their long axes at right angles to the central core, closely resembling the epithelium of the urinary bladder. Generally, such tumours are non-invasive and do not recur when removed.

2. In large papillomas, greater than 1 cm in diameter, the villous processes tend to be shorter and the lining cells show mild atypia and disarray. These tumours are sometimes referred to as *atypical papillomas* and may turn out to be malignant. They may recur following surgical removal, and with each recurrence, they tend to become less differentiated and more aggressive.

Carcinoma

Carcinomas of the urinary passages may be papillary or solid.

1. *Papillary carcinomas* are all transitional-cell carcinomas which arise from benign papillomas. The tumours tend to be flatter and broader than the papillomas, and their processes thicker and shorter. The surface may become necrotic and ulcerating. Malignant change becomes apparent in the cells lining the villous processes and is indicated by a spectrum of histological changes which range from cellular atypia to frank invasion.

2. *Solid carcinomas* may be bulky and polypoid, ulcerating, flat or infiltrating. Most of them are transitional-cell carcinomas of varying degrees of differentiation; occasionally, they may be squamous-cell carcinomas which are considered to have a worse prognosis (Fig. 19.4).

Spread

Tumours of the urinary passages may spread locally along the surface, as seen in some papillary lesions, or by direct invasion of the underlying wall. In the bladder, tumours grow slowly, and the growth is limited to the wall for a considerable period of time. The thin wall of the ureter provides a much less effective barrier,

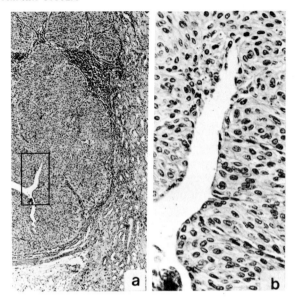

Fig. 19.4 Transitional cell carcinoma of the renal pelvis showing: (a) thickening of the epithelial lining of the pelvis (× 40); (b) the area in the square in (a) is composed of well-differentiated transitional cells (× 240)

and tumours here tend to metastasize earlier than those in the bladder. Direct invasion beyond the bladder, to involve adjacent organs such as the rectum or vagina may occur and may lead to fistula formation. Lymphatic spread occurs first to the regional lymph nodes, and later, to the para-aortic nodes. Blood spread commonly involves the liver, lung and bone.

Prognosis

The chance of successful treatment of carcinoma of the urinary passages is dependent on the site, stage and histological characteristics of the growth. In the bladder, four stages of malignancy are recognized depending on how far the tumour cells have penetrated into the wall.

1. *Stage A tumours* show cellular atypia with no evidence of invasion of the submucosa, but they may recur after removal. These are the atypical papillomas.

2. *Stage B tumours* show invasion of the submucosa and muscle coats. The cells are well-differentiated. Squamous metaplasia may or may not be present.

3. *Stage C tumours* show invasion of the submucosa and muscle coats and invasion of the perivesical fat. The cells are poorly

differentiated but there is no lymph node involvement. Squamous metaplasia may or may not be present.

4. *Stage D tumours* show involvement of the lymph nodes or distant metastases.

FURTHER READING

Bennington, J. L. & Beckwith, J. B. (1975) *Tumors of the Kidney, Renal Pelvis and Ureter*, Fascicle 12, Second series, Washington D.C.: Armed Forces Institute of Pathology.

Case, R. A. M. (1961) Some observations on the alleged casual relationship between infestation with Schistosoma (Bilharzia) haematobium and cancer of the urinary bladder in man. Report to World Health Organization.

Chisholm, G. D. & Roy, R. R. (1971) The systemic effects of malignant renal tumours. *Br. J. Urol.*, **43**, 687.

Holland, J. M. (1973) Cancer of the kidney – natural history and staging. *Cancer*, **32**, 1030.

Jewett, H. J. & Strong, G. S. (1946) Infiltrating carcinoma of the bladder: Relation of depth of penetration of bladder wall to incidence of local extension and metastasis. *J. Urol.*, **55**, 366.

Koss, L. G. (1975) *Tumors of the Urinary Bladder*, Fascicle 11, Second series, Washington D.C.: Armed Forces Institute of Pathology.

Latham, H. S. & Kay, S. (1974) Malignant tumours of the renal pelvis. *Surg. Gynecol. Obstet.*, **138**, 613.

Marshall, V. F. (1952) The relation of preoperative estimate to the pathologic demonstration of the extent of vesical neoplasms. *J. Urol.*, **68**, 714.

Mostofi, F. K. (1973) *International Histological Classification of Tumours No. 10: Histological Typing of Tumours of the Urinary Bladder*. Geneva: World Health Organization.

Oyahu, R. & Hopp, M. L. (1974) The aetiology of cancer of the bladder – collective review. *Surg. Gynecol. Obstet.*, **138**, 97.

Xipell, J. M. (1971) The incidence of benign renal nodules (a clinico-pathologic study). *J. Urol.*, **106**, 503.

20

Tumours of the male genital organs

TUMOURS OF THE TESTIS

Primary tumours of the testis are invariably malignant, but they are rare, accounting for less than 1 per cent of all male cancers. Although testicular tumours can occur at any age, they are most frequent between the ages of 20 and 40 years, and in this age group, they are the most common form of cancer in man. There is a second, but much smaller peak between 60 and 75 years, consisting mainly of lymphomas of the testis. Most testicular tumours present as painless hard swellings of the testis, a small proportion with symptoms attributable to metastases, and a very much smaller fraction with symptoms due to hormone secretion.

Aetiology

The aetiology of testicular tumours is not known. The incidence of tumours in undescended testes is at least 10 times that in normally placed testes, and this incidence is not reduced by bringing the testes to the scrotum surgically. The incidence of malignancy in the remaining testis of patients who have already had one testis removed for cancer is also high. These statistics suggest that the predisposition to malignancy in maldescended testes is probably related to some genetic abnormality rather than to the ectopic position.

Classification

Approximately 95 per cent of testicular tumours arise from germ cells which are pluripotential and capable of differentiating into various types of germ cells. They are invariably malignant. The remaining five per cent arise either from lymphoid or from interstitial cells. The classification of germ-cell tumours of the testis is controversial and still under discussion. At present, several systems are in use, but since only a few tumours need be considered, the following system of nomenclature has been generally adopted:

Tumour	Frequency (%)
Seminoma	45
1. Classical (well differentiated)	
2. Spermatocyctic type	
3. Undifferentiated type (embryonal carcinoma)	
Teratoma	40
1. Well differentiated	
2. Undifferentiated	
3. Choriocarcinoma	
Combined tumours	10
Malignant lymphoma	3
Interstitial-cell tumours	2
1. Leydig	
2. Sertoli-cell tumour	

Seminoma

Macroscopic appearances
This is the most frequent tumour of the testis. It arises from the testicular tubules, and presumably, from the germ cells. Macroscopically it is not encapsulated, but it is well-circumscribed and its cut surface has a homogeneous, creamy-pink colour. Fibrous tissue septa may give the tumour a lobular appearance. In rapidly growing seminomas, yellow areas of necrosis may be present, but they are infrequent (Fig. 20.1).

Histological features
Seminomas are readily recognized, because they are composed of characteristic uniform cells. Three histological types are recognized:

1. *Classical seminoma* is composed of large, round or polyhedral cells, with central dark nuclei. The cytoplasm is usually clear, because it contains glycogen, occasionally it is granular, and the nucleus is hyperchromatic, but mitoses are infrequent. The cells may be arranged in sheets, columns or in tubule formation; they are separated by loose connective tissue which is often infiltrated

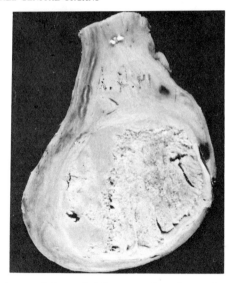

Fig. 20.1   Seminoma of the testis. The cut surface shows a large, solid tumour with a homogeneous appearance

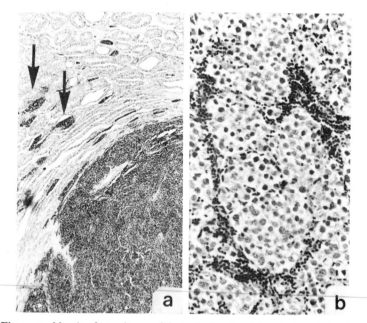

Fig. 20.2   Margin of a seminoma of the testis showing: (a) testicular tubules above and tumour below (the arrows indicate tumour cells in lymphatic vessels) (× 40); (b) tumour composed of two cell types: groups of large, clear cells separated by a scanty stroma containing small dark-staining lymphocytes (× 200)

with lymphocytes. This type of seminoma resembles the dysgerminoma of the ovary (Fig. 20.2).

2. *Spermatocytic seminoma* is usually larger, softer and rather more yellow than the classical type. It is composed of diffuse sheets of medium-sized cells, with round nuclei and eosinophilic cytoplasm. Scattered amongst these cells, there are small lymphocytes, large mononuclear cells and a few giant cells. Mitotic figures are more frequent than in the classical seminoma. The intercellular connective tissue is oedematous, and occasionally, microcysts may be present.

3. *Undifferentiated seminoma* is the most malignant type. The constituent cells are undifferentiated, irregular in form, and have relatively large vesicular nuclei. Some giant cells are present, and mitotic activity is increased. The so-called *embryonal carcinoma* of some authors might be a variant of the undifferentiated seminoma.

Teratoma

Testicular teratoma is a tumour composed of multiple tissues which are foreign to the testis, and unlike the teratoma in the ovary, it is highly malignant. The foreign tissues present are derived from more than one germinal layer, namely ectoderm (squamous epithelium and brain tissue), mesoderm (gastrointestinal, respiratory and urinary structures) and endoderm (cartilage, bone, muscle and lymphoid tissue). In contrast to the uniformity of the seminomas, testicular teratomas show considerable variation in structure, both macroscopically and microscopically.

Macroscopic appearance
The testis is usually enlarged and the tumour may vary in size from 1 to 6 cm in diameter. Although a range of appearances may be seen on the cut surface, these tumours may be divided into two groups: (a) *cystic teratomas*, whose cut surface consists almost entirely of cysts which vary in size, and may contain gelatinous, mucoid or keratohyaline material (Fig. 20.3). This appearance is characteristic of the well differentiated teratomas, and (b) *solid teratomas*, whose cut surface has variegated colour patterns with a yellowish-white background and typically contains large areas of haemorrhage and necrosis. Cystic change is infrequent. This appearance is characteristic of the undifferentiated teratomas which are highly malignant.

Histological features
Because of the multiplicity of tissues in teratomas, many sections

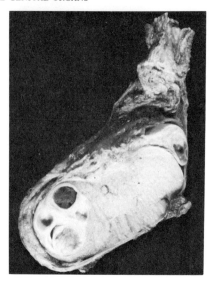

Fig. 20.3   Teratoma of the testis. The cut surface shows a cystic tumour

need to be examined for an adequate assessment of the nature of these tumours. In general, the tissue elements may be mature, embryonic or may show intermediate degrees of differentiation.

1. *Well differentiated teratomas* contain cystic spaces of varying sizes lined by squamous, cuboidal, ciliated columnar or transitional epithelium. The solid tissue between the cysts may contain well developed cartilage, bone, brain, liver, pancreas, muscle fibres etc.

2. *Undifferentiated teratomas* contain areas in which the cells are undifferentiated. Generally, the cells are pleomorphic and show increased mitotic activity. These tumours may resemble carcinomas or sarcomas.

3. *Choriocarcinoma* of the testis is rare (less than 1 per cent of testicular tumours) and is highly malignant. It is usually a small, haemorrhagic tumour which often cannot be palpated. Histologically, it contains epithelial elements of placental tissue (p. 278) growing in a disorderly manner, not as placental villi. They may produce high levels of chorionic gonadotrophins, the presence of which, in the male, are diagnostic of choriocarcinoma (Fig. 20.4).

Combined tumours
In approximately 10 per cent of patients with testicular tumours, two nodules are present in the testis, one resembling a seminoma, the other a teratoma. Each component has the macroscopic and

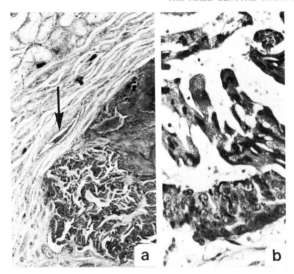

Fig. 20.4 Margin of a teratoma of the testis showing: (a) testicular tubules above and tumour below (the arrows indicate tumour cells in blood vessels) (× 40); (b) tumour composed of trophoblastic tissue characteristic of a choriocarcinoma (× 200)

microscopic features of the respective tumour, and it is generally believed that each tumour arises independently. These tumours are designated combined tumours of the testis.

Malignant lymphoma
Primary malignant lymphomas of the testis are uncommon and account for approximately 3 per cent of testicular tumours. They may occur at any age, but predominantly, they occur in older men, the peak age incidence being at 60 to 75 years. These tumours have a poor prognosis and most patients die within two years. Macroscopically, they vary in size, have no capsule and their cut surface has a solid appearance, with a uniform greyish-tan colour. Lymphocytic, histiocytic and undifferentiated lymphomas occur.

Interstitial-cell tumours
Interstitial cells are derived from the mesenchymal cells of the genital ridge. In the female, they give rise to theca granulosa and luteal cells, and in the male, to the interstitial cells of Leydig and Sertoli. In the testis, interstitial-cell tumours are uncommon (approximately 2 per cent of testicular tumours), but they are an interesting group, because they secrete hormones. Approximately 10 per cent become malignant.

1. *Leydig-cell tumour* is by far the most common stromal tumour in the testis. It occurs at any age, and in 90 per cent of cases, it is unilateral. Macroscopically, it varies in size from 1 to 8 cm in diameter, it is well circumscribed and the cut surface has a uniform, yellow-tan appearance. Microscopically, it is composed of confluent sheets of polygonal cells, with distinct cell outlines and eosinophilic, vacuolated cytoplasm. The nucleus is vesicular, with a dark nucleolus. Intracytoplasmic cigar-shaped bodies (Renke's crystals), best demonstrated with iron-haematoxylin stains, are characteristic features of these tumours.

Normally, Leydig cells secrete testosterone and very little oestrogen, so the Leydig-cell tumours mainly cause masculinization with deepening of the voice, excess pubic and facial hair, and enlargement of the penis. Gynaecomastia is also a common finding and is due to the oestrogen component.

2. *Sertoli-cell tumour* is a rare tumour in man but fairly common in dogs. It occurs at any age as a yellow nodule in the testis and is composed of tall columnar cells, resembling Sertoli cells, arranged in tubules. The cells have large, oval nuclei and a vacuolated cytoplasm containing fat.

THE PROSTATE GLAND

Nodular hyperplasia

This is a very common form of prostatic enlargement affecting older men. Although it is often referred to as benign hypertrophy, the condition is clearly a nodular hyperplasia, involving both glandular and stromal elements and giving rise to multiple adenomas. The condition commences after 45 years of age and then progressively increases in incidence until death. The significance of nodular hyperplasia rests entirely on its tendency to produce bladder neck obstruction, which becomes manifest clinically as a progressive difficulty in urination, with diminution in stream, frequency, chronic retention, dribbling and incontinence. There is no known association with carcinoma of the prostate, but in many cases, it can be difficult to differentiate between the two conditions.

Aetiology

The aetiology of prostatic hyperplasia is uncertain, although it is obvious that age and endocrine disturbances are important. Physiologically, the prostate gland consists of two zones:

1. An inner small zone of simple, short glands which respond to oestrogens.

2. An outer larger zone which contains the prostatic glands proper and which respond to testosterone.

The current view is that all hyperplasias arise from the inner zone and commence at an age when testosterone secretion diminishes. This results in a relative increase in oestrogens due to the persistence of adrenal oestrogen secretion. The paradox is, that whilst prostatic enlargement appears to be testosterone-dependent, it becomes manifest only when the output of testosterone is declining.

Macroscopic appearances

Hyperplasia develops in the inner zones of the lateral and median lobes of the prostate gland.

1. *Middle lobe enlargement* occurs upwards, stretches the internal sphincter, frequently projects into the bladder and acts as a ball-valve which can obstruct the outflow of urine.

2. *Lateral lobe enlargement* compresses the urethra laterally at the neck of the bladder and converts the lumen of the urethra into a vertical slit-like orifice.

Hyperplasia rarely occurs in the anterior or posterior lobes of the prostate gland, the posterior lobe being the common site for carcinoma. The size of the hyperplastic gland varies considerably, depending on the relative amounts of glandular and fibromuscular proliferation. Occasionally it is small, hard and uniform in appearance, but more commonly, it is large, soft and nodular. On section the nodules vary in size, the average being approximately 1 cm in diameter. They have no capsule, yet they are well circumscribed, they are light tan in colour, and when squeezed, a milky exudate oozes out from the cut surface. The nodules arise from the inner zone of the lateral and median lobes, and as they grow, they stretch the outer zone forming an additional capsule, the so-called *surgical capsule* of the prostate gland, which allows easy enucleation of the gland.

Histological features

Half of the normal prostate gland consists of glandular tissue, one quarter of smooth muscle, and one quarter of fibrous tissue. In the hyperplastic gland, all three elements are involved, and the histological pattern in each individual case will depend on the relative amount of each component.

1. *Adenomatous hyperplasia* is composed of collections of glands which are usually large, irregular in size and shape, and lined by cuboidal or columnar epithelium. The lining cells are regular in form, they rest on an intact basement membrane, and frequently

form folds or papillary processes. Corpora amylacea are commonly seen in the lamina of the glands, and lymphocytic infiltrations may be present in the stroma. Squamous metaplasia frequently develops in response to oestrogen therapy, but it may occur in untreated glands.

2. *Stromal hyperplasia* produces solid nodules composed of spindle cells, and may resemble a leiomyoma. Occasionally, small glands are entrapped in the hyperplastic stroma and may be mistaken for adenocarcinoma.

Carcinoma

Carcinoma of the prostate gland is one of the most common malignancies in the middle-aged and elderly male population. The disease is rare under the age of 45 years, the incidence thereafter increases progressively with longevity and reaches a peak in the seventh and eighth decades. The age-adjusted death rate per 100 000 population for carcinoma of the prostate is highest in the negro population of the United States of America and Africa (20 to 25 per 100 000) and lowest in Japan (2 to 5 per 100 000).

Aetiology
The cause of carcinoma of the prostate gland is not known. Three aetiological factors: hormonal disturbances, chemical carcinogens and immunodeficiency are probably significant in the pathogenesis of the disease. Nodular hyperplasia, though often associated, is probably unrelated.

1. *Cadmium* has recently been implicated, because workers exposed to cadmium compounds show an increased risk of developing carcinoma of the prostate gland. Cadmium is a known carcinogen, but its significance in the aetiology of prostatic cancer is not understood. Zinc, which acts as a binding core for the detoxification of metals, is present in high concentrations in normal and hyperplastic glands, but in very low concentrations in prostatic cancer. Since cadmium is a biological competitor for zinc, it is conceivable that high toxic levels of cadmium can develop in the human prostate gland, and be responsible for the development of malignancy.

2. *Hormonal disturbances.* Cancer of the prostate gland is a disease of advancing age when androgen secretion by the testis is diminishing and when the immunological surveillance is declining. It is known that: (a) no examples of carcinoma of the prostate have been recorded in patients subjected to orchidectomy before puberty and (b) that the cells of prostatic cancer are hormone-dependent,

their growth can be inhibited by oestrogen therapy or orchidectomy and promoted by androgens. It is postulated, therefore, that androgens either alone or in combination with other factors play a significant role in the pathogenesis of the disease.

3. *Decline in immunological surveillance*, which occurs with age, also allows the establishment of mutant cells and their development into overt tumours.

Macroscopic appearance

Unlike nodular hyperplasia, carcinoma arises in the outer zone of the posterior lobe of the prostate gland, just under the capsule. It commences as a subcapsular nodule and its chief characteristic is hardness. Rectal examination, therefore, often reveals a firm nodule or a craggy mass occupying all or part of the posterior lobe. A typically malignant nodule is harder, greyer in colour and more difficult to cut than the adjacent hyperplastic tissue. Its cut surface does not bulge or show any lobulation, but it is dry and may show yellow islands of tumour cells. In the early stages of development, it is difficult to recognize the lesion macroscopically; it is only after the tumour has invaded through the capsule and involved adjacent structures that it can be readily identified.

Histological features

Microscopically, prostatic cancers are adenocarcinomas of varying degrees of differentiation:

1. In *the well differentiated type*, the cells are cuboidal or polygonal in shape with prominent, deeply stained, central nuclei and distinct cell outlines. The cells are arranged into small, regular acini with a good stromal-epithelial relationship (*the micro-acinar pattern*). This type of carcinoma is difficult to recognize microscopically, the most unequivocal criteria of diagnosis being invasion and metastasis (Fig. 20.5).

2. *The undifferentiated type*, on the other hand, is easy to identify. There is complete lack of acinar pattern, the cells are hyperchromatic and pleomorphic, the cell outlines are indistinct and there are numerous mitoses present.

Most samples sent for diagnosis are either needle biopsies or transurethal resection specimens, both of which are small fragments of tissue. In these cases, malignancy is assessed on cellular detail, and on whether or not there is invasion of blood vessels or perineural spaces. The tumour cells are often clear or vacuolated, and in some cases, they may form a cribriform or papillary pattern.

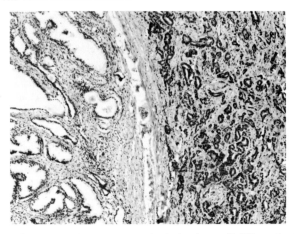

Fig. 20.5 Carcinoma of the prostate gland showing well-differentiated adeno-carcinoma and normal prostatic glands (× 100)

Course and prognosis

Because carcinoma commences in the posterior and peripheral part of the prostate gland, it remains asymptomatic for a long time. First, it spreads locally by invading through the capsule and involving the seminal vesicles, bladder and peritoneum. Distant metastases occur via the lymphatic and blood streams, with early metastases in the vertebrae, pelvis, femora and ribs. Radiologically, bony metastases are predominantly osteoblastic.

The *acid phosphotase* content of the prostate increases at puberty in response to testosterone, but there is very little spill over into the blood stream. Malignant prostatic cells also produce acid phosphotase. Estimation of prostatic acid phosphotase levels in the serum, therefore, is of value both in making a diagnosis and in assessing the extent of spread and the tumour's response to oestrogens. The normal range for serum acid phosphotase in SI units, is 0.1 to 0.6. The levels are raised in almost 100 per cent of patients with distant metastases, in 80 per cent with bony metastases, and in less than 50 per cent of patients with soft tissue invasion. It is important to emphasize that the level of acid phosphotase can be elevated, and remain so for over 24 hours following digital prostatic examination or massage.

The prognosis depends on the degree of histological differentiation and extent of invasion and spread of the disease. Four stages are recognized:

Stage A: Occult nodule recognized only microscopically.

Stage B: The tumour is clinically manifest, but remains intracapsular and the acid phosphotase is not raised.

Stage C: There is extracapsular invasion involving adjacent organs and pelvic glands. The acid phosphotase may or may not be elevated.

Stage D: Bone and extrapelvic metastases. Acid phosphotase is raised.

PENIS AND SCROTUM

The most common tumour of the penis and scrotum is squamous-cell carcinoma. Its incidence varies widely, being very common among Chinese, African negroes and Indians, uncommon among Caucasians, and virtually unknown among Jews who practise circumcision in infancy. The peak incidence occurs between 45 and 70 years of age.

Carcinoma of both penis and scrotum is more common in people with bad living conditions and poor hygiene. The high incidence of carcinoma of the scrotum in chimney sweeps (p. 271) was attributed to soot and poor hygiene. Premalignant lesions of the penis include leukoplakia and Bowen's disease; phimosis and other inflammatory diseases have also been incriminated, but not substantiated.

In the penis, carcinoma usually arises on the dorsum of the glans or prepuce and forms an irregular, warty, fungating mass which is prone to extensive ulceration. This form of cancer may also involve the scrotum. Microscopically, these tumours are squamous-cell carcinomas, usually well differentiated. They spread via the lymphatics to the inguinal lymph nodes. Blood spread occurs only in the advanced stage.

The prognosis is good when inguinal metastases are not present, the five-year survival rate being as high as 95 per cent. The outcome is worse with undifferentiated carcinomas and those that have invaded through to the corpora cavernosa and urethra.

FURTHER READING

Blennerhassett, J. B. & Vickery, A. L. (1966) Carcinoma of the prostate: an anatomical study of tumour location. *Cancer*, **19**, 980.

Cook, W. B. *et al.* (1962) Serum acid phosphotase of prostatic origin in the diagnosis of prostatic cancer: clinical evaluation of 2408 tests by the Fishman–Lerner method. *J. Urol.*, **88**, 281.

Maier, J. G. & Sulak, M. H. (1973) Radiation therapy in malignant testis tumours: seminoma. *Cancer*, **32**, 1212.

Mostofi, F. K. & Price, E. B. (1973) *Tumours of the Male Genital System*, Fascicle 8, Second series, Washington D.C.: Armed Forces Institute of Pathology.

Pugh, R. C. B. (1976) *Pathology of the Testis*. Oxford: Blackwell Scientific Publications.

Willis, R. A. (1967) *Pathology of Tumours*, 4th edn. London: Butterworths.

21

Tumours of the female genital tract

There is considerable variation in the relative frequency of malignant tumours of the female genital organs, but the vast majority occur in the uterus and cervix. The approximate distribution is: vulva (4 per cent), vagina (3 per cent), cervix (70 per cent), corpus uteri (12 per cent), fallopian tubes (1 per cent) and ovaries (10 per cent).

VULVA AND VAGINA

Benign	*Malignant*
Papilloma	Squamous-cell carcinoma
Hidradenoma	Malignant melanoma
	Adenocarcinoma of the vagina

Papillomas
Skin papillomas may grow in the region of the vulva and are commonly due to viral infection or to venereal disease (p. 147).

Hidradenoma
This relatively common benign neoplasm, derived from sweat glands, most commonly forms as an intracystic papillary growth. On occasions, the skin becomes ulcerated, papillary excrescence appears on the surface and the lesion takes the form of a raspberry red, papillomatous growth, rarely exceeding 1 cm in diameter. Despite this appearance, it is a benign lesion.

Squamous-cell carcinoma
This is the common type of malignant tumour of the vulva. It is usually a disease of elderly women and begins on the labia majora, labia minor, the clitoris or the perineum. It may be preceded by a variety of epithelial dysplasias, although frank intra-epithelial malignancies, such as Bowen's or Paget's disease are uncommon.

The common preceding dysplasia often has hyperkeratotic zones which give the clinical appearances of leukoplakia. The tumour generally presents as an ulcer, with raised, rolled-up edges, and when the disease follows leukoplakia, the tumours may be multiple. Histologically it is a keratinising squamous-cell carcinoma. Direct spread is common and often extensive at the time of presentation, and metastases occur in the regional inguinal lymph nodes. On rare occasions, widespread dissemination can occur. Enlargement of lymph nodes in the presence of carcinoma of the vulva may be caused by the associated inflammation, so that histological assessment of enlarged lymph nodes is important in the management of the disease.

Malignant melanoma
Melanoma is a rare primary neoplasm in the vulva. Rarely, it can arise within the vagina, which is not surprising, as the clear cells of Masson are normal components of vaginal epithelium.

Adenocarcinoma
Primary adenocarcinoma of the vagina is also a rare disease. On occasions, a primary squamous-cell carcinoma of the vulva or the cervix can spread extensively to involve the vagina. However, in recent years, there has been a rise in incidence of adenocarcinoma of the vagina, in young women, in their late teens or early twenties. This rise in incidence was recorded in daughters of mothers who had received large doses of stilboestrol during pregnancy, and represents an example of transplacental carcinogenesis.

UTERUS

Benign	*Malignant*

Leiomyoma (fibroma, myoma, 'fibroids')	Carcinoma of the cervix:
	  (a) Squamous-cell carcinoma
	  (b) Adenocarcinoma

Leiomyoma
Leiomyomas of the uterus are very common. They may be single or multiple, and are sub-classified according to their anatomical position.

1. *Submucosal leiomyomas* lie under the mucosa, and project into the uterine cavity.
2. *Intramural leiomyomas* are situated within the muscle wall of the uterus.

3. *Subserosal leiomyomas* lie beneath the peritoneal covering of the uterus and project outwards.

Both submucosal and subserosal myomas may become pedunculated and prone to certain complications, namely: (a) torsion, (b) a submucosal tumour may be extruded through the cervix, (c) because they cause enlargement of the uterus, they may produce symptoms by pressure on adjacent organs, and (d) by increasing the surface area of the endometrium, they can cause heavy periods.

The general shape of the nodules is round, macroscopically well demarcated, but they do not have a capsule. Histologically, the tumours are made up of whorled spindle cells, due to interweaving bundles of muscle fibres, and a variable amount of collagen. During reproductive life, mitotic figures and bizarre nuclear forms can generally be seen, especially adjacent to zones of degeneration or necrosis, and should not be misinterpreted as sarcomatous change.

Hydatidiform mole
Hydatidiform mole is a condition characterized by cystic distension of the chorionic villi of the placenta and by proliferation of the Langhans' and syncytial cells. The condition is relatively rare, being less frequent among Caucasians (1:2 000) than Chinese (1:500) and Filipinos (1:200). Macroscopically, the placenta is converted into a mass of grape-like bodies which vary in size from 1 mm to 2 cm in diameter. Microscopically, the vesicles appear oedematous, as each cyst is a swollen hydropic villus. There are generally no foetal vessels. Approximately 5 per cent of hydatidiform moles become malignant.

Hydatidiform moles secrete large quantities of chorionic gonadotrophic hormone, the level of which progressively increases during the pregnancy and can be detected clinically. Because of the high level of hormone, theca-lutein cysts of the ovary develop in approximately 25 per cent of cases.

Carcinoma of the cervix
Invasive carcinoma of the cervix is a relatively common form of cancer in women. Although occasionally of glandular type, it is most commonly a squamous-cell carcinoma which begins in the region of the squamo-columnar junction of the cervix and which has a peak age-incidence between 40 and 50 years.

Aetiology
In common with other malignant tumours, a specific cause for

carcinoma of the cervix has not been found. Formerly, an aetiological association was drawn between carcinoma of the cervix and
child-bearing, and this relationship was attributed to trauma in-
flicted on the cervix at parturition. Thus 90 per cent to 95 per cent
of cervical carcinomas occur in women who have had one or more
children. Recently, other factors such as early onset of coitus and
promiscuity brought about with the alteration in social attitudes and
the contraceptive pill, have been considered more important. The
aetiological relationship between coitus and the carcinogenic
process is not clear. Carcinogens in smegma, penetration of
cervical epithelial cells by spermatozoa and infection with the genital
strain of Herpes simplex virus type 2 (p. 62) all have their advocates.

The earliest neoplastic changes are covert and precede the epithelial disarrays (dysplasia, carcinoma *in situ* and early stromal
invasion). Dysplasia and carcinoma *in situ* often occur together, but
appear at least a decade earlier than invasive cancer, and women
with such epithelial dysplasias develop invasive cancer significantly
more frequently than women without dysplasias (Fig. 21.1). Experimentally, there is good evidence that many of these lesions regress,
but it is not possible, in our present state of knowledge, to predict
in any one patient the outcome of a particular dysplasia. It seems
likely that, though many of the dysplasias may regress, few of the
carcinoma *in situ* lesions do so. Although progression is important,

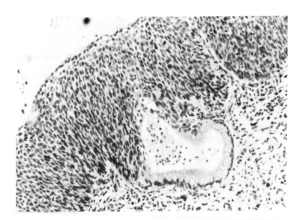

Fig. 21.1 Carcinoma *in situ* of the cervix uteri showing disarray of cell layers,
loss of surface stratification and considerable proliferation of basal cells which are
pleomorphic, hyperchromatic and have dark-staining cytoplasm. The expanding
epithelium is lifting off the epithelial lining of a cervical gland but is not invasive.
The basal layer of cells is clearly demarcated from the adjacent stroma by a well-
defined basement membrane (× 320)

the possibility of regression must never be forgotten before indulging in potentially dangerous, crippling treatment.

Pathology
Carcinoma of the cervix may take on an ulcerating, infiltrating or fungating form. A carcinomatous ulcer has rolled-up edges, and the cervix is usually indurated and infiltrated by tumour cells. It is friable and tends to bleed on touch. The cancer extends locally to invade adjacent organs and spreads by lymphatics to the regional nodes. Eventually metastases can be established at any site. Death may be due to renal failure because of constriction of the ureters by direct invasion of the structures in the broad ligament.

Microscopically, the vast majority of carcinomas of the cervix are squamous-cell carcinomas showing various degrees of differentiation (Fig. 21.2). Occasionally, the growth arises in the glandular epithelium lining the endocervical canal and is an adenocarcinoma.

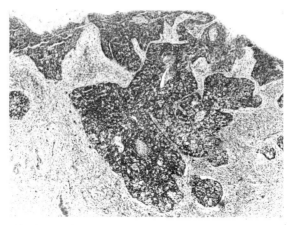

Fig. 21.2 Carcinoma of the cervix uteri showing invasion of the adjacent stroma by well differentiated carcinoma (× 40)

Adenocarcinoma of the endometrium

Clinically, this tumour usually presents later in life than carcinoma of the cervix as post-menopausal bleeding in a nulliparous, hypertensive, obese woman who may also have diabetes. Although there is no direct association between endometrial hyperplasia and adenocarcoma, there is evidence that an atypical hyperplasia may precede or be associated with an adenocarcinoma. Endomentrial carcinoma arises from a broad area of endometrium, and usually presents as an elevation in the region of the fundus. From there it spreads in two directions:

1. Over the surface of the endometrium to involve almost the entire endometrium until it is arrested at the isthmus.
2. Through the myometrium to penetrate the wall of the uterus and involve the peritoneum and adjacent pelvic organs.

Direct spread is common, but infiltration of the myometrium, lymphatics or blood spread occur late and the prognosis is, in general, much better than that associated with carcinoma of the cervix.

Choriocarcinoma

This is a rare and biologically unique neoplasm. It is formed from tissue genetically different from that of the host, because it is derived from placental trophoblast where half the genes in the cells are derived from the mother and half from the father. Approximately half the cases of choriocarcinoma arise following a hydatidiform mole, the other half, are equally distributed between a normal pregnancy or an abortion. The condition is uncommon in most Western countries, but it is comparatively common in the Orient.

A normal physiological characteristic of trophoblast is invasion of blood vessels. Choriocarcinoma, therefore, is characterized by widespread bloodborne metastases, and nearly all the deposits, whether primary or secondary, are macroscopically and microscopically haemorrhagic. Histologically, there are no villi, but the neoplasm is generally made up of an intimate mixture of both cytotrophoblast and syncytiotrophoblast. The syncytial type of trophoblastic cells are large and pleomorphic, and contain large pale nuclei, whereas the cytotrophoblastic cells are clearly defined cuboidal cells. The growth pattern of the tumour is more important in diagnosis than cellular detail because trophoblast is normally undifferentiated and active in appearance.

Choriocarcinoma tissue is almost invariably associated with secretion of chorionic gonadotrophic hormone which is excreted in the urine. Estimation of the level of hormone is not only valuable in diagnosis, but it also serves as a measure of the amount of viable tumour tissue in the body following therapy. In the past, the condition was invariably fatal, death resulting from multiple pulmonary metastases or from intracerebral deposits. In recent years, use of cytotoxic drugs and folic acid antagonists have greatly improved survival rates.

THE OVARIES

During reproductive life, the ovaries undergo a monthly cyclical change, with development of follicular cysts, extrusion of the ovum and development of a corpus luteum which, if pregnancy occurs, enlarges to form the corpus luteum of pregnancy. Cystic distension of some of these structures can form lumps (follicular cysts or corpus luteum cysts), but these are not tumours, they are simple cysts and rarely give rise to clinical symptoms. Within the ovary, there are three basic types of cells capable of giving rise to tumours:

1. *Surface coelomic epithelium* has the capacity to differentiate into serous, ciliated columnar or non-ciliated mucus-secreting columnar cells.
2. *Stromal cells* can give rise to theca, granulosa or luteal cells.
3. *Germ cells* which are totipotential.

Therefore, the array of tumours that can occur in the ovaries is great, and a complete classification of such tumours is necessarily complicated. In this section a simplified, working classification is used:

Benign tumours	*Malignant tumours*
(a) Cystic –	(a) Cystic –
Cystic teratoma	Mucinous cystadenocarci-
('dermoid')	noma
Mucinous cystadenoma	Papillary serous
Papillary serous cysta-	cystadenocarcinoma
denoma	
(b) Solid –	(b) Solid –
Fibroma	Adenocarcinoma
Adenofibroma	Dysgerminoma
Thecoma	Granulosa-cell tumour
	Malignant teratoma
	Mixed Mullerian tumour

Cystic teratoma

In the ovary, benign cystic teratomas are common, often bilateral (25 per cent) and, because of the preponderance of skin appendages within the tumours, they are incorrectly called 'dermoid cysts'. The cyst is generally filled with a tangled mass of hair and sebaceous material which tends to make the tumour heavy, and because of its heaviness, it may lie in front of the uterus and cause symptoms during pregnancy. On removal of sebaceous material, there is usually a papilla covered by skin, which may contain teeth or portions of bone which can be seen in a plain X-ray of the abdomen. Histologically, apart from skin and skin appendages, the most frequent component is nervous tissue which may be well differentiated. On rare occasions, the preponderant tissue present is thyroid gland, sometimes called *struma ovarii*. The thyroid follicles can be functional and may cause symptoms of hyperthyroidism.

Mucinous and papillary serous cystadenomas

These are common, and together make up more than 50 per cent of all ovarian tumours. The terms *mucinous* or *serous* are given because of the character of the fluid within the cysts and this, in turn is dependent on the lining epithelium which is either tall mucin-secreting columnar epithelium or a cuboidal, sometimes ciliated, epithelium which forms papillae. Such cysts can be very large and yet remain entirely benign. There is a report of a mucinous cystadenoma which weighed over 140 kg. Each variety of cystadenoma is equally common, and both usually present in the third or fourth decade. The mucinous cystadenomas are often unilateral and nearly always multilocular, whereas the serous cystadenomata are often bilateral and generally have few loculi, but are nearly always papilliferous. Mucinous cystadenomata may perforate spontaneously or be damaged during removal with subsequent implantation of mucin-secreting epithelium throughout the peritoneum, giving rise to one form of *pseudomyxoma peritonei*. Papillary serous cystadenomata may have papillae on the external surface, and may seed throughout the peritoneum without losing histological characteristics of benignity. In such neoplasms, it may be very difficult to relate the histological appearances with the clinical course.

Fibroma

Approximately 2 per cent to 5 per cent of ovarian tumours are fibromas. Such tumours are generally of moderate size, unilateral and generally spherical, with a characteristic white, faintly whorled cut surface. They are almost invariably benign. Meigs pointed out that such tumours might be associated with ascites and hydrothorax, features commonly associated with malignant tumours. The importance of *Meig's syndrome* is that clinical characteristics most often associated with malignant ovarian tumours may be found with a benign tumour, such as a fibroma of the ovary. The mechanism whereby fluid accumulates is not certain, but it is generally thought to be a function of the fibroma itself.

Adenofibroma

These are generally benign, bilateral, lobulated, semi-solid and semi-cystic tumours of the ovary. Macroscopically, apart from their lobulated appearance, they resemble a fibroma in which there are small cysts or slit-like spaces. Histologically, there is a fibrous stroma in which there are small cysts lined by cuboidal epithelium which often forms papillary projections.

Thecoma

This tumour closely resembles the fibroma, but is distinguished from it by: (a) the yellow colour macroscopically, (b) the demonstration of fat within and between the tumour cells histologically, and (c) clinically, by the common association of hyperoestrinism.

Cystic carcinomas

Both mucinous cystadenocarcinoma and papillary serous cystadenocarcinoma can be identified, and particularly in the mucinous type, a histological gradient can be traced from benign mucinous lesions, through proliferating lesions, to adenocarcinomas. Both can disseminate widely and usually present late. Papillary serous cystadenocarcinomas have a tendency to spread throughout the peritoneal cavity causing a severe, distressing ascites.

Adenocarcinomas

Such neoplasms are solid and not derived from mucinous or papillary serous tumours. They have a range of histological patterns and characteristics, but all have a bad prognosis and not infrequently present late in the course of the disease.

Dysgerminoma

Histologically, the dysgerminoma of the ovary is similar to the seminoma of the testis. Macroscopically, it is a rubbery, solid, white tumour usually hormonally inert. Like the seminoma, it consists of acinar or tubular structures composed of large, round cells with clear cytoplasm and round nuclei (Fig. 21.3). Usually there are very few mitoses present, and occasionally, giant cells may be seen. Between the tubules, there is a fine connective tissue stroma which contains large numbers of lymphocytes. Because of its preponderance in the second and third decade, it is sometimes called the carcinoma of young girls (*carcinoma puellarum*). Such a neoplasm has been reported in women with chromosomal abnormalities, but mostly it is found in normal women. Like the seminoma, it tends to

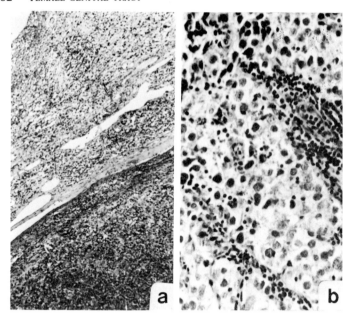

Fig. 21.3 Dysgerminoma of the ovary showing: (a) ovarian tissue above and tumour below (× 40); (b) tumour composed of large round cells with clear cytoplasm and lymphocytes (× 200). Compare with seminoma (p. 262)

respond well to radiotherapy. When the tumour is confined to one ovary, prognosis is good, but if it has spread, the prognosis is poor.

Granulosa-cell tumour

The term granulosa-cell tumour, rather than granulosa-cell carcinoma, is frequently used because of the difficulty in relating histological appearances with subsequent clinical courses. Granulosa-cell tumour is usually unilateral, varies greatly in size and the cut surface usually shows a semi-solid, semi-cystic tumour with distinctly yellow zones. Histologically, the tumour is made up of sheets of small, darkly staining cells which tend to take up a follicle-like pattern, and generally resembles the granulosa cells of a ripening follicle (Fig. 21.4). Indicative also of the origin of the cell is the fact that this tumour is frequently associated with hyper-oestrinism. The neoplasm may present at all ages. Like the dysgerminoma, when the tumour is unilateral, the prognosis may often be good, but when spread has occurred, the prognosis is poor. Granulosa-cell tumour is one of the neoplasms associated with metastases many years after the removal of the primary tumour.

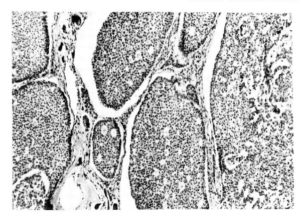

Fig. 21.4 Granulosa cell tumour of the ovary composed of small dark-staining cells tending to form follicle-like patterns (× 100)

Malignant teratoma

In contrast to the testis, the vast majority of teratomas of the ovary are cystic and benign. Malignant transformation is rare in the cystic teratoma, and when it does occur, it is seen only in one tissue element, usually the skin, with the formation of squamous-cell carcinoma. A primary, solid, malignant teratoma can occur but this also is very rare. It generally presents as a lump in the late teens or early twenties. Macroscopically, it has no specific characteristics, but microscopically, it is made up of a mixture of primitive tissues which show varying degrees of differentiation. The tumour tends to spread widely; it produces metastatic deposits in many organs and responds poorly to treatment.

Mixed Mullerian tumours

This term is used to cover a group of highly malignant tumours which, histologically, are made up of a mixture of tissues, most commonly of carcinosarcomatous type, but having, on rare occasions, readily demonstrable cartilage or other tissues present. Such tumours are rare; they tend to occur either in the vagina and cervix of children, presenting as the so-called *sarcoma botryoides*, or in the endometrium of post-menopausal women. Rarely, they may arise in the ovary. Mixed Mullerian tumours are highly malignant, metastasize widely, and the metastatic deposits may show a change of histological pattern.

Secondary tumours of the female genital tract

The female genital tract can be involved by direct spread from tumours arising in the bladder, colon, rectum, or more rarely, from malignant tumours arising in the bones of the pelvis. The uterus and ovaries can also be involved, at a late stage, in the course of any disseminated malignancy, but most·commonly, in association with primary carcinomas of the breast or malignant melanomas.

Krukenberg tumours of the ovary

Under the name *fibrosarcoma muco-cellulare carcinomatodes*, Krukenberg, in 1896, described bilateral, solid, kidney-shaped tumours of the ovary which he considered to be primary and sarcomatous. In fact, Krukenberg tumours are secondary carcinomas characterized, histologically, by a mucin-filled, signet ring cell set in a fibrous tissue stroma. Clinically, such neoplasms may be the presenting features of an otherwise latent gastric or colonic carcinoma.

FURTHER READING

Avarette, H. E. *et al.* (1975) Staging of cervical cancer. *Clin. Obstet. Gynecol.*, **18**, 215.

Frick, A. C. *et al.* (1973) Carcinoma of the endometrium. *Am. J. Obstet. Gynecol.*, **115**, 663.

Herbst, A. L. *et al.* (1972) Clear cell adenocarcinoma of the genital tract in young females: Registry report. *N. Engl. J. Med.*, **287**, 1259.

Louis, C. J. (1960) A histochemical study of the epithelial tumours of the cervix and uterus. *Am. J. Obstet. Gynecol.*, **79**, 336.

Louis, C. J. (1966) Some aspects of hydatidiform mole and choriocarcinoma. *Med. J. Aust.*, **1**, 334.

Riotton, G. & Christopherson, W.M. (1973) *International Histological Classification of Tumours No. 8: Cytology of the Female Genital Tract.* Geneva: World Health Organization.

Serov, S. F. & Scully, R. E. (1973) *International Histological Classification of Tumours No. 9: Histological Typing of Ovarian Tumours.* Geneva: World Health Organization.

Willis, R. A. (1967) *Pathology of Tumours*, 4th edn. London: Butterworths.

22

Tumours of the nervous system

Tumours are relatively common within the nervous system. They account for approximately 10 per cent of primary tumours in man and are responsible for 2 per cent of deaths. They may be arbitrarily divided into: (a) tumours of the central nervous system (CNS), which include tumours of the brain and spinal cord, and (b) tumours of the peripheral nerves.

Intracranial tumours disclose their whereabouts partly by interfering with the function of the adjacent part of the brain and partly by taking up space within the rigid cranium (p. 97). The raised intracranial pressure compresses the brain as a whole, and may cause brain shifts by herniation of intracranial contents from compartments of high pressure into compartments of lower pressure. Consequently, the clinical features produced consist of:

1. Localizing symptoms and signs.
2. Features due to raised intracranial pressure.
3. Evidence of brain shifts.

The vast majority (95 per cent) of space-occupying lesions are neoplasms, and of these, approximately one half are primary tumours, and one half, metastatic deposits. The metastases are mainly secondary carcinomas, predominantly from the lung and breasts, some are melanomas, and the rest, sarcomas and lymphomas. A small fraction (5 per cent) of space-occupying lesions is made up of abscesses, aneurysms, granulomas, chronic subdural haematomas and hydatid cysts.

Most primary tumours are neuroglial in origin, and are called *gliomas*. Mature neurons do not give rise to tumours, although their precursors, the neuroblasts, probably do in the form of embryonal tumours. Tumours arising from the arachnoid cells in the meninges or dura are called *meningiomas*, and those arising from Schwann cells in the nerve sheaths, *Schwannomas* or *neuromas*. Finally, there are the pituitary gland adenomas and some rare developmental tumours (pinealoma, craniopharyngioma, chordoma, epidermoid cyst and tuberose sclerosis).

Aetiology

As with tumours of other organs, the cause of brain tumours in man is not known. Some gliomas are common in young children and often show a higher incidence in some families, but no genetic markers have been identified and the significance of a familial tendency is not understood. It is possible that carcinogens such as nitrosamines, taken during pregnancy (p. 51), cross the placental barrier and may be responsible for some brain tumours seen in young children. The majority of brain tumours, however, occur in adults, and it is assumed that malignant transformation is acquired after birth.

Over the years, many attempts have been made to identify specific aetiological agents which might account for the cause of brain tumours, and the results obtained recently with the N-Nitroso compounds and viruses may have some relevance to man. Some of these are shown in Table 22.1.

Table 22.1   Induction of brain tumours

	Route of administration	Animal	Period	Tumours induced
Chemical carcinogens				
2-Acetylaminofluorene	Oral	Rat	300 days	Gliomas, meningiomas Schwannomas
Dibenzanthracene	Intravenous	Newborn Hamsters	300 days	Gliomas
N-Nitroso compounds				
Methylnitrosourea	Intragastric Intravenous	Rats	200 days	Cerebral gliomas and medulloblastomas
Ethylnitrosourea	Intragastric Intravenous	Pregnant Rats	200 days	Variety of tumours in brain, cranial nerves, spinal cord and peripheral nerves
Viruses				
Rous sarcoma virus	Intracerebral	Dogs and Hamsters	15 days	Gliomas
Polyoma virus	Intracerebral	Dogs and Hamsters	30 days	Gliomas, ependymomas, choroid plexus papilloma
Adenovirus	Intracerebral	Dogs and Hamsters	30 days	Gliomas

THE GLIOMAS

The gliomas are a mixed group of tumours which occur in different frequencies and different sites in children and adults. They are twice as common in males as in females. Histologically, they are classified on the predominant cell type, and anatomically, on whether they are located above or below the tentorium cerebelli. In adults, 75 per cent of primary brain tumours are supratentorial, whereas in children, 75 per cent are infratentorial in the posterior fossa. Gliomas occur at all ages, but in children under 15 years of age, they rank first among solid tumours. The following list shows the different types of gliomas and some of their characteristics:

	Frequency of gliomas		Age incidence (years)	
	Adults (%)	Children (%)	Range	Peak
Astrocytoma	25	48	20–60	45
Glioblastoma Multiforme	55	—	30–70	55
Oligodendroglioma	5	—	25–60	45
Ependymoma	5	8	3–30	10
Medulloblastoma	10	44	5–25	12

Astrocytoma

Astrocytoma is a slow-growing tumour derived from astrocytes, and can occur in practically any part of the central nervous system. It accounts for approximately 25 per cent of intracranial gliomas in adults, and 48 per cent in children. In children, astrocytoma commonly occurs below the tentorium and is found in the cerebellum, usually in the wall of the 4th ventricle, whereas in adults, it is predominantly supratentorial, found in the cerebral cortex. Two histological types of astrocytoma may be recognized:

1. *The protoplasmic-cell astrocytoma*, in which the constituent cells and their processes do not contain glial fibres. This type tends to occur in the grey matter and has a soft consistency.

2. *The fibrillary astrocytoma* is composed of cells which contain fibrillae. This type occurs in the white matter and is the more slow-growing variety. Fibrillary astrocytoma is smooth and hard: its cut surface has a pale, yellow-white colour, and its edge which tends to merge with the surrounding white matter may be particularly difficult to define.

Probably, because of the scanty blood supply, both types of astrocytoma often show degenerative change and occasionally cyst formation. Cysts may be single or multiple, and in children, they may grow to a considerable size; they have a smooth wall and contain clear yellow fluid, with a high content of albumin which may coagulate on fixation. A solid nodule of tumour tissue (*mural nodule*) may be found in the wall protruding into the lumen of the cyst. Benign astrocytomas usually occur in adults under the age of 40 years. They grow slowly and have a tendency to infiltrate the surrounding brain substance. Malignant astrocytomas typically occur after the age of 40, and although malignancy may develop in a previously benign tumour, most are malignant from the start. Their rapid growth causes oedema of the surrounding brain substance and expansion of the hemisphere, and their cut surface often shows haemorrhages, yellow areas of necrosis, cyst formation and well-defined margins.

Microscopic features
Astrocytomas are composed entirely of astrocytes which may vary in size, shape and density, from area to area. In some areas, the cells are spindle-shaped, densely packed and closely related to thin-walled blood vessels; in other areas, the tumour is sparsely cellular and may contain microcysts. The nuclei are regular in form and mitotic figures are rare, areas of necrosis and haemorrhage are uncommon, but foci of calcification and perivascular cuffs of lymphocytes are often present (Fig. 22.1).

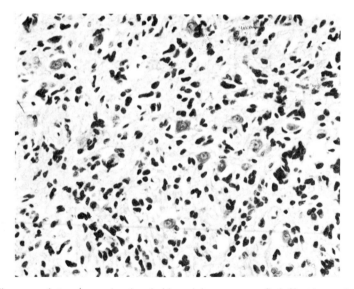

Fig. 22.1 Astrocytoma showing darkly staining tumour cells infiltrating arot neurones (× 200)

Normally, astrocytomas do not show histological features of malignancy, but they are capable of doing so at any stage of their development. Four grades of malignancy are described depending on the microscopic appearances, Grade 1 being the least and Grade 4 the most malignant.

Glioblastoma multiforme

This is the commonest type of primary malignant brain tumour. It represents approximately 55 per cent of all gliomas, tends to occur in middleage, most cases occurring between 45 and 65 years with a peak age incidence at 55 years, and is twice as common in males as in females. It is rare in children. Glioblastoma tends to occur in the white matter, predominantly in the cerebral hemispheres, and much less frequently in the brain stem and cerebellum. It is a rapidly fatal tumour, the average survival period after the appearance of symptoms being less than twelve months.

Macroscopic appearance

Glioblastoma can reach a very large size. It grows rapidly, destroying a large part of one or even both hemispheres. The cut surface shows characteristic variegated colour patterns due to areas of fatty degeneration which are yellow, necrosis (grey) and haemorrhages of various stages (brown to red). The surrounding brain tissue is oedematous, and the adjacent surface convolutions may be flattened and discoloured. Metastases within the C.N.S. commonly occur through the C.S.F., but metastases in distant organs are exceptionally rare (Fig. 22.2).

Microscopic features

Glioblastoma multiforme is a cellular tumour in which, as its name implies, the cells are undifferentiated and exhibit great diversity in size, shape and arrangement. Usually the cells are small, with round to ovoid dark staining nuclei, and intermingled with these cells are larger cells and giant cells with multiple or multilobed nuclei and abundant cytoplasm. Mitotic figures are common. Occasionally, there are primitive glial cells which are spindle shaped and resemble unipolar or bipolar astrocytes. In addition to the cells, there are areas of haemorrhage and necrosis, cyst formation, phagocytic cells containing fat vacuoles, and proliferation of the endothelial cells of small blood vessels and capillaries.

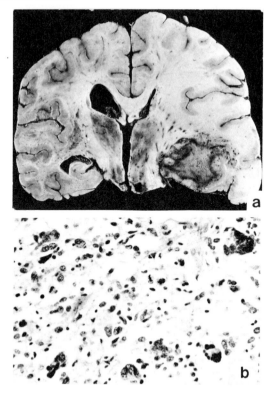

Fig. 22.2 Expanding malignant brain tumour involving the temporal lobe: (a) shows distortion of the ventricular system and upward displacement of the Sylvian fissure; (b) histologically the tumour is a glioblastoma multiforme consisting of pleomorphic cells, giant cells, inclusion bodies and mitotic figures (× 200)

Oligodendroglioma

This is a relatively uncommon tumour which accounts for less than five per cent of all gliomas. Like the astrocytoma, it is a slow-growing tumour which usually occurs in the white matter of the frontal lobe. It is rare in the cerebellum. Oligodendroglioma occurs predominantly in adults and has a peak incidence in the fifth decade.

Macroscopic appearance

It is usually a well circumscribed tumour which varies in size from one to several centimetres in diameter. Its cut surface has a grey to pink colour, and commonly shows foci of calcification and haemorrhage.

Microscopic features

Oligodendroglioma is composed of masses of small, uniformly distributed and closely packed cells, on a vascular connective tissue stroma. Characteristically, the cells have small, round, dark-staining nuclei, surrounded by clear cytoplasm and have been likened to fried eggs. Mitotic figures are rare. Occasionally, astrocytes may be intermingled with the oligodendrocytes (Fig. 22.3).

Ependymoma

The ependymoma arises from the ependymal cells lining the ventricular system, especially the fourth ventricle and the central canal of the spinal cord, and less frequently, in the lumbosacral enlargement and the filum terminale (ependyma of the cauda equina). Like the oligodendroglioma, it is slow-growing, relatively uncommon and represents approximately five per cent of all gliomas. Macroscopically, two types are described:

1. *Intraventricular ependymoma* occurs in adults, usually found in the fourth ventricle and is attached to the floor of the ventricle; it varies in size from 1 to 8 cm in diameter, is relatively well circumscribed and has a somewhat firm consistency. The cut surface often shows foci of calcification and cyst formation. In the spinal cord,

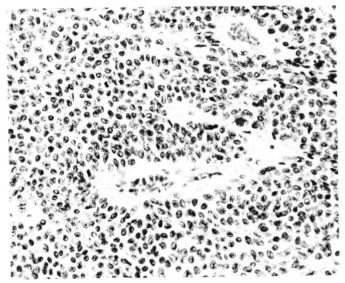

Fig. 22.3 Oligodendroglioma composed of closely packed cells with uniform spheroidal nuclei (× 200)

it assumes the shape of a pencil and extends over several segments.

2. *Extraventricular ependymoma* nearly always occurs in children in the central hemisphere adjacent to the lateral ventricle. It is the commonest supratentorial tumour in children.

Microscopically, these tumours are composed of ependymal cells which vary in their arrangement, but two basic varieties are distinguished:

1. *Papillary ependymoma* is usually found in the spinal cord and filum terminale. It consists of small papillary processes composed of a core of connective tissue stroma lined by ependymal cells. The stroma may undergo myxomatous change.

2. *Cellular ependymoma* is commonly found in the cerebral hemispheres and in the posterior fossa. It is composed of irregular groups of closely packed ependymal cells, lying in apparently clear spaces with no stromal support. Sometimes, the cells are arranged in rosettes round a central clear space or round small blood vessels (Fig. 22.4).

Generally, the ependymoma is a benign tumour, but malignant varieties do occur, and when they do, they spread directly via the C.S.F., or they may recur following excision.

Papilloma of the choroid plexus

These are rare tumours occurring predominantly in children and accounting for less than 0.5 per cent of all gliomas. They are found in those parts of the ventricular system which contain choroid plexus, particularly in the fourth ventricle, and occasionally, in the lateral and third ventricles.

The tumours are well circumscribed, friable in consistency and they vary in size; in the lateral ventricles, they may reach a size of 5 to 8 cm in diameter, but in other sites, they range from 1 to 2 cm in diameter. Some papillomas are functional; they secrete excessive amounts of C.S.F. and are frequently associated with hydrocephalus. Microscopically, the papillary processes have a core of loose vascular connective tissue lined by a single layer of uniform cells. The cells differ from ependymal cells in that they do not possess cilia.

Although most choroid papillomas are benign and their structure closely resembles that of choroid plexus, in rare cases, frank malignant changes occur, and tumour seedlings are seen elsewhere in the ventricular system and in the subarachnoid space.

Colloid cyst of the third ventricle

This is a rare developmental cyst, commonly found in the anterior part of the third ventricle. It is not a true tumour.

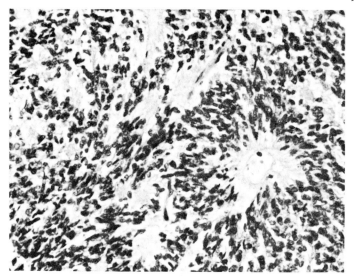

Fig. 22.4 Ependymoma showing typical perivascular rosettes with elongated fibrillated cells (× 200)

It is a spherical, pedunculated cyst, which hangs from its attachment on the roof of the third ventricle, in close relationship to the interventricular foramina. It varies in size from 1 to 4 cm in diameter, has a thin, smooth wall, and contains a greenish colloid fluid which often coagulates after fixation. The wall of the cyst is lined by a single layer of cells supported by a vascular connective tissue capsule. The cells are regular in form, vary from cuboidal to tall ciliated columnar, and there are many goblet cells present containing PAS-positive mucin.

Although developmental in origin, the cysts do not present until adult life. They tend to block the foramen of Monro, causing intermittent obstruction to the flow of C.S.F. and resulting in hydrocephalus and severe postural headaches.

Medulloblastoma
This a malignant embryonal tumour which occurs predominantly in children. It has a peak age incidence between five and twelve years, and accounts for approximately 44 per cent of all gliomas in this age group. Medulloblastoma nearly always arises in the cerebellar vermis, in the anterior part of the fourth ventricle, the area concerned predominantly with the function of walking and balance. Other sites are rare.

Macroscopic appearance
The vast majority of medulloblastomas in children are midline tumours which tend to fill the cavity of the fourth ventricle. It is well circumscribed, soft and friable, and its cut surface is mainly grey in colour with areas of necrosis, but haemorrhages, calcification and cyst formation are uncommon. In adults, the tumour tends to be laterally situated in one lobe of the cerebellar cortex. In both children and adults, medulloblastoma tends to invade and infiltrate the adjacent brain tissue and into the cavity of the fourth ventricle. Metastatic spread via the C.S.F. within the skull and spinal cord is common, but distant metastases to other organs are very rare.

Histological features
Medulloblastoma consists of small, ovoid, undifferentiated cells which are irregular in shape, and have dark-staining nuclei. Numerous mitotic figures are usually present. The distinguishing feature of medulloblastoma, is the presence of *carrot-shaped* cells (medulloblasts), with ovoid nuclei, scanty cytoplasm and indistinct cell outlines. Generally, these cells are irregularly arranged, but often, they exhibit pseudo-rosette formation with the tails of the cells pointing inwards, and no central cavity.

The histogenesis of medulloblastomas is not yet resolved and they are only loosely classified as gliomas. Since the tumour is sometimes present at birth, it is considered to be embryonic in origin, and is believed to arise from: (a) the external granular layer of the cerebellum which is present at birth and disappears at an early age, and (b) nests of primitive cells persisting in the inferior medullary velum.

MENINGIOMA

Meningioma is a relatively common tumour, next in frequency to the glioma, and is responsible for approximately 15 per cent of intracranial and 25 per cent of intraspinal tumours. It is believed to arise from arachnoid fibroblasts which form the core of the arachnoid villi, or from displaced arachnoid cells in the dura. The tumour may occur at any age, but it is predominantly found in adults; 80 per cent occur between the ages of 30 and 60 years, the peak age incidence being 45 years. It is twice as common in females as in males, and as a rule, it is a slow growing benign tumour which does not recur after complete removal.

Site
The incidence of meningiomas in certain sites of the C.N.S. corresponds to the incidence of arachnoid granulations at those sites. Thus, (a) 50 per cent are found in the convexity (parasaggital sinus and falx cerebri, (b) 40 per cent are basal (olfactory groove, lesser wing of the sphenoid and sella turcica), and (c) 10 per cent in the posterior fossa and foramen magnum. In the spinal cord, they occur in the lateral compartments of the subdural space, being most common in the thoracic segment. Very occasionally, meningiomas may be intraventricular.

Macroscopic appearances
Meningiomas vary in size, some are small and symptomless and are found incidentally at necropsy, other are large and may reach 7 to 8 cm in diameter. They are round, hard, encapsulated nodules embedded in brain substance and, except for the rare intraventricular tumours, they are always attached to the dura. The cut surface is grey-white in colour. Foci of calcification are common, and are often sufficiently dense to be rendered visible in plain X-rays of the skull.

Histological features
Many histological variants of meningiomas have been described, but the different appearances give little indication as to their rate of growth or tendency to recur after excision.

1. *Syncitial (Endotheliomatous) meningioma* is the most characteristic. It consists of clusters of cells separated by strands of connective tissue containing blood vessels. The cells are polygonal or spindle-shaped, with granular cytoplasm, indistinct cell outlines and large, pale, vesicular nuclei. Within the clusters, the cells are commonly arranged in onionskin-like whorls, especially around small blood vessels. The centres of the whorls often undergo hyaline degeneration and may become calcified to form *psammoma bodies* (psammos = sand) or brain-sand particles (Fig. 22.5).

2. *Fibroblastic meningioma* resembles a small fibroma because it is composed of elongated cells. Occasionally, whorls and psammoma bodies are seen, but they are not common.

TUMOURS OF NERVE SHEATHS

Neuromas (Schwannomas)
These are benign tumours arising from Schwann cells and,

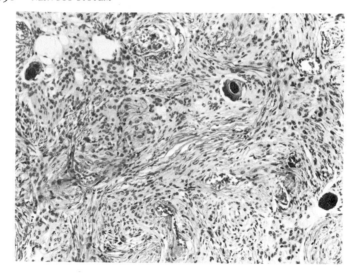

Fig. 22.5 Meningioma composed of spindle-shaped cells forming whorls. Note three psammoma bodies (× 120)

therefore, may be found on cranial nerves, spinal nerve roots, peripheral nerve trunks and at nerve endings. They are usually unilateral and solitary, but when bilateral, they are nearly always part of the syndrome of multiple neurofibromatosis or *von Recklinghausen's* disease. Macroscopically, neuromas are smooth, well-encapsulated tumours with a firm, rubbery consistency, and their cut surface shows a reddish-grey to yellow colour. Histologically, the tumours are surrounded by a fibrous tissue capsule and consist of bundles of elongated cells separated by connective tissue. The cells are long and narrow with cigar-shaped nuclei and very little cytoplasm. They may be arranged in whorls or they may show palisading of the nuclei (Fig. 22.6). Electron microscopy has identified these cells as Schwann cells.

1. *Acoustic Neuroma* (The cerebello-pontine-angle tumour) is the most common neuroma, representing approximately eight per cent of intracranial tumours. As a rule, it is a single tumour which arises from the sheath of the eighth nerve, as it emerges from the internal auditory meatus in the cerebello-pontine angle. It is an encapsulated and slow-growing tumour, but as it grows, it indents the lateral aspect of the pons, medulla and adjacent cerebellum, and stretches and compresses the nerves in the cerebello-pontine angle. At first, the tumour causes tinnitus because the eighth nerve is involved, later, deafness results. Eventually, compression of the

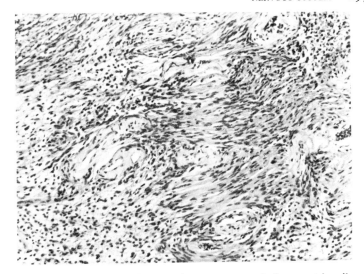

Fig. 22.6 Schwammoma of the acoustic nerve composed of compact bundles of thin elongated cells. Note tendency of the nuclei to form palisades (× 120)

fifth and seventh nerves results in loss of the corneal reflex and facial weakness respectively, and sooner or later, signs of increased intracranial pressure becomes evident.

2. *Neuromas of spinal nerve-roots* are situated mainly on the dorsal sensory nerve roots of the thoracic segments, and less frequently, in the cervical and lumbar segments, and cauda equina. Small tumours are generally confined within the subdural space. As they increase in size, they grow through the intervertebral foramina, and continue to enlarge both within and outside the vertebral canal, giving rise to the *spinal dumb-bell tumour.*

TUMOURS OF THE PITUITARY GLAND

Pituitary tumours are not of nervous tissue origin; they all arise in the epithelial portion of the anterior part of the hypophysis which develops as an outgrowth of the buccal mucosa (Rathke's pouch). They form approximately 18 per cent of intracranial tumours, and most of them are adenomas. Carcinomas occur occasionally, but they are difficult to distinguish from metastatic carcinomas arising in other organs.

Pituitary tumours occur mainly in adults between the ages of 20 and 50 years, and are more common in men than in women. They are round, red-brown, encapsulated tumours, usually contained in the sella turcica, but occasionally, they are much larger in size, destroy the sella and give rise to local manifestations. Traditionally, they are classified histologically according to the predominant cell type, as identified in haematoxylin and eosin stained sections. Three types are recognized:

1. *Chromophobe adenoma* is the most common and largest type, accounting for approximately 70 per cent of pituitary tumours. It is composed of cells with clear cytoplasm in which no granules can be demonstrated.

2. *Acidophil adenoma* is much less frequent and smaller than chromophobe adenoma. It consists of polyhedral cells containing red granules in the cytoplasm.

3. *Basophil adenoma* is a rare tumour characterized by blue granules in the cytoplasm of the tumour cells. More often, a tumour is not visible macroscopically and only foci of basophil cell hyperplasia are present.

As with tumours of other endocrine glands, the pituitary adenomas may be functional or nonfunctional. The pituitary gland secretes approximately 10 different hormones, and tumours that arise in the pituitary may secrete one or a mixture of these hormones. Since chromophobe adenoma is the most common tumour, it is likely to be the most functional, its clear cytoplasm presumably representing a phase of degranulation associated with activity.

The traditional classification of pituitary tumours, therefore, is unsatisfactory. A new classification is being developed based on recent advances on the biology and structure of the normal pituitary cell. Using electron microscopy and immunohistochemical staining techniques, it is possible both to differentiate between functional and nonfunctional adenomas and to identify the specific hormones that the tumours secrete. The following list compares the traditional with the new functional classification:

Adenoma

Functional type		Conventional type	Syndrome
Somatotropic	(STH)	Acidophil Chromophobe	Acromegally
Mammotropic	(Prolactin)	Chromophobe	Amenorrhoea Galactorrhoea
Corticotropic	(ACTH)	Chromophobe Basophil	Cushing's Disease
Thyrotropic	(TSH)	Basophil Chromophobe	Thyrotoxicosis
Gonadotropic	(FSH & LH)	Basophil Chromophobe	
Melanotropic	(MSH)	Basophil Chromophobe	Cushing's Disease

FURTHER READING

Harkin, J. C. & Reed, R. J. (1969) *Tumours of the Peripheral Nervous System*, Fascicle 3, Second series, Washington, D.C.: Armed Forces Institute of Pathology.

Rubinstein, L. J. (1972) *Tumours of the Central Nervous System*, Fascicle 6, Second series, Washington, D.C.: Armed Forces Institute of Pathology.

Russell, D. S. & Rubinstein, L. J. (1976) *Pathology of Tumours of the Nervous Systeh*, 4th ed. London, Edward Arnold.

Zimmerman, H. M. (1973) Brain Tumours. *Methods in Cancer Research*, **10**, 105.

Zülch, K. K. (1975) *Atlas of Gross Neurological Pathology*, Berlin, Heidelberg, New York, Springer-Verlag.

23

Tumours of soft tissues

The soft tissue tumours described in this chapter are those derived from the following non-epithelial, extra-skeletal tissues: connective tissue, muscle and blood vessels. They may be benign or malignant. Benign tumours are common, but it is rare for them to undergo malignant change, whereas malignant tumours are rare, their overall incidence being less than two per 100 000 population. Soft tissue sarcomas mainly occur between the ages of 40 and 70 years and are equally distributed between the sexes.

The classification of soft tissue tumours is based on the type of tissue of which the tumour is composed. In cases where the type of tissue cannot be evaluated by routine histological stains, the following special stains are of help.

1. *Van Gieson stain* distinguishes between collagen fibres (red) and muscle fibres (yellow).

2. *Fat stain*, on frozen sections, helps identify lipoblasts.

3. *Alcian blue* for mucin.

4. *PTAH* (phosphotungstic acid haematoxylin) enhances muscle striations.

5. *Reticulin stains* for reticulin fibres.

6. *Silver stains* for nerve fibres.

TUMOURS OF CONNECTIVE TISSUE

Tissue	Benign tumour	Malignant tumour
Fibrous tissue	Fibroma	Fibrosarcoma
Adipose tissue	Lipoma	Liposarcoma
Mucoid tissue	Myxoma	Myxosarcoma

Connective tissue tumours may arise either from differentiated connective tissue cells, or from mesenchymal cells present in the loose connective tissue around capillaries. Perivascular connective tissue is found in every part of the body, so that connective tissue tumours also can occur in every part of the body. Proliferating mesenchymal cells have two important properties:

1. They are pluripotential and capable of producing almost all types of connective tissue that embryonic mesenchyme can produce.

2. Differentiated mesenchymal cells have a great potential for metaplasia. Tumours arising in these cells, therefore, may show more than one kind of connective tissue, namely: mucoid change, fatty change, cartilage and bone.

The tumour cells of connective tissue tumours differ from those of epithelial tumours in that they are separated by intercellular material which is produced by the cells themselves. Diagnosis of the type of tumour is largely dependent on the recognition of the intercellular material, so that in the histological diagnosis of these tumours, special stains are often necessary.

Fibroma

Fibroma is a ubiquitous tumour. It is found in: (a) the skin and subcutaneous tissues, (b) fascia and fibrous tissue of the dura mater, peritoneum, tendons and nerve sheaths, and (c) the stroma of organs, especially the kidneys, ovary and uterus. Minute fibromas (or neurofibromas) may form in enormous numbers in connection with fibrous sheaths of cutaneous nerves (*von Recklinghausen's disease*). Fibromas arising in the dermis, adjacent to the epidermis are called *dermatofibromas*. *Desmoid tumour* is a variant of the fibroma which mainly occurs within the rectus sheath of parous women, possibly as a result of damage to the muscle during pregnancy.

Macroscopically, fibromas vary in size from 2 to 3 mm up to several centimetres in diameter, the very large tumours often weighing several kilograms. The majority are encapsulated, and their cut surface shows a glistening white fibrillar pattern which may have a whorled appearance. In hollow organs, fibromas may become pedunculated. Histologically, they resemble normal fibrous tissue and, depending on their cellularity and collagen content, two types are described.

1. *Hard fibromas* are slow growing and are composed of dense fibro-collagenous tissue.

2. *Soft fibromas* are cellular tumours with little collagen formation. They grow more rapidly than the hard variety.
Hard and soft areas may be present in the same tumour. Malignant change is rare.

In some connective tissue tumours, the main cell present is the histiocyte. These tumours are called *histiocytomas*. Histologically, they show: (a) histiocytic cells and large pale nuclei and abundant pale cytoplasm in which no fat can be demonstrated, (b) fibroblast-like cells arranged in various patterns producing collagen, and (c) Touton-type giant cells.

Lipoma

Lipoma is the commonest and most easily identified benign connective tissue tumour. It occurs between 40 and 60 years of age in the subcutaneous tissues about the neck, shoulder, back or buttock. Although mostly solitary, multiple lipomas sometimes occur, and one or two of them might be painful (*lipoma dolorosa*). Macroscopically, a lipoma resembles normal adipose tissue, except that it may be paler in colour. It is well defined and its cut surface shows a thin capsule which sends in septa, dividing the tumour into lobules. Microscopically, the main difference from normal fatty tissue lies in the irregular size of the cells. The cells are arranged in lobules separated by delicate fibrous septa which carry the blood vessels.

The true nature of lipomas is not clear; there is some controversy as to whether they are true tumours or hamartomas. Malignant change is rare.

Myxoma

This tumour is composed of round or stellate cells containing mucin, and giving the appearance of primitive mesenchyme or of mucoid connective tissue of the umbilical cord (Wharton's jelly). A pure myxoma is rare; its presence might represent a metaplasia in a fibroma, chondroma etc. The usual sites are the left ventricle, subcutaneous and submucous tissues, muscle sheaths and retroperitoneal tissues. The tumours are sometimes diffuse and spread widely, but do not give rise to secondary growths.

Fibrosarcoma

Fibrosarcoma is the commonest sarcoma of connective tissue. It occurs predominantly in adult life and has a peak incidence between 30 and 50 years of age. It has a widespread distribution, the commonest sites being the limbs and retroperitoneal tissues.

Macroscopically, it is a large, soft, irregular tumour. Its cut surface has a characteristic fleshy appearance with areas of haemorrhage and necrosis.

The histological features are not characteristic. Some tumours are well differentiated, consisting of mature fibroblasts which show slight pleomorphism and very few mitotic figures. Collagen and reticulin fibres can be demonstrated between the cells. The cells and collagen fibres form bands which may run in parallel, interlace or form whorls. In less differentiated tumours, the cells are pleomorphic, arranged haphazardly and many are in mitosis. Tumour giant cells, with one large or two to three irregular nuclei, are often present. The blood vessels are numerous, and unlike those in fibromas, they are thin-walled, often appearing as endotheliallined spaces, and easily rupture causing haemorrhages.

In general, fibrosarcomas grow slowly, metastasize late and may reach a very large size before the patient seeks attention. As they are radioresistant, the treatment of choice is surgical.

Liposarcoma

In contrast to lipoma, liposarcoma is a very rare tumour which tends to appear after the age of 50 years. Common sites are the retroperitoneal region, mesentery of the gut, buttocks, thighs and popliteal spaces. Generally, it is a large, lobulated tumour, devoid of a capsule, and tends to infiltrate through cleavage plains and invade neighbouring structures. Satellite nodules around the main tumour mass are often present. The cut surface shows grey-white bands of fibrous tissue separating lobules of yellow fat. Foci of necrosis, mucoid change, haemorrhages and cystic spaces are common.

The histological structure of liposarcoma varies considerably, and at times, diagnosis can be extremely difficult.

1. In the *well differentiated type*, there is a mixture of fat cells and immature mesenchymal cells which are fusiform in shape and contain minute vacuoles of fat (lipoblasts) (Fig. 23.1).

2. *Undifferentiated tumours* have a complex structure. They may show various amounts of: (a) myxomatous tissue containing bizarre giant cells, with large irregular pyknotic nuclei and vacuolated cytoplasm (b) mononuclear polyhedral cells, with finely vacuolated cytoplasm, crowding around the giant cells, (c) fibrosarcomatous areas, and (d) metaplastic changes showing foci of cartilage and bone.

In common with other sarcomas, the blood vessels are ill-formed, and areas of haemorrhage and necrosis may be present. Frozen sections stained for fat are helpful in making a diagnosis.

Liposarcomas usually grow slowly, but there is a wide variation in their degree of malignancy. The treatment of choice is wide surgical excision.

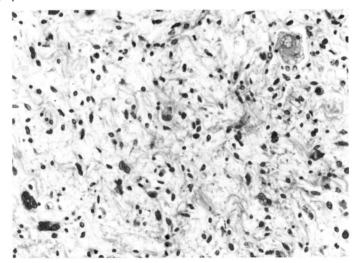

Fig. 23.1 Liposarcoma of the thigh showing vacuolated cells, spindle cells, lipoblasts and bizarre giant cells

TUMOURS OF MUSCLE

Tissue	Benign tumour	Malignant tumour
Smooth muscle	Leiomyoma	Leiomyosarcoma
	(a) Superficial	
	(b) Vascular	
	(c) Bizarre	
Striated muscle	Rhabdomyoma	Rhabdomyosarcoma
		(a) Adult
		(b) Juvenile

Leiomyoma

Leiomyomas are common tumours, especially in the uterus and gastrointestinal tract. They also occur in the walls of arteries, in the skin, where they arise either from the *erectores pilorum* muscles of the dermis or from smooth muscle cells in the walls of arteries, and in the retroperitoneal tissues such as mesentery, kidney and bladder. They may be solitary or multiple and may vary in size from a few millimetres to several centimetres in diameter.

Histologically, they are composed of bundles of smooth muscle cells with cigar-shaped nuclei which are frequently arranged in palisade formation. The bundles of muscle cells are supported by varying amounts of fibrous tissue which contain the blood vessels.

The main histological criterion of smooth muscle cells is the demonstration of myofibrils by special stains.

There are three types of leiomyoma:

1. *Superficial leiomyoma* which occurs in the skin and arises from the erectores pilorum muscles.

2. *Vascular leiomyoma* arises from muscle cells in the walls of blood vessels. This type tends to be more vascular and may occur in the skin or deeper tissues.

3. *Bizarre leiomyoma* occurs in the wall of the gastrointestinal tract (p. 201).

Leiomyosarcoma

These are uncommon tumours. They usually arise *de novo*, although some may arise in a pre-existing leiomyoma. The macroscopic and microscopic distinction between leiomyoma and leiomyosarcoma is not easy. Macroscopically, they vary in size from 2 to 10 cm in length, the larger ones generally occur in the retroperitoneum and omentum. Areas of haemorrhage and necrosis are common in the large, but uncommon in the small tumours. Histologically, well differentiated leiomyosarcomas resemble benign leiomyomas, but they tend to be more cellular. In less differentiated tumours, the nuclei become irregular, mitotic figures are increased in number and tumour giant cells may be present.

Rhabdomyoma

It is doubtful whether benign tumours of striated muscle exist, a view in keeping with the inability of striated muscle cells to regenerate. In any case, rhabdomyoma is a very rare tumour. Rhabdomyomas have been described in the tongue of children, in the kidney and in the myocardium, where they constitute part of the tuberose sclerosis syndrome and are considered developmental in nature.

Rhabdomyosarcoma

These are rare, but highly malignant tumours of striated muscle. They are regarded as embryonic tumours arising from immature myoblasts or mesenchymal cells, not from mature muscle cells. Two types of rhabdomyosarcoma are recognized:

1. *Adult rhabdomyosarcoma* usually occurs after middle age, and approximately 90 per cent in the limbs, back and retroperitoneum. It represents 75 per cent of all rhabdomyosarcomas. Macroscopically, it is large, soft and fleshy, with areas of haemorrhage

and necrosis. Microscopically, the cells are characteristically pleomorphic and undifferentiated, showing a variety of sizes and shapes: (a) cigar-shaped cells with irregular, hyperchromatic nuclei and peripheral vacuolation (*spider-web cells*), (b) cells shaped like tennis racquets, and (c) groups of *strap-cells*, which probably represent rhabdomyoblasts because they frequently contain striations. Sometimes, striations are evident in haematoxylin and eosin sections, at other times, they can be made visible with special stains (PTAH). The demonstration of muscle striations is essential for the diagnosis of rhabdomyosarcoma (Fig. 23.2).

2. *Juvenile rhabdomyosarcoma* occurs in children, especially in the bladder, head and neck, orbit and viscera. Macroscopically, they resemble adult rhabdomyosarcoma, but they are smaller, and microscopically, the cells are less pleomorphic. Tumours in the genital tract or nasopharynx, often present as large, grape-like

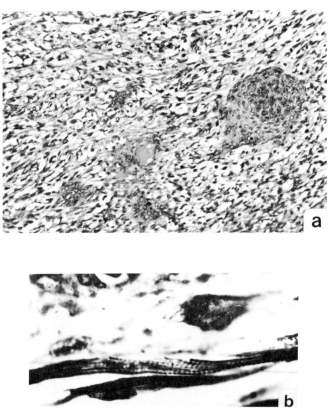

Fig. 23.2 Rhabdomyosarcoma showing: (a) typical giant cells with different shapes (× 100); (b) a PTAH stain demonstrating striations in a strap cell (× 1000)

masses (*botryoid rhabdomyosarcoma*). They consist of round, oval or strap cells arranged in nests or rosettes. Sometimes, they are supported on an alveolar framework with neoplastic cells filling the alveolar spaces (*alveolar rhabdomyosarcoma*).

Areas of rhabdomyoblastic tissue occur on a number of tumours such as mixed mesenchymal tumours, hepatoblastoma, nephroblastoma and teratoma.

TUMOURS OF BLOOD VESSELS

Angiomas are composed either of blood vessels (*haemangiomas*) or lymphatic vessels (*lymphangiomas*). Both types are essentially similar in structure, the main difference being that whilst haemangiomas are filled with blood, lymphangiomas contain lymph-like fluid with a few lymphocytes. Tumours of blood vessels are classified according to their histological structure; those composed of widely dilated spaces (venous channels) are called *cavernous haemangiomas*, whereas those composed of capillary-size spaces, capillary haemangiomas. Many haemangiomas contain a mixture of the cavernous and capillary types.

Cavernous haemangioma

These are hamartomas, not true tumours. They occur on the face, lips, mucous membranes, skeletal muscles, brain, liver and bone Histologically, they consist of large, irregular, interconnecting spaces lined by endothelium and filled with blood (Fig. 23.3a).

Capillary haemangioma

Capillary haemangiomas commonly occur as birth marks in the skin and subcutaneous tissues of the face, neck, scalp and in the mucous membranes. Most of them are small, but occasionally, large lesions are seen such as the *port-wine stain*. They are composed of a mesh of endothelium-lined spaces of capillary size. The different histological types of haemangiomas are based on the type and distribution of the proliferating cells, and in this connection, the structure of the capillary wall needs to be stressed.

Histologically, the capillary wall is made up of three components:

1. *Endothelial cells* lining the lumen of the vascular space.

2. *Reticulin fibres* forming a supporting sheath for the endothelial cells. This sheath is demonstrated with reticulin stains.

3. *Pericytes*, which are mesenchymal cells with long branching processes, are attached to the outer surface of the reticulin sheath. They do not possess contractile properties.

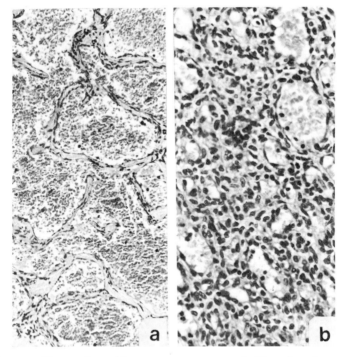

Fig. 23.3 Haemangioma: (a) cavernous type composed of large irregular spaces lined by endothelium and filled with blood (× 60); (b) capillary type composed of capillaries (× 100)

Common capillary haemangioma

The common type of capillary haemangioma has no definite pattern. It is composed of discrete masses of small capillaries arranged haphazardly (Fig. 23.3b).

Occasionally, capillary haemangiomas exhibit regressive changes, possibly as a result of trauma and haemorrhage. This results in a pale or tan nodule which shows varying amounts of fibrosis, collagen formation, lipid and haemosiderin-containing histiocytes, and thin-walled blood vessels. Such nodules go under various names: *sclerosing haemangioma*, *dermatofibroma* or *histiocytoma*.

Benign haemangioendothelioma

This is composed of capillary-size channels lined by two or three layers of endothelial cells. The cells are round in shape and often obscure the lumen of the capillaries. Silver stains which outline the reticulin sheath of the capillary show that the proliferating cells are located inside the sheath.

Benign haemangiopericytoma

This tumour is composed of proliferating pericytes. The cells are arranged around vascular spaces which are lined by a single layer of endothelial cells (Fig. 23.4). There is a collar of connective tissue separating the endothelial cells from the proliferating pericytes. Silver stains show that the connective tissue collar is, in fact, the reticulin sheath of the capillary, and that the pericytes are situated outside this sheath. It is not easy to predict the course of these tumours on histological grounds.

Glomas tumour (glomangioma)

This is a rare but very interesting tumour. Presumably, it arises from the glomus body, which contains islands composed of chemoreceptor cells, pericytes, and unmyelinated nerve fibres between the pericytes and the chemoreceptor cells. The glomus

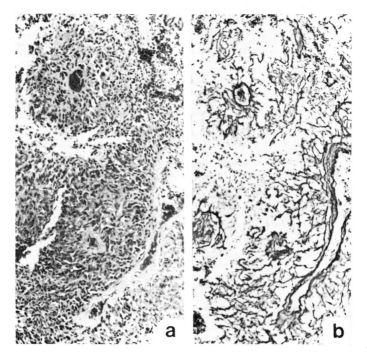

Fig. 23.4 Haemangiopericytoma showing: (a) proliferating cells (pericytes) around small blood vessels; (b) a silver stained section demonstrating the pericytes are situated outside the reticulin sheath (× 100)

body controls the blood flow and temperature, particularly through the fingers and toes.

The glomus tumour is a very tender, blue coloured tumour, usually situated subcutaneously at the ends of the fingers and toes. It is a variant of the haemangiopericytoma in that it is composed of cells (presumably pericytes) outside the reticulin sheath. Silver stains show numerous nonmyelinated nerve fibres between the capillaries.

Angiosarcoma

Angiosarcomas are rare tumours which have been reported in soft tissues, liver and spleen. They may arise from pre-existing angiomas, but most probably, they arise *de novo*. The cause of angiosarcoma is not known, although recent epidemiological studies have shown that exposure to *vinyl chloride* appears to predispose to the otherwise rare haemangiosarcoma of the liver.

Angiosarcomas appear as white or pink lobulated masses with areas of haemorrhage. Microscopically, they are composed of narrow vascular channels lined by large cells in which many mitotic figures can be seen. Groups of similar cells without visible vascular spaces are also present. In both cases the tumour cells are inside the reticulin sheaths.

Malignant haemangiopericytoma

There is no characteristic feature which will distinguish between benign and malignant haemangiopericytomas.

Kaposi's sarcoma

This condition consists of multiple blue-red nodules and plaques in the skin of the legs and arms, and in the viscera. It appears after the age of 50 years; it is common in coloured races (African and American negroes), and is more frequent in males than in females. The nature of this lesion is not understood; the early lesion resembles a granuloma, but later, it simulates an angiosarcoma.

FURTHER READING

Enzinger, F. M. (1969) *International Histological Classification of Tumours No. 3: Histological Typing of Soft Tissue Tumours*. Geneva: World Health Organization.

Stout, A. P. & Lattes, R. (1967) *Tumours of Soft Tissues*, Fascicle 1, Second series, Washington D.C.: Armed Forces Institute of Pathology.

Willis, R. A. (1967) *Pathology of Tumours*, 4th edn. London: Butterworths.

24

Tumours of cartilage and bone

The skeleton consists of bone, cartilage, fibrous tissue, marrow and adipose tissue, all of which are capable of giving rise to tumours. According to Dahlin, the approximate percentages of tumours arising in each of these tissues are as follows: haemopoietic, 37 per cent; cartilage, 24 per cent; bone, 20 per cent; fibrous tissue, 4 per cent; unknown, 10 per cent. In this chapter, only the tumours listed below will be discussed, the remainder are dealt with elsewhere:

	Tumour	
Type of tissue	*Benign*	*Malignant*
Cartilage	Osteochondroma	Chondrosarcoma
	Chondroma	
	Chondroblastoma	
	Chondromyxoid fibroma	
Bone	Osteoma	Osteosarcoma
	Osteoid osteoma	
	Benign osteoblastoma	
Unknown	Giant cell tumour of bone	
Marrow		Myeloma
		Ewing's tumour

Bone and cartilage arise from undifferentiated mesenchymal cells, capable of giving rise to a variety of tissues. Some authorities consider that the fibroblast, a differentiated mesenchymal cell, can differentiate into osteoblasts and chondroblasts. Mesenchymal cells growing in tissue culture, for example, (a) if subjected to tension, differentiate into fibroblasts, (b) if subjected to compression and low oxygen tension, differentiate into chondroblasts, and (c) if subjected to compression and good oxygen supply, they become osteoblasts. It is necessary to bear these facts in mind in order to understand the variety of tissues that can occur in tumours arising in bone and cartilage.

As with other tissues, tumours in bone may be primary or

secondary, benign or malignant. Primary malignant tumours are relatively uncommon, accounting for less than 1 per cent of all deaths from cancer. The most common malignancies in bone are metastases, especially from carcinoma arising in the breast, bronchus, thyroid gland, kidney and prostate gland.

Most bone tumours present as painful swellings, worse at night. X-rays are essential to establish the diagnosis and localize the lesion; they do not only show the presence of a tumour, but also give useful suggestions on the probable type of tumour. Biopsy is essential for an accurate diagnosis, which is based on histological structure; but histology alone is not always sufficient, and in special cases, supplementary histochemical tests are necessary.

1. *Alkaline phosphatase* is present in osteoblasts and is of help in distinguishing osteosarcoma from secondary carcinoma.

2. *Acid phosphatase* identifies secondary prostatic cancer.

3. *PAS-stain* demonstrates intracellular glycogen which distinguishes Ewing's tumour from other types of small round cell sarcoma.

4. *Metachromasia* indicates the presence of acid mucopolysaccharides and suggests a cartilaginous matrix.

Electron microscopy is of little value in the diagnosis of bone tumours.

CARTILAGE FORMING TUMOURS

These tumours are benign, growing either (a) on the surface of long bones (*ecchondromas*), in young adults, or (b) in the interior of smaller bones (*enchondromas*) which occur at any age. They grow by expansion and destroy the bone in consequence. Such tumours often show a myxomatous change which tends to give rise to cyst formation, and occasionally, they may show areas of ossification. Parts of these tumours may undergo malignant change, and the chondrosarcomas so formed may invade veins and lymphatics giving rise to distant metastases. There are five important cartilaginous tumours:

Osteochondroma (ecchondroma)

This is the most common type of benign bone tumour. It occurs between the ages of 10 and 25 years, and is slightly more common in males than in females (3:2). Osteochondroma arises predominantly in the metaphyses of long bones, especially in the region of the knee joint, although it may occur in any bone (ileum, scapula, ribs and lower spine). Basically, it is an exostosis with a broad attachment to the host bone, and consists of a bony framework with a cap of cartilage (*cartilage-capped exostosis*). Radiologically, the mass is characteristically a lobulated bony outgrowth which is usually much denser than the shaft. It continues growing until the epiphyses fuse. Resumption of growth of these tumours in adult life is strongly suggestive of malignant change.

Chondroma (enchondroma)

Chondroma is also a benign tumour, but unlike osteochondroma, it grows within bones. It is mainly found in the small bones of the hands and feet, the hands rather than the feet and phalanges rather than the metacarpals. It also occurs within the pelvic bones, ribs, scapulae and vertebrae, but it is rare in long bones. Multiple tumours occur in about 5 per cent of patients (Ollier's disease). Chondromas occur at any age and they are equally distributed between the sexes.

The tumour is usually less than 1 cm in diameter, is embedded in bone, and as it grows by expansion, it tends to erode the cortex. Its cut surface shows a typically blue cartilaginous appearance, and a distinct lobular outline. In X-ray films, there is a large area of bone rarefaction which balloons the cortex, the translucent area being trabecular and showing foci of ossification. Microscopically, the tumour lobules consist of hyaline cartilage, separated by thin bands of vascular connective tissue. Areas of myxomatous change and foci of ossification are common.

Because of their erosive character, chondromas cause pain and may result in a pathological fracture. In small bones, they are always benign; in long bones, they occasionally become malignant and may recur after removal, but in the pelvis, they are frequently malignant.

Chondroblastoma

Chondroblastoma is a rare cartilaginous tumour which, like the giant cell tumour of bone, always arises in an epiphysis, especially of a long bone. For this reason, it is sometimes referred to as *benign epiphyseal chondroblastoma*. It mainly occurs between the ages of 10 and 20 years, and is equally frequent in males and females. Chondroblastoma is usually larger than the chondroma, but resembles the chondroma in appearance, although there may be foci of necrosis and haemorrhage.

Microscopically, it consists of chondroblasts supported on a matrix of chondromucin. The cells are well differentiated, but there may be increased numbers of mitotic figures and multinucleated giant cells, containing as many as 50 nuclei which resemble the nuclei of chondroblasts. Foci of calcification are common. The presence of a chondromucinous matrix distinguishes chondroblastoma from giant cell tumour of bone.

Chondromyxoid fibroma

This tumour is as rare as chondroblastoma. Like the latter, it occurs predominantly at the ends of long bones, especially the upper end of the tibia and lower end of the femur. It occurs between the ages of 10 and 30 years, and may grow to a size of 5 cm in diameter. Microscopically it differs from chondroma in containing fibrous zones in addition to cartilaginous and myxomatous areas. Cell pleomorphism is common and makes the distinction from a chondrosarcoma a difficult one.

Chondrosarcoma

This is a malignant cartilaginous tumour which accounts for approximately 10 per cent of bone tumours. It usually arises *de novo*, but occasionally, it may complicate a pre-existing chondroma (secondary chondrosarcoma). Chondrosarcoma has a peak age incidence between 40 and 70 years. It is uncommon under 30 years of age and is slightly more common in males than in females (3:2). It occurs predominantly in the trunk and the upper ends of the femur and humerus.

Macroscopic appearances

The tumour varies in size from 1 to 10 cm in diameter, a diameter greater than 4 or 5 cm being usually indicative of malignancy. It is distinctly lobular in outline, and on section, the lobules show a blue-grey colour, often with necrotic and cystic centres and with areas of calcification and ossification. These features give rise to characteristic radiological appearances on X-ray films, namely: (a) destruction of bone due to the expansile growth, and (b) mottled densities due to calcification and ossification.

Histological features

Microscopically, chondrosarcomas show a wide variation in structure, from well differentiated hyaline cartilage to undifferentiated myxomatous areas. Cellular atypia and an abnormal matrix are the distinguishing features. In the obviously malignant cases, the cells are undifferentiated, spindle-shaped, pleomorphic and may show giant-cell formation; the stroma is myxomatous and resembles that of the foetus. These cases do not present a diagnostic problem.

The majority of chondrosarcomas, however, are composed of well differentiated hyaline cartilage and mature cells, and resemble the benign chondroma. In these cases, unless several sections from different areas are examined, it might be impossible to distinguish them from a benign lesion. The main distinguishing features are, a greater cellularity, the presence of pleomorphic, plump and bi-nucleate cells, and myxomatous changes in the matrix; but these are not fixed criteria. Often, the clinical, radiological, macroscopic and microscopic evidence all needs to be assessed before a diagnosis can be made.

Prognosis
In adequately excised cases, the prognosis is generally good. More cures are obtained with chondrosarcomas than any other bone malignancy. Blood spread occurs late in the disease and metastases, when they appear, are in the lung first and rarely in other organs.

BONE FORMING TUMOURS

Osteoma
Like the chondromas, the osteomas occur as exostoses and eno-stoses. The exostoses grow out near the end of the shaft of long bones and are formed in fibrous tissue or cartilage. Exostoses and ecchondromas are much the same thing. They have a cap of cartilage and stop growing when the epiphyses unite. They are frequently multiple, symmetrical and are regarded by some authorities as hamartomas rather than true tumours. The osteomas are sub-divided into two groups:

1. *The ivory osteoma* is composed of compact bone. It is a rare tumour which mostly occurs at the base of the skull or in the bones forming the sinuses (hyperostosis frontalis interna).

2. *The spongy osteoma* is composed of cancellous bone. This type is more frequent than the ivory osteoma, and found in connection with muscle attachments.

Osteoid osteoma
The current feeling is that osteoid osteoma is a true benign neoplasm. It occurs as a very painful swelling in the shafts of long bones, particularly the femur and tibia, between the ages of 10 and 25 years, and is three times more common in males than in females. The tumour is usually less than 1 cm in diameter, red-brown in colour due to its vascularity, and embedded in cortical bone. Microscopically, it is composed of closely packed osteoid

trabeculae, separated by a highly vascular connective tissue stroma. The nodule is surrounded by a zone of reactive bone. It is a benign lesion and does not recur following surgical removal.

Benign osteoblastoma
This is a very rare benign tumour which mostly occurs in the vertebral column. It resembles the osteoid osteoma in colour and histological structure but differs from it in being much larger (2 to 10 cm in diameter). For this reason, it is also known as giant osteoid osteoma.

Osteosarcoma (osteogenic sarcoma)
Osteosarcoma arises from periosteal or endosteal osteoblasts capable of forming osteoid and bone. It is a rare tumour, but it is the most malignant primary tumour of bone; it affects males more frequently than females, and over 75 per cent of patients are between the ages of 10 and 25 years. The condition is rare after the age of 40 years, except in patients suffering with Paget's disease of bone. Apart from ionizing radiations (p. 70), the cause of osteosarcoma is not known.

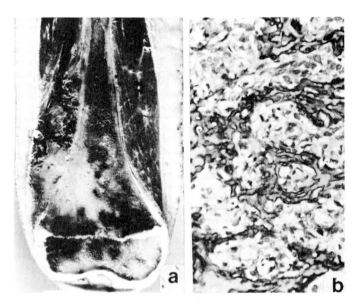

Fig. 24.1 Osteosarcoma of the lower end of the femur: (a) pale tumour tissue just proximal to the epiphyseal plate lifting the periosteum and invading bone; (b) photomicrograph showing osteoid and malignant osteoblasts (× 120)

The favourite sites for osteosarcoma are the actively growing ends of long bones (the metaphyses). The lower end of the femur and upper end of the tibia together account for approximately 50 per cent of all cases of osteosarcoma. Other common sites include the upper ends of the femur and humerus, the pelvic bones, skull, scapula, vertebrae and ribs. Extraskeletal osteosarcomas do occur, but they are rare.

Macroscopic appearance
Typically, the tumour appears as a spindle-shaped, painful swelling over the end of a long bone. Its consistency may be soft or hard, depending on the amount of bone formation, and accordingly, it is sub-divided into osteoblastic and osteolytic types. Longitudinal and transverse sections through bone and tumour show that the bulk of the tumour lies between the periosteum and cortex, and tends to spread up, down and round the shaft. It tends to erode the bone and infiltrate the marrow cavity, but the periosteum usually remains intact until the latter stages of the disease. The cut surface of the tumour is generally grey in colour but may show yellow areas of necrosis, bluish areas of cartilage, haemorrhages and white areas of new bone formation. As the periosteum is elevated, it tends to rejoin the shaft by forming a wedge of bone which can be seen in X-ray films (*Codman's triangle*), a typical but non-specific appearance. Other radiological signs are determined by the rate of growth of the tumour and its ability to form bone.

1. *Osteolytic osteosarcoma*, if rapidly-growing, causes bone erosion. If slow-growing, it gives rise to characteristic spicules due to formation of bone along the walls of the vessels which extend from the shaft to the elevated capsule (the *sun-ray pattern*).

2. In *osteoblastic osteosarcoma*, the spicules of bone fuse forming an irregular mass which surrounds and masks the erosion of the host bone.

Histological features
The microscopic appearances of osteosarcoma show extraordinary variability in both the tumour cells and stroma.

1. *The tumour cells* are typically pleomorphic and may consist of: (a) small, spindle-shaped cells with hyperchromatic nuclei and poorly defined cytoplasm, (b) larger polyhedral cells which may show excessive mitotic activity, and (c) giant cells which may be of the tumour or foreign body type (p. 8).

2. *The stroma* is equally variable and may contain fibrous, cartilaginous, myxomatous, osteoid and osseous areas. Osteoid and

bone formation are essential for diagnosis. A distinction between tumour and normal bone can be difficult, but as a rule, tumour bone tends to blend with the stroma and is not lined by osteoblasts. The stroma contains many poorly formed blood vessels.

Course and prognosis

Because of its vascularity, blood spread occurs early and mainly to the lungs, liver and bones. The prognosis is not good, and according to Dahlin, the five-year survival rate is approximately 20 per cent and the 10-year, 17 per cent. An elevated serum alkaline phosphatase is present in a high proportion of patients with osteosarcoma. The level drops to normal following amputation.

Giant cell tumour of bone

This is a rare tumour of obscure origin, characterized by the presence of large numbers of giant cells. Unlike other bone tumours, it is slightly more common in females than in males and has a peak age incidence between 20 and 50 years. Over 50 per cent of cases occur in the region of the knee joint, the lower end of the femur and upper end of the tibia, 30 per cent in the pelvic bones and upper end of the femur, and the remaining 20 per cent is approximately equally distributed to all the other bones.

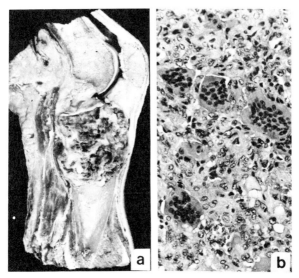

Fig. 24.2   Giant cell tumour of upper end of tibia: (a) the tumour involves the epiphysis; (b) photomicrograph of the tumour showing a stroma of spindle cells and giant cells with numerous uniform nuclei ($\times$ 120)

Macroscopic appearance

In long bones, the tumour is nearly always located at the ends in the region of the epiphyses, but as it grows, it may involve the metaphysis, never the joint cartilage. As a general rule, if a tumour does not involve the epiphysis, it is unlikely to be a giant cell tumour. It is usually central in origin, well circumscribed and encapsulated. The cut surface has a variegated appearance with solid and cystic areas, haemorrhages, yellow areas of necrosis and fibrous intersections extend from the capsule into the interior of the tumour. The overall colour resembles liver. Larger tumours cause destruction and expansion of bone. An irregular, infiltrative margin is presumptive evidence of malignant change.

Histological features

The distinguishing feature of giant cell tumour of bone is the presence of large numbers of foreign body type giant cells, with abundant cytoplasm and numerous nuclei which are regular in form. The giant cells are set in a stroma containing spindle-shaped cells and many thin-walled blood vessels. Cysts, areas of scarring and haemorrhages are common, but osteoid and bone formation are rare. The nature of the giant cells is not known; they resemble osteoclasts, and because of this, the tumour is sometimes erroneously referred to as *osteoclastoma*, implying that the osteoclasts are the neoplastic component. It should be stressed that, in cases of malignancy, it is the stromal cells that represent the malignant component, and that the more malignant the tumour, the less frequent are the giant cells.

Course and prognosis

Most patients with giant cell tumour of bone present with swelling and pain. As these tumours occur mainly in adults, the age of the patient is an important factor in making a diagnosis. Ordinarily, giant cell tumour may be considered a benign growth, and in 60 per cent of cases, the outcome is good, irrespective of whether the tumour is treated or not. Approximately 30 per cent will recur after simple excision, and the remaining 10 per cent may give rise to metastases. Those arising in the bones of the pelvis are more likely to be malignant.

MARROW TUMOURS

Tumours arising in the marrow and presenting as primary bone lesions include myeloma, lymphoma and Ewing's tumour. Of these, the lymphomas are discussed in Chapter 13.

Myeloma

This is a highly malignant tumour which is composed of proliferating plasma cells and which represents approximately 50 per cent of malignant primary bone tumours. The disease is more common in females than in males, and most cases are seen in the middle-aged and elderly, between 55 and 80 years of age, with a peak at 65 years.

Myeloma may be present for a long time before tumour masses become apparent in bones, and indeed, only a small percentage (20 per cent) of cases show X-ray evidence of bone destruction. In most cases, therefore, diagnosis depends upon: (a) marrow puncture showing proliferation of mature plasma cells, and (b) other methods of investigation which are based on the fact that the plasma cells, in myeloma, retain their capacity to synthesize globulins (myeloma proteins). The less differentiated tumours produce α-globulins while the differentiated tumours produce immunoglobulins. The additional investigations, therefore, include:

1. *Haematological tests.* The blood usually shows an anaemia, a rapid ESR, coagulation defects with a bleeding diathesis and a predisposition to infection. The blood film shows rouleau formation, and sometimes, plasma cells.

2. *Biochemical tests.* Bence–Jones proteins in the urine are diagnostic, but are only present in 50 per cent of cases.

3. *Abnormal serum protein.* Approximately 95 per cent of patients have a raised serum globulin, and in these patients, serum electrophoresis enables identification of the abnormal globulin fraction. Of these: (a) 1 per cent of patients have no abnormal protein, (b) 25 per cent show elevation of the light chain fraction, (c) 55 per cent show elevation in IgG, and (d) 20 per cent show elevation in IgA.

Tumour masses, when present, may appear simultaneously over widespread areas throughout the skeleton, suggesting the possibility of a multifocal origin, hence the name *multiple myeloma*. Occasionally, a solitary tumour is present. X-ray films show numerous, rounded areas of bone destruction, which vary in size from 0.5 to 5 cm in diameter and which have a smooth, almost punched-out appearance. No periosteal reaction is present. Such lesions are widespread and involve all marrow-containing bones, the skull, spine, ribs, pelvis and long bones. Macroscopically, these areas are soft, grey and friable.

Microscopically, the tumours are composed of sheets of closely-packed plasma cells, with very little intercellular material. The cells are large with granular, basophilic cytoplasm, and a distinct cell membrane. The nucleus is characteristically cart-wheel in appearance, eccentric in position and may contain two or three nucleoli. These cells may also be seen in 50 per cent of blood smears.

Course and prognosis
The outlook of patients with myeloma is poor. Less than 10 per cent survive five years and the majority die within two years of diagnosis. Anaemia, infections, spinal cord involvement and renal failure from amyloid deposits are the major contributing causes.

Ewing's tumour

It is now generally accepted that Ewing's tumour is a specific entity – a highly malignant, small round-cell sarcoma of obscure origin. It is a rare tumour which accounts for approximately 7 per cent of malignant tumours of bone. Essentially, Ewing's tumour is a disease of childhood, in that over 80 per cent of cases occur before 25 years of age, and males are affected twice as frequently as females. The most common sites are the metaphyses of long bones and the pelvis, although any bone may be involved. Macroscopically, the tumour is a jelly-like mass with foci of haemorrhage on its cut surface. Microscopically, it is made up of sheets of densely packed, undifferentiated, small round cells, divided into small groups or nests by fibrous-tissue septa. The cells have a round nucleus with prominent nucleoli, but indistinct cell outlines. There are usually many mitoses present. Because the cells are undifferentiated, these tumours may easily be confused with metastases from other undifferentiated cancers, and in fact, Willis maintains that Ewing's tumour represents a solitary metastasis in bone from a neuroblastoma. The cells of Ewing's tumour contain glycogen which can be demonstrated as PAS-positive intracellular material, whereas the cells of neuroblastoma are PAS-negative because they do not contain glycogen.

Ewing's tumour metastasizes early to the lung, liver and bones, and has a poor prognosis. The five-year survival rate is less than 15 per cent.

FURTHER READING

Dahlin, D. C. (1967) *Bone Tumors*, 2nd edn. Springfield, Charles C. Thomas.

Spjut, J. H. *et al.* (1971) *Tumors of Bone and Cartilage*, Fascicle 5, Second series, Washington D.C.: Armed Forces Institute of Pathology.

Schajowicz, F. *et al.* (1972) *International Histological Classification of Tumours No. 6: Histological Typing of Bone Tumours*. Geneva: World Health Organization.

Willis, R. A. (1967) *Pathology of Tumours*, 4th edn. London: Butterworths.

Index